AF688811

Migraine and Headache: A Comprehensive Clinical Guide

Migraine and Headache: A Comprehensive Clinical Guide

Edited by Sienna West

AMERICAN
MEDICAL PUBLISHERS
www.americanmedicalpublishers.com

American Medical Publishers,
41 Flatbush Avenue,
1st Floor, New York,
NY 11217, USA

Visit us on the World Wide Web at:
www.americanmedicalpublishers.com

© American Medical Publishers, 2022

This book contains information obtained from authentic and highly regarded sources. Copyright for all individual chapters remain with the respective authors as indicated. All chapters are published with permission under the Creative Commons Attribution License or equivalent. A wide variety of references are listed. Permission and sources are indicated; for detailed attributions, please refer to the permissions page and list of contributors. Reasonable efforts have been made to publish reliable data and information, but the authors, editors and publisher cannot assume any responsibility for the validity of all materials or the consequences of their use.

ISBN: 978-1-63927-304-1

Trademark Notice: Registered trademark of products or corporate names are used only for explanation and identification without intent to infringe.

Cataloging-in-Publication Data

Migraine and headache : a comprehensive clinical guide / edited by Sienna West.
p. cm.
Includes bibliographical references and index.
ISBN 978-1-63927-304-1
1. Migraine. 2. Headache. 3. Migraine--Treatment. 4. Headache--Treatment.
5. Cluster headache. I. West, Sienna.
RC392 .M54 2022
616.849 12--dc23

Table of Contents

Preface

Headache is the pain in the face, head or neck. There are different types of headaches which can be classified as either primary or secondary headaches based on their symptoms and severity. Primary headaches are generally tension headaches or migraines. Secondary headaches are caused by underlying infections, brain bleed, tumors, head injury or vascular disorders. Severe headaches can sometimes cause depression. Migraine is a type of primary headache that causes moderate to severe headaches. The headaches that occur in migraine are of pulsating nature and affect half of the head. The causes of migraine include environmental and genetic factors. This book unravels the recent studies associated with migraine and headache. It is a valuable compilation of topics, ranging from the basic to the most complex aspects of this area of study. This book is a resource guide for experts as well as students.

All of the data presented henceforth, was collaborated in the wake of recent advancements in the field. The aim of this book is to present the diversified developments from across the globe in a comprehensible manner. The opinions expressed in each chapter belong solely to the contributing authors. Their interpretations of the topics are the integral part of this book, which I have carefully compiled for a better understanding of the readers.

At the end, I would like to thank all those who dedicated their time and efforts for the successful completion of this book. I also wish to convey my gratitude towards my friends and family who supported me at every step.

Editor

1

Case-control study of *GRIA1* and *GRIA3* gene variants in migraine

Jie Fang[1], Xingkai An[1], Shuai Chen[2], Zhenzhen Yu[1], Qilin Ma[1,2*] and Hongli Qu[1*]

Abstract

Background: As the most abundant excitatory neurotransmitter in the central nervous system, glutamate has been accepted to play a major role in the pathophysiology of migraine. The previous studies have reported the glutamate receptor ionotropic *GRIA1* and *GRIA3* genes variants associated with migraine. The project aims to investigate the polymorphisms in both genes for their association with migraine in the Chinese Han population.

Methods: A Han-Chinese case-control population, including 331 unrelated female migraine patients and 330 matched controls, was studied. Variants in genes (*GRIA1* and *GRIA3*) were genotyped by Multiplex SNaPshot assay.

Results: In the group of patients, the frequency of allele C was 84.1 % (557 C alleles) and allele T was 15.9 % (105 T alleles) for the *GRIA1* (rs2195450) in migraineurs, this was significantly as compared with the controls ($P = .001$, OR = 1.786, 95 % CI: 1.28–2.49). And an association was also seen in the migraine with aura (MA) subtype ($P = .012$, OR = 2.092, 95 % CI: 1.17–3.76) and migraine without aura (MO) subtype ($P = .002$, OR = 1.737, 95 % CI: 1.23–2.45). However, no evidence was found that *GRIA1* (rs548294) or *GRIA3* (rs3761555) is associated with migraine.

Conclusion: Our data of this study confirmed the association of *GRIA1* (rs2195450) to female migraine (MA, MO) susceptibility in the Chinese Han population. The result provides evidence that the glutamatergic system is implicated in the pathophysiology of migraine.

Keywords: Migraine, GRIA1, GRIA3, Gene variant, Glutamate

Background

Migraine, characterized by recurrent attacks of severe headache, is a complex debilitating neurovascular disorder accompanying with nausea, vomiting, photophobia and phonophobia, which can cause temporary incapacitation in the migraineur. It is divided into two common forms: migraine with/or without aura (MA and MO), and diagnosed according the ICHD-III(HIS 2013) [1]. Epidemiological studies have shown that migraine prevalence accounts for 12 % in Caucasian populations [2] and 9.3 % in mainland of China [3]. With severe influence on the patient's physical and mental health, and even their normal social function, this disorder is seemed as a heavy burden for patents.

The exact causes and pathophysiological mechanisms that underlie migraine is elusive. It is generally considered to be associated with the genetic factors, about 50 % of affected individuals have a first-degree relative also suffering from migraine [4], with family and twin studies reporting heritability estimates from 34 to 57 % [5]. Current research suggests that the trigeminovascular system also plays an important role in migraine [6, 7], and neurotransmitters in this system include: serotonin, dopamine and glutamate implicated in migraine pathogenesis. The implication of glutamate in trigeminovascular activation, central sensitization and cortical spreading depression(CSD) [8–10] as well as the assessment of glutamate concentration in plasma, platelets and cerebrospinal fluid in clinical studies [11] argue for a significant role of the glutamatergic neurotransmission in the pathophysiology of migraine. Genetic association studies have mostly investigated variants in serotonin and dopamine receptor genes. Nevertheless, fewer studies have

* Correspondence: qilinma@yeah.net; xmhongliqu@hotmail.com
Jie Fang and Xingkai An contributed equally to this work as first authors.
[1]Department of Neurology, The First Affiliated Hospital of Xiamen University, Xiamen, China
Full list of author information is available at the end of the article

been done in relation to the genetics of the Glutamatergic system in migraine [12]. The study by Formicola et al. [13] who found a positive association with 2 SNPs in *GRIA1* and 1 SNP in the *GRIA3* in an Italian population of 250 migraineurs and 260 controls [13]. Recently, genome-wide association studies (GWAS) also support a correlation between migraine and variants in glutamatergic system genes [14–16].

However, involved in regulating neuronal glutamate signals lipoprotein receptor *LRP1* (rs11172113) gene variation, the gene mutation of *LRP1* has not been found in the Han population-based study [17]. Therefore, further research into the glutamate system is necessary to ascertain the gene variation in Han-population. Therefore, to determine if these variations in the *GRIA1* and *GRIA3* genes contribute to migraine susceptibility in an Chinese Han population case-control cohort, we report the findings of our association study of the 3 SNPs with a large sample involving 661 female individuals from southern Fujian province of China.

Methods

Subjects

Based on previous experience our study involves a relatively larger sample size. The study group comprised 331 Han-Chinese female migraine patients from outpatient of the Department of Neurology at the First Affiliated Hospital of Xiamen University during the period between September 2013 and May 2015. All of the migraine patients were diagnosed as having either migraine with (MA) or migraine without (MO) aura, by two headache specialists after neurological examination, direct interview, computed tomography (CT), or magnetic resonance imaging (MRI), according to the diagnostic criteria set by the International Headache Society (international classification of headache disorders,3rd edition, 2013) [1]. The control group comprised 330 non-headache healthy female volunteers, who were recruited from the same regional background (southern Fujian province), and matched for age and gender with the study group. Familial Hemiplegic Migraine, tumor, depression and other comorbid psychiatric disorders were excluded from the study. The Ethics Committee of the First Affiliated Hospital of Xiamen University approved this study, and informed consent was obtained from all participants and volunteers.

Genetic analysis

Genomic DNA from each participant was extracted from peripheral blood with ethylene diamine tetraacetic acid (EDTA) anticoagulant. Genomic DNA was prepared by a standard extraction method using the QiaAmp DNA Mini Kit (Qiagen, Hilden, Germany) and the DNA samples were stored at −20 °C before being used. The three SNPs were selected for this study rs548294 and rs2195450 in *GRIA1*, rs3761555 in *GRIA3* were genotyped using Multiplex SNaPshot technique (Applied Biosystems by Life Technologies, Foster City, CA, USA). Table 1 shows the primers of PCR and SNaPshot reaction. PCR reactions containing 25 μl final volume mixture (50 mM $MgCl_2$, 10 mM dNTP, 1 μM primers, 5 units Platinum Taq DNA polymerase). The PCR conditions used were: 95 °C denaturation for 2 min, amplification reaction for 33 cycles (95 °C for 20s, 55 °C for 20s, 72 °C for 40s), with a final extension step of 72 °C for 5 min. The PCR products were examined on a 1.5 % agarose gel whose fragments indicate successful experiment. SNaPshot reaction contains 5 μl final volume mixture (Reaction mix 2.5 μl, PCR products 1.5 μl, Probe Mix 1.0 μl). SNaPshot reaction procedure is as following: amplification reaction for 25 cycles (96 °C for 10s, 50 °C for 5 s, 60 °C for 30s), with a final extension step of 60 °C for 1 min. DNA sequencing: a 10 μl final volume mixture (SNaPshot purified product 1 μl, Formamide Deionized 8.5 μl, GeneScan-120 LIZ Size Standard 0.5 μl). 95 °C denaturation 5 min, and sequenced using an ABI PRISM 3730 DNA Sequencer (Applied Biosystems by Life Technologies, Foster City, CA, USA). All sequence analyses were performed using it's own DNA Sequencing Analysis software, GeneMapper4.0.

Statistical analysis

To assess the deviation of each polymorphism from the Hardy-Weinberg equilibrium (HWE), the public statistics web tool (http://ihg.gsf.de/cgi-bin/hw/hwa1.pl) was employed. All statistical analyses were performed using the statistical package SPSS version 20.0 for Windows (SPSS, Inc., Chicago, IL, USA). The Chi-squared test or t-test was used to compare age and sex among the groups, allele and genotype frequencies were compared using the Chi-squared test. P values were adjusted for multiple testing using the Bonferroni correction, therefore, we used $P < .05/3 \approx .017$ as a threshold for significance.

Table 1 PCR and SNaPshot Probe Primer Sequences

Polymorphisms	Primers	Product size	Sequence 5′ → 3′
GRIA1	Forward	297bp	CACCCCAAGTTTTCACTGCT
rs548294	Reverse	297bp	GAACCTAAAAGATCCCCAGGT
	Probe	63bp	37Ts+CTTAACTCTTAGGCTCTAATA
GRIA1	Forward	259bp	GCTGGAGGAGTCCAGAACAG
rs2195450	Reverse	259bp	TGCTTGGTAGATGGTGCTTG
	Probe	70bp	45Ts+CCCCTCACTCCTTCTTCT
GRIA3	Forward	373bp	TGCCAGTGTAAAGCGAACTG
rs3761555	Reverse	373bp	GGGGATGACCAACCTTACCT
	Probe	56bp	35Ts+TTCAAAATGGAGACAAAAGAT

Results

General information

This study involved a total of 331 female migraine patients and 330 female controls. The mean age of the migraine patients was 35.0 ± 7.6 years, and the controls were 34.4 ± 7.2 years. The migraine patients and the controls were matched with respect to age and gender ($P = .255/1.00$). There are 47 MA and 284 MO included in the migraine patients group. Two SNPs (rs548294 and rs2195450) in the *GRIA1* gene and one SNP (rs3761555) in the *GRIA3* gene that have previously demonstrated positive association to migraine in the study by Formicola et al. were selected and tested in our study [13]. All the genotypic distributions analyzed in patients and controls were in accordance with the Hardy-Weinberg equilibrium ($P > .05$).

GRIA1 polymorphisms

No significant difference in genotypic and allelic distribution was observed in the polymorphisms of rs548294 between migraine cases and controls. And also, difference was not observed for any of the migraine subtypes (MA, MO) tested (Tables 2 and 3).

The frequencies of the genotypes of the SNP rs2195450 marker showed significant difference between migraine cases and controls ($P = .004$), and also a positive association with the allelic distribution was observed with an overrepresentation of the T allele (Tables 2 and 3). In the group of patients, the frequency of allele C was 84.1 % (557 C alleles) and allele T was 15.9 % (105 T alleles) for the *GRIA1* (rs2195450) in migraineurs, this was significantly as compared with the controls ($P = .001$, OR = 1.786, 95 % CI: 1.28–2.49). And an association was also seen in the MA subtype ($P = .012$, OR = 2.092, 95 % CI: 1.17–3.76) and MO subtype ($P = .002$, OR = 1.737, 95 % CI: 1.23–2.45).

Table 2 Genotype frequencies of gene polymorphism in Chinese population

Gene	SNP	Group	Genotype n(%)			P
GRIA1	rs548294		GG	GA	AA	
		Migraine	159(48.0)	130(39.3)	42(12.7)	.642
		MA	28(59.6)	16(34.0)	3(6.4)	.280
		MO	131(46.1)	114(40.1)	39(13.7)	.494
		Control	157(47.6)	138(41.8)	35(10.6)	
	rs2195450		CC	CT	TT	
		Migraine	238(71.9)	81(24.5)	12(3.6)	.004*
		MA	31(66.0)	15(31.9)	1(2.1)	.027
		MO	207(72.9)	66(23.2)	11(3.9)	.011**
		Control	272(82.4)	53(16.1)	5(1.5)	
GRIA3	rs3761555		GG	GA	AA	
		Migraine	135(40.8)	154(46.5)	42(12.7)	.564
		MA	21(44.7)	19(40.4)	7(14.9)	.864
		MO	114(40.1)	135(47.5)	35(12.3)	.470
		Control	134(40.6)	145(43.9)	51(15.5)	

Abbreviations: *MA* migraine with aura, *MO* migraine without aura, *SNP* single nucleotide polymorphisms

*All female migraine patients compared with controls by genotype: $P < .017$

**MO compared with controls by genotype: $P < .017$

Table 3 Allele frequencies of gene polymorphism in Chinese population

Gene	SNP	Group	Allele n(%)		P
GRIA1	rs548294		G	A	
		Migraine	448(67.7)	214(32.3)	.752
		MA	72(76.6)	22(23.4)	.110
		MO	376(66.2)	192(33.8)	.394
		Control	452(68.5)	208(31.5)	
	rs2195450		C	T	
		Migraine	557(84.1)	105(15.9)	.001*
		MA	77(81.9)	17(18.1)	.012**
		MO	480(84.5)	88(15.5)	.002***
		Control	597(90.5)	63(9.5)	
GRIA3	rs3761555		G	A	
		Migraine	424(64.0)	238(36.0)	.579
		MA	61(64.9)	33(35.1)	.663
		MO	363(63.9)	205(36.1)	.629
		Control	413(62.5)	247(37.4)	

Abbreviations: *MA* migraine with aura, *MO* migraine without aura, *SNP* single nucleotide polymorphisms, *CI* confidence interval

*All female migraine patients compared with controls by allele: odds ratio =1.786, 95 % CI: 1.28–2.49, $P < .017$

**MA compared with controls by allele: odds ratio =2.092, 95 % CI: 1.17–3.76, $P < .017$

***MO compared with controls by allele: odds ratio =1.737, 95 % CI: 1.23–2.45, $P < .017$

GRIA3 polymorphisms

No significant difference in genotypic and allelic distribution was observed in the polymorphisms of rs3761555 between migraine cases and controls. And also, difference was not observed for any of the tow migraine subtypes tested (Tables 2 and 3).

Discussion

Glutamate is the most abundant excitatory neurotransmitter in the brain,glutamate and the receptors are intimately involved in trigeminovascular activation, central sensitization and cortical spreading depression. Alterations in the function or expression of components of this system may be involved in migraine susceptibility [12]. Biochemical, preclinical experiments and pharmacological studies also support involvement of glutamate in migraine [18–20].

In addition, the previous studies have reported the significant role of glutamatergic gene variants played in the pathophysiology of migraine. GWAS supported that genetic variants (rs1835740 at 8q22.1 and rs11172113 in *LRP1*)associated with migraine [16, 21, 22], and both of these tow genetic variants were involved in the regulation of glutamatergic system [23]. Another association analysis on Italian population have reported two genes that code for subunits of the ionotropic AMPA receptors *GRIA1* and *GRIA3* have been implicated in migraine [13]. Although a number of studies have reported associations between particular glutamatergic gene variants and migraine susceptibility, replication studies to confirm previous findings are generally lacking [24]. For instance, as for the *LRP1* gene variation, our previous results [17] and another research-based Chinese Han population [25] both failed to replicate the association between rs11172113 and migraine. The present study is the first reported case-control association study to independently replicate the variations in the *GRIA1* and *GRIA3* genes in Chinese Han population.

In our present study, a statistically significant finding is that the *GRIA1* rs2195450 variant is a potential genetic risk factor for female migraine in the Chinese Han population from the southern Fujian province of China. In the subgroup analysis, the variant indicates association with the MA, MO subtype. This result was not as same as the previous reports. In 2010, Formicola and colleagues first reported the rs2195450 SNP of *GRIA1* gene was associated with the MA subgroup of migraineurs in Italian Caucasian population [13]. However, the SNP rs2195450 was in Hardy-Weinberg disequilibrium (DHW) both in controls and in patients, suggesting the possibility in the study of inappropriate population stratification and selection or other confounding factors.

Subsequently, two independent studies in Australia [26] and Italy Caucasian population [27] have both failed to identify the association of rs2195450 with migraine, either MA or MO. But it should be noted that the study in Australia population, the rs2195450 SNP was in DHW in the control group, and the study in Italy Caucasian population only included 186 patients. Compared with previous studies, our study involves a relatively larger sample size. Moreover, the rs2195450 SNP was found in HWE both in controls and in patients. Nonetheless, an even larger scale case-control study in populations of different origin should be performed to evaluate the association of the *GRIA1* rs2195450 variant to migraine susceptibility.

However, no association of the other SNP (rs548294) of *GRIA1* gene with migraine was found in our study, even in the subtype's analysis. Although the previous results manifests that rs548294 SNP was significantly associated with migraine (MO and Female) in Italian Caucasian population [13]. But subsequent replication studies of this variant carried out in Italian Caucasian population failed to identify the association of rs548294 with migraine. Furthermore, when the two Italian Caucasian population studies were combined for pooled analysis, none of the genetic models testes provided a significant association between rs548294 polymorphism and MO risk [27]. In addition, another study in Australia population reported no evidence of association between rs548294 and risk of migraine [26]. Existing studies indicates that this variant may be not a risk factor for migraine.

Similarly, the rs3761555 SNP of *GRIA3* gene was also found no association with MA or MO in our study. This result was opposite to the previous two findings. The two former studies have showed the same results that rs3761555 SNP was significantly associated with migraine (MA and Female) [26, 27]. These controversial results may be caused by ethnic differences, environmental effects, and limited sample size.

Conclusions

This study is the first report of rs2195450 SNP in *GRIA1* gene associated with female migraine (MA, MO) in Chinese Han population. The result also provides evidence that the glutamatergic system, particularly the *GRIA1* gene, is implicated in the pathophysiology of migraine. Further research into the glutamatergic system is necessary to ascertain the mechanism in the aetiology of migraine.

Competing interests
The authors declare that they have no competing interests.

Authors' contributions
JF and XA carried out the molecular genetic studies, performed the statistical analysis and drafted the manuscript. SC and ZY carried out the acquisition of data. QM and HQ conceived of the study, and participated in its design and coordination and helped to draft the manuscript. All authors read and approved the final manuscript.

Acknowledgments
We would like to thank all the patients and control subjects who participated in this study. We gratefully acknowledge Professor Jean-Marc Burgunder for his help in the section of language and statistics. This work was supported by the National Natural Science Foundation of China (No.81400912), Fujian Medical Technology Innovation Programs (No.2014-CXB-33), Xiamen Important Joint Research Project of Major Diseases (No.3502Z20149028), Science and Technology Program of Xiamen (No.3502Z20154014).

Author details
[1]Department of Neurology, The First Affiliated Hospital of Xiamen University, Xiamen, China. [2]The First Clinical Medical College of Fujian Medical University, Fuzhou, China.

References

1. Headache Classification Committee of the International Headache S (2013) The international classification of headache disorders, 3rd edition (beta version). Cephalalgia 33(9):629–808
2. Lipton RB, Bigal ME, Diamond M, Freitag F, Reed ML, Stewart WF et al (2007) Migraine prevalence, disease burden, and the need for preventive therapy. Neurology 68(5):343–349
3. Yu S, Liu R, Zhao G, Yang X, Qiao X, Feng J et al (2012) The prevalence and burden of primary headaches in China: a population-based door-to-door survey. Headache 52(4):582–591

4. Schurks M (2012) Genetics of migraine in the age of genome-wide association studies. J Headache Pain 13(1):1–9
5. Mulder EJ, Van Baal C, Gaist D, Kallela M, Kaprio J, Svensson DA et al (2003) Genetic and environmental influences on migraine: a twin study across six countries. Twin Res 6(5):422–431
6. Lambert GA, Zagami AS (2009) The mode of action of migraine triggers: a hypothesis. Headache 49(2):253–275
7. Parsons AA, Strijbos PJ (2003) The neuronal versus vascular hypothesis of migraine and cortical spreading depression. Curr Opin Pharmacol 3(1):73–77
8. Moskowitz MA (2007) Genes, proteases, cortical spreading depression and migraine: impact on pathophysiology and treatment. Funct Neurol 22(3):133–136
9. Andreou AP, Goadsby PJ (2009) Therapeutic potential of novel glutamate receptor antagonists in migraine. Expert Opin Investig Drugs 18(6):789–803
10. Vikelis M, Mitsikostas DD (2007) The role of glutamate and its receptors in migraine. CNS Neurol Disord Drug Targets 6(4):251–257
11. Ramadan NM (2003) The link between glutamate and migraine. CNS Spectr 8(6):446–449
12. Gasparini CF, Griffiths LR (2013) The biology of the glutamatergic system and potential role in migraine. Int J Biomed Sci 9(1):1–8
13. Formicola D, Aloia A, Sampaolo S, Farina O, Diodato D, Griffiths LR et al (2010) Common variants in the regulative regions of GRIA1 and GRIA3 receptor genes are associated with migraine susceptibility. BMC Med Genet 11:103
14. Anttila V, Stefansson H, Kallela M, Todt U, Terwindt GM, Calafato MS et al (2010) Genome-wide association study of migraine implicates a common susceptibility variant on 8q22.1. Nat Genet 42(10):869–873
15. Chasman DI, Schurks M, Anttila V, de Vries B, Schminke U, Launer LJ et al (2011) Genome-wide association study reveals three susceptibility loci for common migraine in the general population. Nat Genet 43(7):695–698
16. Freilinger T, Anttila V, de Vries B, Malik R, Kallela M, Terwindt GM et al (2012) Genome-wide association analysis identifies susceptibility loci for migraine without aura. Nat Genet 44(7):777–782
17. An XK, Ma QL, Lin Q, Zhang XR, Lu CX, Qu HL (2013) PRDM16 rs2651899 variant is a risk factor for Chinese common migraine patients. Headache 53(10):1595–1601
18. Andreou AP, Goadsby PJ (2011) Topiramate in the treatment of migraine: a kainate (glutamate) receptor antagonist within the trigeminothalamic pathway. Cephalalgia 31(13):1343–1358
19. Bigal M, Rapoport A, Sheftell F, Tepper D, Tepper S (2008) Memantine in the preventive treatment of refractory migraine. Headache 48(9):1337–1342
20. Marin JC, Goadsby PJ (2010) Glutamatergic fine tuning with ADX-10059: a novel therapeutic approach for migraine? Expert Opin Investig Drugs 19(4):555–561
21. de Vries B, Frants RR, Ferrari MD, van den Maagdenberg AM (2009) Molecular genetics of migraine. Hum Genet 126(1):115–132
22. Ligthart L, de Vries B, Smith AV, Ikram MA, Amin N, Hottenga JJ et al (2011) Meta-analysis of genome-wide association for migraine in six population-based European cohorts. Eur J Hum Genet 19(8):901–907
23. Kai-Kai MA, Howe R (1991) Glutamate-immunoreactivity in the trigeminal and dorsal root ganglia, and intraspinal neurons and fibres in the dorsal horn of the rat. Histochem J 23(4):171–179
24. Cutrer FM, Smith JH (2013) Human studies in the pathophysiology of migraine: genetics and functional neuroimaging. Headache 53(2):401–412
25. Fan X, Wang J, Fan W, Chen L, Gui B, Tan G et al (2014) Replication of migraine GWAS susceptibility loci in Chinese Han population. Headache 54(4):709–715
26. Maher BH, Lea RA, Follett J, Cox HC, Fernandez F, Esposito T et al (2013) Association of a GRIA3 gene polymorphism with migraine in an Australian case-control cohort. Headache 53(8):1245–1249
27. Cargnin S, Viana M, Mittino D, Bellomo G, Tassorelli C, Nappi G et al (2014) Lack of association between GRIA1 polymorphisms and haplotypes with migraine without aura or response to triptans. Neurol Sci 35(3):421–427

2

Differences in central facilitation between episodic and chronic migraineurs in nociceptive-specific trigeminal pathways

Jong-Hee Sohn*, Chul-Ho Kim and Hui-Chul Choi

Abstract

Background: The trigeminal nociceptive system plays a pivotal role in the pathophysiology of migraines. The present study investigated whether there are differences between patients with episodic migraine (EM) and patients with chronic migraine (CM) in trigeminal pain processing at the brainstem and cortical levels using the nociceptive blink reflex (nBR) and pain-related evoked potentials (PREP).

Methods: This study assessed 68 female migraineurs (38 EM patients and 30 CM patients) and 40 age-matched controls using simultaneous recordings of nBR and PREP during the interictal period.

Results: In terms of the nBR, EM patients displayed significantly decreased latencies and larger amplitudes and area-under-the-curve (AUC) values for the R2 component, whereas CM patients showed significantly prolonged latencies and smaller amplitudes and AUC values for the R2 component ($p < 0.05$). In terms of PREP, both the EM and CM patients had decreased latencies (N1, P1), with larger amplitude compared with the controls ($p < 0.05$), which indicates facilitation at the cortical level. Additionally, the amplitude and AUC values of the R2 component exhibited a negative correlation, whereas the latency of the R2 component for the nBR showed a positive correlation, with the frequency of headaches in migraineurs ($p < 0.01$).

Conclusions: In the present study, the facilitation in the trigeminal nociceptive pathway of the EM group suggests the occurrence of migraine-specific hyperexcitability. Additionally, the suppression of R2 at the brainstem level in the CM group may relate to impaired or dysfunctional descending pain modulation. These findings suggest that there are adaptive or maladaptive responses due to the chronification of migraine attacks.

Keywords: Chronic migraine, Episodic migraine, Nociceptive blink reflex, Pain-related evoked potential, Trigeminal pathway

Background

Chronic migraine (CM) is a disabling neurological condition, accepted by the main body of the current beta version of the International Classification of Headache Disorders-3 (ICHD-3β) [1]. This classification indicates that the chronicity of the disorder is not a complication of migraine, but rather a transformation from an episodic to a chronic disorder. Approximately 3 % of individuals with episodic migraine (EM) progress to CM over the course of a year [2]. Despite the spectrum conceptualization of migraine, there are important distinctions between EM and CM. Several studies have provided data on differences in symptoms, comorbidity profiles, disabilities, and treatment responses of CM versus EM [3–6]. Moreover, differences in pathophysiology and functional correlates observed in electrophysiological and imaging studies have been noted [7]. Although the precise mechanisms underlying headache chronification from EM to CM are not fully understood, the central sensitization and dysfunctional pain control systems are thought to be involved [8].

The trigeminal nociceptive system plays a pivotal role in the pathophysiology of migraine. The use of neurophysiological methods to explore pain-related circuits is

* Correspondence: deepfoci@hallym.or.kr
Department of Neurology, Chuncheon Sacred Heart Hospital, Hallym University College of Medicine, 153 Gyo-dong, Chuncheon-si, Gangwon-do 200-704, Republic of Korea

an important aid in headache research. To increase nociceptive sensitivity, previous studies have developed a novel technique of selective electrical transcutaneous nociceptive fiber stimulation using a custom concentric planar electrode. The concentric electrode allows quantitative measurements of trigeminal nociception transmission and is highly sensitive to changes in trigeminal nociception [9–13]. Investigations of trigeminal nociceptive pathways during ictal phases have been recorded in EM, and these data suggest temporary and specific sensitization of central trigeminal neurons during acute migraine attacks [9, 14]. In addition, the possibility that increased excitability of the trigeminal pathways may persist during the interictal period has been proposed in EM [15]; however, investigations of trigeminal sensory pathways in CM, particularly in regard to nociceptive processing, are rare. One previous study did not observe any changes [16], whereas other studies observed abnormal excitability [13, 17]. These inconsistencies may result from the use of different study techniques, such as the conventional blink reflex, or different study groups, such as in individuals with combined medication-overuse headaches. It has been assumed that these abnormalities would be more marked in CM, and that there are distinctions between EM and CM.

Thus, we hypothesized that the nociceptive trigeminal pathway may be altered to varying degrees in patients with EM and CM. We assessed trigeminal nociceptive processing in patients with EM and CM during the interictal period compared to healthy controls to investigate the presence or absence of facilitation processes in the patient group. To determine whether there were differences in trigeminal pain processing at the brainstem and cortical levels, we used the nociceptive blink reflex (nBR) and pain-related evoked potentials (PREP) in EM and CM patients.

Methods

Subjects

This study collected data from patients with EM and CM treated in the headache clinic of a university hospital between October 2014 and June 2015. All participants were between 20 and 60 years of age, and only females were included to eliminate age and gender bias. They were examined and classified according to the ICHD-3β by a board-certified neurologist based on patient history, a neurologic examination, and neuroimaging study. Additionally, patients were required to have at least a 1-year migraine history prior to enrollment, to exclude other primary headaches. 30 patients with CM and 38 patients with EM were investigated in a case–control design. The control group consisted of 40 age-matched female volunteers. We recruited the control group via advertisements such as posted notices in the hospital. Control participants had to be devoid of headaches for at least 3 months prior to enrollment, have no personal or family history of migraine, and have no more than an occasional mild headache (<5 times per year); we also included only those participants who had not sought medical treatment for headaches. Exclusion criteria included subjects with prophylactic daily medication to prevent headaches, concomitant medication-overuse headache based on ICHD-3β, neurological disorders, any other systemic disease, history of Bell's palsy, somatic or psychiatric illness (e.g., depression, anxiety disorder), use of oral contraceptives, and pregnancy.

The patients with migraine were asked to complete a headache questionnaire during the last one month. Headache frequency (days/month) by the number of days with headaches for a month, duration (hours/day) by the sum of the total hours of headaches per attack, and intensity (numeric rating scale [NRS]: 0 = no pain to 10 = unbearable pain) by calculating the mean of the NRS for the days with headaches were described. All participants were instructed to refrain from caffeine, nicotine, and alcohol for at least 24 h prior to testing. This study protocol and informed consent form were reviewed and approved by the local Institutional Review Board (Institutional Review Board/Ethics Committee of Hallym University Chuncheon Sacred Heart Hospital). Written informed consent was obtained from all participants prior to enrollment in the study.

Experimental procedure

The recording sessions were conducted at the same time of day (2–5 PM) by expert neurophysiologists (J-H, J) blind to the clinical diagnosis of the subjects. Recordings were performed using a Nicolet EDX EMP/EP machine (Natus Neurology, Middleton, WI, USA). Patients with migraine underwent testing during headache-free days. Specifically, recordings in EM patients were obtained interictally at least 2 days after the last and before the next migraine attack. All CM patients underwent the recordings in the interictal period (at least 2 days before and after a typical migraine attack), but a current background mild headache (NRS < 3) was allowed. Following the test, patients were contacted by telephone and excluded from the study if they had experienced a migraine attack within 2 days of the recording. The participants were in a lying position with their eyes closed during the recordings. Two planar concentric surface stimulating electrodes were used for nociceptive stimulation (inomed Medizintechnik GmbH, Emmendingen, Germany, http://www.inomed.com).

Individual sensory (Is) and pain (Ip) perception thresholds were defined as the minimum stimulation intensity perceived as tactile and painful, respectively. We first determined sensory and pain threshold on both sides of the forehead using ascending and descending single pulses in 0.1 mA steps, with a duration of 0.5 ms and an interstimulus interval of 15–20 s (randomized interval). For patients' comfort and to avoid a lengthy procedure, we performed unilateral stimulation for the nBR and PREP recordings. The concentric electrode was placed on the left lower forehead, approximately 10 mm above the supraorbital foramen, to stimulate the supraorbital nerve. nBR and PREP were recorded simultaneously following trigeminal stimulation of the forehead A fixed stimulation intensity (SI) of 1.5 × Ip was used to evoke the nBR and PREP. Trains of electrical stimulation composed of three pulses (each 0.5 ms in duration) with a 5 ms interpulse interval were applied to further increase nociceptive specificity [12], and stimulation intensities > 2 mA were excluded to minimize the risk of Aβ fiber co-activation [10]. Repeated stimulation of the train pulse was delivered at random intervals of 18–22 s to obtain at least 11 consecutive responses. Surface recording electrodes for nBR were placed on the infraorbital area (active) and at the base of the nose with a 2 Hz to 1 kHz band-pass filter (sampling rate 2.5 kHz, 150 ms sweep length, 200 ms analysis time, and 100 μV sensitivity), which was used for recording. PREP was recorded with electrodes placed at Cz linked to both earlobes (A1–A2) based on the international 10–20 system.

Analysis

An investigator who was blind to the diagnosis performed signal analyses. All recordings were averaged offline using the Synergy Reader software, version 20.1 (Natus Neurology). The first recording was excluded from signal analysis to avoid contamination with startle response.

For the nBR recording, the 10 responses were rectified and averaged offline. The onset latency was visually determined as the initial point from the baseline (ms), and the AUC was determined between 27 ms and 87 ms of the R2 component (mV*ms) [18]. The following parameters were measured: the onset latency (ms), the mean amplitude of the root mean square (RMS, μV), and the area under the curve (AUC, mV*ms) values from the ipsilateral and contralateral R2 (iR2 and cR2).

For the PREP recording, the 10 responses were averaged offline. The negative (N1) and positive (P1) peak latencies and peak-to-peak amplitudes (PPA) were analyzed. The following parameters were measured: the peak latency of N1 and P1 (ms) and the mean of the PPA (μV).

Statistics

Statistical analyses were performed using SPSS software ver. 21.0 for Windows (SPSS, Inc., Chicago, IL, USA). All values are reported as means and standard deviations. The Kruskal-Wallis test was used to compare the thresholds and parameters of nBR and PREP between groups. The Mann–Whitney *U* test for multiple comparisons was performed for the *post-hoc* analyses. Spearman's correlation analysis was used to explore the relationship between electrophysiologic parameters and headache parameters (i.e., frequency, duration, and intensity). Results were considered significant at a p-value < 0.05.

Results

Clinical characteristics

No significant differences in age were noted (EM: 40.95 years, CM: 43.07 years, controls: 43.73 years). The frequency of headaches and the duration of the headaches according to the headache questionnaire were 4.81 days/month and 14.71 h/day, in patients with EM and 20.03 days/month and 16.00 h/day, respectively, in patients with CM. The mean intensity per episode (NRS) was 7.74 in patients with EM and 7.96 in patients with CM. The duration of having the headache condition was 9.93 years and 14.13 in patients with EM and CM, respectively (Table 1).

Sensory and pain thresholds

The mean values for sensory and pain perception thresholds (mA) were as follows: 0.20 ± 0.09, 0.78 ± 0.30 in EM, 0.19 ± 0.05, 0.77 ± 0.26 in CM, and 0.20 ± 0.10, 0.84 ± 0.35 in controls. Patients with CM displayed lower sensory and pain perception thresholds during the recording; however, no significant differences were noted

Table 1 Demographic data and headache features

	EM *n* = 38	CM *n* = 30	Control *n* = 40	*P*-value
Age (years)	40.95 ± 10.00	43.07 ± 11.09	43.73 ± 11.75	NS
Frequency (days/month)	4.81 ± 3.30	20.03 ± 4.39	-	0.00
Duration (hours/day)	14.71 ± 8.44	16.00 ± 8.46	-	NS
Intensity (NRS: 0–10)	7.74 ± 1.91	7.96 ± 1.67	-	NS
Disease duration (years)	9.93 ± 9.06	14.13 ± 10.00	-	0.07

Values are expressed as mean ± standard deviation
CM chronic migraine, *EM* episodic migraine, *NS* not significant, *NRS* numeric rating scale

between subject groups. The mean values for pain stimulation intensity of each group was 1.17 (confidence interval, CI, 0.32–1.98) in EM, 1.16 (CI, 0.59–1.95) in CM, and 1.27 (CI, 0.32–1.98) in controls.

Nociceptive blink reflex

The nBR results related to trigeminal nociceptive processing at the brainstem level are summarized in Table 2. Examples of an nBR recording from a patient with EM, a patient with CM, and a healthy control are shown in Fig. 1. The mean amplitude (RMS) and AUC values from the ipsilateral and contralateral R2 components (iR2 and cR2) were significantly lower in CM patients than in control and EM patients. Additionally, significantly prolonged latencies of the R2 component were seen in patients with CM (iR2 in CM vs. controls, iR2 and cR2 in CM vs. EM, $p < 0.05$). However, EM patients displayed significantly decreased latencies and larger amplitudes and AUC values of both R2 components in nBR ($p < 0.05$).

Pain-related evoked potentials

The PREP results regarding trigeminal nociceptive processing at the cortical level are summarized in Table 3. Examples of a PREP recording from patients with EM and CM and a healthy control are shown in Fig. 1. EM patients displayed significantly decreased latencies (both N1 and P1), with larger right amplitude (PPA), compared with controls ($p < 0.05$). Additionally, CM patients showed significantly decreased latencies (left N1, left and right P1), with larger right amplitude (PPA), compared with controls ($p < 0.05$). However, no significant differences were found in the PREP parameters between patients with EM and CM.

Correlations between headache parameters and electrophysiologic parameters

To explore possible clinical–electrophysiological correlations, we examined the correlations between headache parameters, including frequency, duration, and intensity, and nBR and PREP parameters. Although the latency of the R2 component in the nBR was positively correlated with the frequency of headache, the amplitude and AUC from the R2 component in the nBR were negatively correlated with the frequency of headache parameters in the migraine group ($p < 0.01$) (Table 4). However, apart from these, no significant correlations were noted between nBR and PREP parameters and other headache parameters.

Discussion

Our results showed R2 suppression at the brainstem level (nBR) and facilitation at the cortical level (PREP) of trigeminal pain processing in CM patients, and facilitation at both the brainstem and cortical levels in EM patients. In addition, for the nBR, a significant correlation between headache frequency and R2 suppression (prolonged latency, low amplitude, low AUC) was demonstrated in migraineurs.

A variety of nociceptive stimuli are able to elicit PREP at the cortical level and can be used to assess spinothalamocortical pain-temperature pathways [19, 20]. Previous clinical studies have demonstrated the facilitation of the trigeminal nociceptive system in a pain-free state with event-related potentials following CO_2 laser stimulation (LEP) in CM and chronic tension-type headache [21, 22]. In patients with medication overuse headache, activation of trigeminal and somatic PREP, but not of nBR was also found [13]. However, these central facilitation changes at the cortical level have not been observed in other chronic headache disorders, such as hypnic headache [23]. Thus, it is not clear whether this observed phenomenon is the cause or the consequence of the headache chronification.

In our study, facilitation of trigeminal PREP during the inter-ictal period was observed in both the EM and CM groups. The cingulate cortex has been thought to play a major role in cortical plasticity as the main generator of PREP or LEP [24, 25]. Patients with EM have shown deficient habituation with LEP represented by an abnormal excitability of cortical areas during interictal phase [26]. Several studies have shown modulation of the habituation deficit in LEP induced by preventive medication and by high-frequency repetitive transcranial magnetic stimulation [27, 28]. This deficient habituation in the LEP was also

Table 2 Nociceptive blink reflex parameters

	iR2 of nBR			cR2 of nBR		
	Latency (ms)	Amplitude (μ)	AUC (mV *ms)	Latency (ms)	Amplitude (μ)	AUC (mV *ms)
EM	42.76 ± 3.90**, ***	306.50 ± 126.17**, ***	3.50 ± 1.87**, ***	44.96 ± 3.69**, ***	238.55 ± 85.95**, ***	2.84 ± 1.28**, ***
CM	48.44 ± 5.04*, ***	154.56 ± 41.66*, ***	1.59 ± 0.54*, ***	51.02 ± 5.89***	111.78 ± 43.73*, ***	1.11 ± 0.37*, ***
Controls	45.47 ± 3.92	198.68 ± 75.01	2.24 ± 1.00	48.18 ± 4.16	177.81 ± 86.04	2.16 ± 1.30

*$p < 0.05$ between CM and controls; **$p < 0.05$ between EM and controls; ***$p < 0.05$ between CM and EM. *P*-values were determined using the Mann–Whitney *U* test

All values are expressed as means and standard deviations. *EM* episodic migraine, *CM* chronic migraine, *nBR* nociceptive blink reflex, *iR2* ipsilateral R2 component, *cR2* contralateral R2 component, *AUC* area under the curve

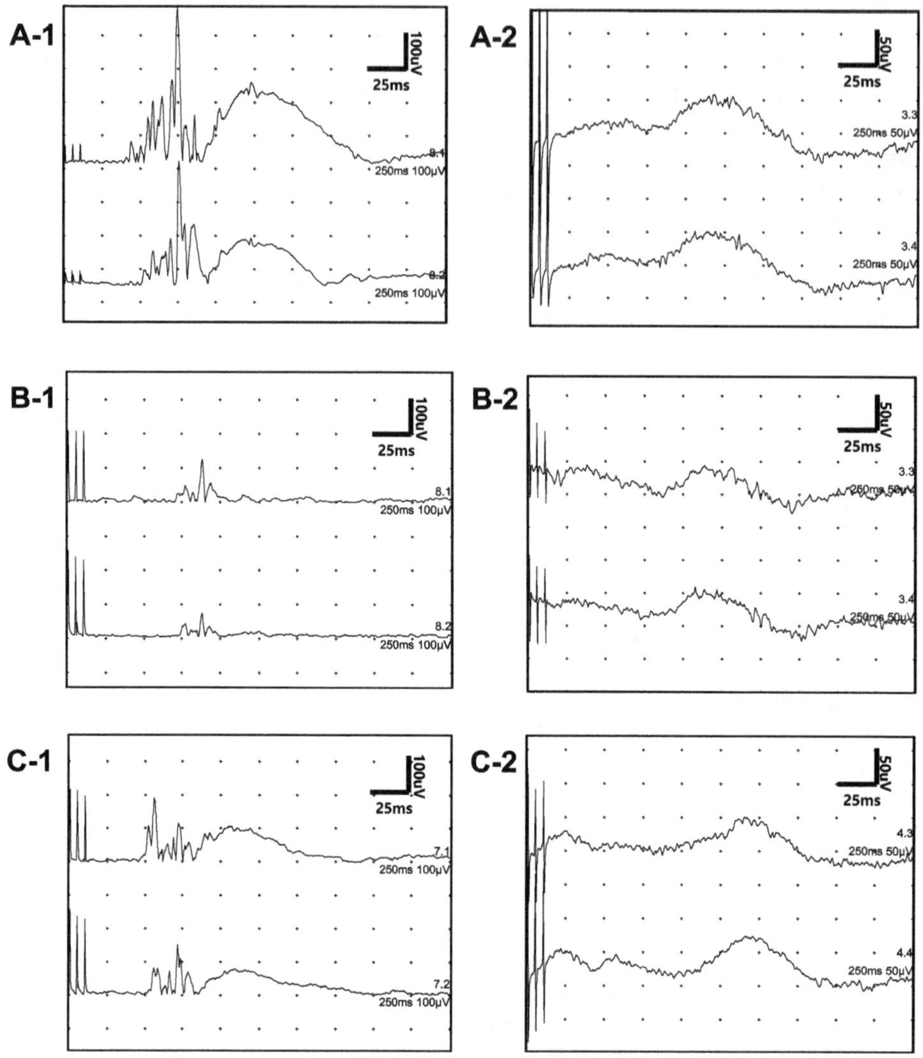

Fig. 1 Examples of the nBR and PREP in patients with episodic and chronic migraine and controls. **A-1** nBR in an EM patient, **A-2** PREP in an EM patient, **B-1** nBR in a CM patient, **B-2** PREP in a CM patient, **C-1** nBR in a control patient, **C-2** PREP in a control patient. nBR, nociceptive blink reflex; PREP, pain-related evoked potential; EM, episodic migraine; CM, chronic migraine

partly restored after treatment of medication overuse headache [29]. These experimental studies reflect a modification in pain-processing pathways, which may constitute an important dysfunction, that probably forms the background in migraineurs. Thus, the facilitation of trigeminal nociception at the cortical level may be specific to migraineurs rather than to the chronification of pain.

The R2 component of the blink reflex reflects the excitability of brainstem interneurons and the function of synaptic transmission in the brainstem [30]. Previous studies have reported that the R2 component of the nBR

Table 3 Pain-related evoked potential parameters

	Left PREP			Right PREP		
	N1 latency (ms)	P1 latency (ms)	PPA (μ)	N1 latency (ms)	P1 latency (ms)	PPA (μ)
EM	122.62 ± 9.71**	169.82 ± 9.70**	63.76 ± 13.22	121.37 ± 10.09**	169.56 ± 10.61**	63.75 ± 13.35**
CM	125.25 ± 8.71*	172.83 ± 10.43*	61.05 ± 15.65	125.95 ± 8.46	172.47 ± 10.43*	59.13 ± 15.74*
Controls	130.71 ± 6.84	179.10 ± 8.50	59.48 ± 14.25	130.14 ± 6.94	178.59 ± 8.05**	54.63 ± 13.91

*$p < 0.05$ between CM and controls; **$p < 0.05$ between EM and controls; there are no statistical differences between CM and EM for PREP parameters. *P*-values were determined using the Mann–Whitney *U* test. All values are expressed as means and standard deviations

EM episodic migraine, *CM* chronic migraine, *PREP* pain-related evoked potential, *PPA* peak-to-peak amplitude, *AUC* area under the curve

Table 4 Correlation coefficients between headache characteristics and parameters of the nBR and the PREP in migraineurs

	Correlation coefficient (*r*) for the nBR parameters		
	Latency	Amplitude	AUC
Frequency of headache attacks (days)	0.497 (iR2)**	−0.588 (iR2)**	−0.521 (iR2)**
	0.469 (cR2)**	−0.634 (cR2)**	−0.626 (cR2)**
Duration of headache attacks (hours)	NS	NS	NS
Pain intensity of headache attacks (NRS)	NS	NS	NS

Spearman's correlation test (*r*), ***p* < 0.01. *EM* episodic migraine, *CM* chronic migraine, *PREP* pain-related evoked potential, *NRS* numeric rating scale, *NS* non-significant, *nBR* nociceptive blink reflex, *iR2* ipsilateral R2 component, *cR2* contralateral R2 component, *AUC* area under the curve, *PREP* pain-related evoked potential, *PPA* peak-to-peak amplitude

by nociceptive stimuli was more than six times greater during migraine attacks [9]; these facilitation changes are specific to episodic migraines and act as the central driving force for migraine attacks [14]. Several studies using neurophysiologic tools to explore the trigeminal system during the interictal period found that patients with EM have a lack of habituation of nBR and enhanced R2 recovery of BR and corneal reflex abnormality [15, 31, 32]. Our results showing R2 facilitation of nBR between attacks in EM patients are consistent with these findings. These phenomena suggest that sensitization of the trigeminal system may persist interictally. Another interesting finding is that asymptomatic individuals with a family history of migraine present the same nBR abnormalities as patients with full-brown migraine between attacks [33]. On the other hand, another study found normal the R2 recovery curves between attacks in EM patients and these results do not support persistent interictal sensitization in the spinal trigeminal sensory system [34].

However, in terms of the nBR, R2 suppression occurred in the CM group, which differed from the EM group in our study in this regard. Additionally, each parameter of the nBR (latency, amplitude, and AUC) was positively or negatively correlated with headache frequency in migraineurs. Thus, the degree of R2 suppression seems to be correlated with the number of headache days. Brainstem interneuronal excitability is assumed to be under the control of rostral structures, and the R2 component of the blink reflex is largely influenced by suprasegmental control, that comes mainly from the cerebral cortex and basal ganglia [35, 36]. The descending pain modulation system might be responsible for keeping the primary value of the nBR within certain physiological boundaries with respect to homeostatic neuronal plasticity [37]. These networks of cortical and subcortical structures with modulatory nociceptive and antinociceptive functions become abnormally activated during, or even between, migraine attacks [38]. During repeated migraine attacks, modification of this network can occur. Therefore, excessive R2 suppression at the brainstem level may be related to an impaired or dysfunctional descending pain modulation system. These findings may relate to adaptive or dysregulated/maladaptive mechanisms within the context of the allostatic load model [39].

Excitability changes in the blink reflex circuit can also occur as a consequence of damage in the neural structures along the blink reflex circuit [36]. Several neuroimaging studies on migraineurs reported morphological and functional abnormalities in the brainstem [40–43]. In particular, EM patients demonstrated activation of the rostral brainstem during the interictal phase in functional MRI and exhibited increased density in the periaqueductal gray matter in structural imaging using voxel-based morphometry [42, 43]. MRI findings of iron accumulation in the brainstem have been correlated with both duration of illness and frequency of attacks in migraineurs [44]. Additionally, CM patients showed persistent brainstem dysfunction in positron emission tomography evaluations and brainstem atrophy in high-resolution anatomical MRI images [45, 46]. A functional imaging study using ^{1}H-magnetic resonance spectroscopy showed an increased N-acetyl aspartate/creatinine (NAA/Cr) ratio suggestive of neuronal hypertrophy at the dorsal pons in EM compared with controls. Headache frequency and intensity were negatively correlated with the NAA/Cr ratio. These findings suggest that after an initial response of hypertrophy in EM, there may be neuronal loss in CM in these regions [47]. Thus, these plastic structural changes according to migraine status may influence the R2 facilitation or suppression of the nBR in migraineurs. Repeated episodes of central sensitization may be associated with neuronal damage at the brainstem level, with resultant poor modulation of pain, and migraine progression [48]. However, it is currently unclear whether these structural brain changes seen in migraineurs are the cause or the result of headaches.

Our study had several limitations. Patients at a specialized headache clinic were recruited, and the size of the sample was small. Additionally, the study used a cross-sectional design that provided limited information. To further understand the differences between EM and CM, longitudinal electrophysiological follow-up studies are warranted. Moreover, we used only unilateral stimulation for recording to avoid an excessively lengthy procedure and to enhance patients' comfort. We believe that these decisions are probably not relevant to the interpretation of our results, because none of our patients had fixed unilateral migraine attacks, and there were no side differences in stimulus detection and pain threshold measurements. In addition, only females were included in the present study because of potential effects of sex on the blink reflex [49]; therefore, we are unable to generalize to men. A larger study sample will be required for a better and improved understanding of the relationship between measured electrophysiological factors and clinical findings.

Conclusions

In conclusion, this study provides electrophysiological evidence that excitability of nociceptive-specific trigeminal pathways is different between EM and CM. Facilitation of trigeminal nociceptive processing was observed in EM, whereas R2 suppression at the brainstem level and additional central facilitation changes at the cortical level were seen in CM. Facilitation along trigeminal nociceptive processing in EM patients was associated with migraine-specific hyperexcitability due to intrinsically increased excitability or impaired intra-inhibitory mechanisms. In CM, additional R2 suppression at the brainstem level may be related to impaired or dysfunctional descending pain modulation. These changes in CM are suggestive of adaptive or maladaptive responses due to repetitive episodes of migraine attacks.

Abbreviations

AUC: area under the curve; CM: chronic migraine; cR2: contralateral R2 component; EM: episodic migraine; ICHD-3β: beta version of the International Classification of Headache Disorders-3; Ip: pain perception threshold; iR2: ipsilateral R2 component; Is: sensory perception threshold; N1: negative peak; nBR: nociceptive blink reflex; NRS: numeric rating scale; P1: positive peak; PPA: peak-to-peak amplitude; PREP: pain-related evoked potentials; RMS: root mean square; SI: stimulation intensity.

Competing interests

The authors declare that they have no competing interests.

Authors' contributions

Conception and design of the experiments: JHS. Performance of experiments: CHK, HCC, and JHS. Data analysis: JHS. Writing of the manuscript: JHS. All authors read and approved the final manuscript.

References

1. Headache Classification Committee of the International Headache Society (2013) The international classification of headache disorders, 3rd edition (beta version). Cephalalgia 33:629–808
2. Bigal ME, Lipton RB (2008) Concepts and mechanisms of migraine chronification. Headache 48(1):7–15
3. Blumenfeld AM, Varon SF, Wilcox TK, Buse DC, Kawata AK, Manack A, Goadsby PJ, Lipton RB (2011) Disability, HRQoL and resource use among chronic and episodic migraineurs: results from the International Burden of Migraine Study (IBMS). Cephalalgia 31(3):301–315
4. Buse D, Manack A, Serrano D, Reed M, Varon S, Turkel C, Lipton R (2012) Headache impact of chronic and episodic migraine: results from the American Migraine Prevalence and Prevention study. Headache 52(1):3–17
5. Ferrari A, Leone S, Vergoni AV, Bertolini A, Sances G, Coccia CP, Ottani A, Pinetti D, Sternieri E (2007) Similarities and differences between chronic migraine and episodic migraine. Headache 47(1):65–72
6. Katsarava Z, Manack A, Yoon MS, Obermann M, Becker H, Dommes P, Turkel C, Lipton RB, Diener HC (2011) Chronic migraine: classification and comparisons. Cephalalgia 31(5):520–529
7. Aurora SK, Kulthia A, Barrodale PM (2011) Mechanism of chronic migraine. Curr Pain Headache Rep 15(1):57–63
8. Coppola G, Schoenen J (2012) Cortical excitability in chronic migraine. Curr Pain Headache Rep 16(1):93–100
9. Kaube H, Katsarava Z, Przywara S, Drepper J, Ellrich J, Diener HC (2002) Acute migraine headache: possible sensitization of neurons in the spinal trigeminal nucleus? Neurology 58(8):1234–1238
10. Kaube H, Katsarava Z, Kaufer T, Diener H, Ellrich J (2000) A new method to increase nociception specificity of the human blink reflex. Clin Neurophysiol 111(3):413–416
11. Katsarava Z, Ellrich J, Diener HC, Kaube H (2002) Optimized stimulation and recording parameters of human 'nociception specific' blink reflex recordings. Clin Neurophysiol 113(12):1932–1936
12. Giffin NJ, Katsarava Z, Pfundstein A, Ellrich J, Kaube H (2004) The effect of multiple stimuli on the modulation of the 'nociceptive' blink reflex. Pain 108(1–2):124–128
13. Ayzenberg I, Obermann M, Nyhuis P, Gastpar M, Limmroth V, Diener HC, Kaube H, Katsarava Z (2006) Central sensitization of the trigeminal and somatic nociceptive systems in medication overuse headache mainly involves cerebral supraspinal structures. Cephalalgia 26(9):1106–1114
14. Katsarava Z, Lehnerdt G, Duda B, Ellrich J, Diener HC, Kaube H (2002) Sensitization of trigeminal nociception specific for migraine but not pain of sinusitis. Neurology 59(9):1450–1453
15. Sandrini G, Proietti Cecchini A, Milanov I, Tassorelli C, Buzzi MG, Nappi G (2002) Electrophysiological evidence for trigeminal neuron sensitization in patients with migraine. Neurosci Lett 317(3):135–138
16. Brooks JB, Fragoso YD (2013) The blink reflex test does not show abnormalities in a large group of patients with chronic migraine. Arq Neuropsiquiatr 71(11):862–865
17. De Marinis M, Pujia A, Colaizzo E, Accornero N (2007) The blink reflex in 'chronic migraine. Clin Neurophysiol 118(2):457–463
18. Ellrich J, Treede RD (1998) Characterization of blink reflex interneurons by activation of diffuse noxious inhibitory controls in man. Brain Res 803(1–2): 161–168
19. Arendt-Nielsen L, Andersen OK (2006) Electrophysiological assessment of pain. Suppl Clin Neurophysiol 59:241–249
20. Kakigi R, Inui K, Tamura Y (2005) Electrophysiological studies on human pain perception. Clin Neurophysiol 116(4):743–763
21. de Tommaso M, Libro G, Guido M, Sciruicchio V, Losito L, Puca F (2003) Heat pain thresholds and cerebral event-related potentials following painful CO2 laser stimulation in chronic tension-type headache. Pain 104(1–2):111–119
22. de Tommaso M, Valeriani M, Guido M, Libro G, Specchio LM, Tonali P, Puca F (2003) Abnormal brain processing of cutaneous pain in patients with chronic migraine. Pain 101(1–2):25–32
23. Holle D, Gaul C, Krebs S, Naegel S, Diener HC, Kaube H, Katsarava Z, Obermann M (2011) Nociceptive blink reflex and pain-related evoked potentials in hypnic headache. Cephalalgia 31(11):1181–1188
24. Bromm B (2004) The involvement of the posterior cingulate gyrus in phasic pain processing of humans. Neurosci Lett 361(1–3):245–249
25. Kakigi R, Watanabe S, Yamasaki H (2000) Pain-related somatosensory evoked potentials. J Clin Neurophysiol 17(3):295–308
26. Valeriani M, de Tommaso M, Restuccia D, Le Pera D, Guido M, Iannetti GD, Libro G, Truini A, Di Trapani G, Puca F, Tonali P, Cruccu G (2003) Reduced habituation to experimental pain in migraine patients: a CO(2) laser evoked potential study. Pain 105(1–2):57–64
27. de Tommaso M, Brighina F, Fierro B, Francesco VD, Santostasi R, Sciruicchio V, Vecchio E, Serpino C, Lamberti P, Livrea P (2010) Effects of high-frequency repetitive transcranial magnetic stimulation of primary motor cortex on laser-evoked potentials in migraine. J Headache Pain 11(6):505–512
28. Di Clemente L, Puledda F, Biasiotta A, Vigano A, Vicenzini E, Truini A, Cruccu G, Di Piero V (2013) Topiramate modulates habituation in migraine:

evidences from nociceptive responses elicited by laser evoked potentials. J Headache Pain 14:25
29. Ferraro D, Vollono C, Miliucci R, Virdis D, De Armas L, Pazzaglia C, Le Pera D, Tarantino S, Balestri M, Di Trapani G, Valeriani M (2012) Habituation to pain in "medication overuse headache": a CO2 laser-evoked potential study. Headache 52(5):792–807
30. Ellrich J (2000) Brain Stem Reflexes: Probing Human Trigeminal Nociception. News in Physiol Sci 15:94–97
31. Katsarava Z, Giffin N, Diener HC, Kaube H (2003) Abnormal habituation of 'nociceptive' blink reflex in migraine–evidence for increased excitability of trigeminal nociception. Cephalalgia 23(8):814–819
32. Shibata K, Yamane K, Iwata M (2006) Change of excitability in brainstem and cortical visual processing in migraine exhibiting allodynia. Headache 46(10):1535–1544
33. Di Clemente L, Coppola G, Magis D, Fumal A, De Pasqua V, Di Piero V, Schoenen J (2007) Interictal habituation deficit of the nociceptive blink reflex: an endophenotypic marker for presymptomatic migraine? Brain 130(Pt 3):765–770
34. Coppola G, Di Clemente L, Fumal A, Magis D, De Pasqua V, Pierelli F, Schoenen J (2007) Inhibition of the nociceptive R2 blink reflex after supraorbital or index finger stimulation is normal in migraine without aura between attacks. Cephalalgia 27(7):803–808
35. Esteban A (1999) A neurophysiological approach to brainstem reflexes. Blink reflex. Neurophysiol Clin 29(1):7–38
36. Valls-Sole J (2012) Assessment of excitability in brainstem circuits mediating the blink reflex and the startle reaction. Clin Neurophysiol 123(1):13–20
37. Bienenstock EL, Cooper LN, Munro PW (1982) Theory for the development of neuron selectivity: orientation specificity and binocular interaction in visual cortex. J Neurosci 2(1):32–48
38. Welch KM (2003) Contemporary concepts of migraine pathogenesis. Neurology 61(8 Suppl 4):S2–S8
39. Borsook D, Maleki N, Becerra L, McEwen B (2012) Understanding migraine through the lens of maladaptive stress responses: a model disease of allostatic load. Neuron 73(2):219–234
40. Weiller C, May A, Limmroth V, Juptner M, Kaube H, Schayck RV, Coenen HH, Diener HC (1995) Brain stem activation in spontaneous human migraine attacks. Nat Med 1(7):658–660
41. Bahra A, Matharu MS, Buchel C, Frackowiak RS, Goadsby PJ (2001) Brainstem activation specific to migraine headache. Lancet 357(9261):1016–1017
42. Moulton EA, Burstein R, Tully S, Hargreaves R, Becerra L, Borsook D (2008) Interictal dysfunction of a brainstem descending modulatory center in migraine patients. PLoS ONE 3(11), e3799
43. Rocca MA, Ceccarelli A, Falini A, Colombo B, Tortorella P, Bernasconi L, Comi G, Scotti G, Filippi M (2006) Brain gray matter changes in migraine patients with T2-visible lesions: a 3-T MRI study. Stroke 37(7):1765–1770
44. Welch KM, Nagesh V, Aurora SK, Gelman N (2001) Periaqueductal gray matter dysfunction in migraine: cause or the burden of illness? Headache 41(7):629–637
45. Aurora SK, Barrodale PM, Tipton RL, Khodavirdi A (2007) Brainstem dysfunction in chronic migraine as evidenced by neurophysiological and positron emission tomography studies. Headache 47(7):996–1003, discussion 1004–1007
46. Bilgic B, Kocaman G, Arslan AB, Noyan H, Sherifov R, Alkan A, Asil T, Parman Y, Baykan B (2015) Volumetric differences suggest involvement of cerebellum and brainstem in chronic migraine. Cephalalgia. doi:10.1177/0333102415588328
47. Lai TH, Fuh JL, Lirng JF, Lin CP, Wang SJ (2012) Brainstem 1H-MR spectroscopy in episodic and chronic migraine. J Headache Pain 13(8):645–651
48. Bigal ME, Lipton RB (2006) When migraine progresses: transformed or chronic migraine. Expert Rev Neurother 6(3):297–306
49. Peddireddy A, Wang K, Svensson P, Arendt-Nielsen L (2006) Influence of age and gender on the jaw-stretch and blink reflexes. Exp Brain Res 171(4):530–540

3

Quantitative neuromagnetic signatures of aberrant cortical excitability in pediatric chronic migraine

Kimberly A. Leiken[1*], Jing Xiang[1,2], Emily Curry[1], Hisako Fujiwara[1], Douglas F. Rose[1,2], Janelle R. Allen[3], Joanne E. Kacperski[1,2], Hope L. O'Brien[1,2], Marielle A. Kabbouche[1,2], Scott W. Powers[2,3] and Andrew D. Hershey[1,2]

Abstract

Background: Reports have suggested that abnormal cortical excitability may be associated with acute migraines. The present study quantitatively assesses the degree of cortical excitability in chronic migraine as compared to acute migraine and healthy controls within the pediatric population.

Methods: We investigated 27 children suffering from chronic migraine, 27 children suffering from acute migraine, and 27 healthy controls using a magnetoencephalography (MEG) system, recording at a sampling rate of 6000 Hz. All groups were age-matched and gender-matched. Neuromagnetic brain activation was elicited by a finger-tapping motor task. The spatiotemporal and spectral signatures of MEG data within a 5–2884 Hz range were analyzed using Morlet wavelet transform and beamformer analyses.

Results: Compared with controls, the chronic migraine group showed (1) significantly prolonged latencies of movement-elicited magnetic fields (MEFs) between 5 and 100 Hz; (2) increased spectral power between 100 and 200 Hz, and between 2200 and 2800 Hz; and (3) a higher likelihood of neuromagnetic activation in the ipsilateral sensorimotor cortices, supplementary motor area, and occipital regions. Compared with acute migraine group, chronic migraine patients showed (1) significantly higher odds of having strong MEFs after 150 ms; and (2) significantly higher odds of having neuromagnetic activation from the deep brain areas.

Conclusions: Results demonstrated that chronic migraine subjects were not only different from the healthy controls, but also different from acute migraine subjects. The chronification of migraines may be associated with elevated cortical excitability, delayed and spread neural response, as well as aberrant activation from deep brain areas.

Keywords: Migraine, Magnetoencephalography (MEG), Pediatric, High frequency oscillations, Deep brain sources, Wavelet transform

Background

The prevalence rate of chronic migraine in the general population is 2–4 % [1]. Each year, approximately 2.5 % of patients with episodic migraines eventually develop new-onset chronic migraines [2]. Migraines are defined as "chronic" when a patient has headaches on 15 or more days per month with migraine features for at least 3 months [3–11]. Diagnoses come, in part, from subjective descriptions of patients' episodic headache or pain, leaving few clues for objectively investigating the cerebral mechanism underlying chronic migraine.

Recent reports have found that the alteration of cortical excitability plays a key role in *acute* migraine [12–16], crucial information for diagnosis and treatment. However, it remains unclear whether there is a similar association between cortical abnormalities and *chronic* migraines. Therefore, the present study will address this. Magnetoencephalography (MEG) is well suited for objectively investigating the cerebral

* Correspondence: Kimberly.leiken@cchmc.org
[1]Division of Neurology, Cincinnati Children's Hospital Medical Center, 3333 Burnet Avenue, MLC 2015, Cincinnati, OH 45220, USA
Full list of author information is available at the end of the article

mechanisms underlying migraine for several reasons [17–19]. First, MEG has outstanding temporal resolution to capture brain signals from low- to very high-frequency ranges [20, 21], superior to the capabilities of functional magnetic resonance imaging (fMRI). Therefore, MEG can be used to reveal the abnormality of brain activity in migraine with millisecond-level resolution. Second, MEG has high spatial resolution to assess where and to what degree altered cortical excitability is occurring in migraine, which is superior to that of electroencephalography (EEG) [22].

The objective of the present study was to quantitatively assess the spatiotemporal and spectral signatures of aberrant brain activation in chronic migraine during headache attacks with MEG. To better understand the spatiotemporal and spectral features of chronic migraine, we compared MEG data from chronic migraine subjects to acute migraine subjects and healthy controls. To our knowledge, this is the first report using both low- and high-frequency neuromagnetic signals to spatially and spectrally assess cortical excitability in pediatric chronic migraine. This study provides quantitative information about the location and nature of the neuromagnetic abnormalities associated with chronic migraine that are not present in typically developing children. Furthermore, this study also reveals neuromagnetic biomarkers for distinguishing chronic migraine from acute migraine. These findings are useful for refining existing treatments, for developing novel diagnosis and treatment protocols for migraines, and for determining preventative strategies for the chronification of migraines [23–27].

Methods

Subjects

Twenty-seven chronic migraine subjects (15 females, 12 males; mean (μ) = 13.5 years; standard deviation (SD) = ±3.1 years), 27 acute migraine subjects (19 females, 8 males; μ = 14.2 years; SD = ±2.4 years), and 27 healthy controls (15 females, 12 males; μ = 13.4 years; SD = ±3.2 years) were recruited from the Headache Center at Cincinnati Children's Hospital Medical Center (CCHMC). Inclusion criteria for migraine participants were: (1) migraine with or without aura as defined in the International Classification of Headache Disorders, 2nd Edition (ICHD-II) [28, 29]; (2) no other neurological disorder and (3) being naïve to medication. Controls were recruited to match the subjects diagnosed with chronic migraine for age and gender. Control subjects met inclusion criteria of: (1) healthy without history of neurological disorder, headache or brain injury; (2) age-appropriate hearing, vision, and hand movement. Exclusion criteria for all participants were: (1) presence of an implant, such as a cochlear implant, a pacemaker or neuro-stimulator, or any other devices containing electrical circuitry, generating magnetic signals, or having other metal that could produce visible magnetic noise in the MEG data; (2) noticeable anxiety regarding participation (e.g., expressing worry about the tests with noticeable physical trembling or sweating); and/or (3) inability or unwillingness to readily communicate with personnel operating the MEG equipment. The research protocol (IRB#: 2010-2438) was reviewed and approved by the Institutional Review Board (IRB) at CCHMC. Informed consent was obtained from each subject prior to testing.

Both chronic and acute migraine subjects were diagnosed and pre-screened by pediatric neurologists of the CCHMC Headache Center. The clinical characteristics of migraine subjects were preliminarily assessed with a questionnaire that is collected as a routine clinical procedure for the Headache Center's patients, and has also been employed in previously published research studies [30]. The questionnaire assesses headache frequency, duration, severity, and information about prophylactic and treatment medication [29]. If migraine subjects met the criteria of the present study during screening at their clinical appointment, a MEG researcher would then discuss the study with them and obtain signatures on the IRB consent forms. MEG data from the migraine subjects were recorded during their headache attacks. That is, for patients diagnosed with acute migraine, MEG recordings were performed during acute attacks. As chronic migraine patients are consistently suffering from migraine symptoms, MEG recordings were performed in conjunction with these. For all migraine patients, MEG recordings were performed prior to the initiation of either acute or long-term treatment.

Sound cue task

Participants were instructed to press a button immediately after hearing a 500Hz square wave tone cue. Similar to previous reports [17, 18], subjects used the index finger that was ipsilateral to the tone presented, while keeping other body parts still, and with eyes open and fixed to an arbitrary target during the tests. A trigger from the response button was sent to the MEG system for each button press to align the time course of the behavioral data with the neuromagnetic recordings. The stimuli consisted of 200 trials of tone-button press pairings; 100 tones per ear, which were presented randomly through plastic tubes and earphones. Stimulus presentation and response recording were performed using BrainX software, which is based on DirectX (Microsoft Corporation, Redmond, WA, USA) [17, 18].

MEG recording

The MEG signals were recorded in a magnetically shielded room (Vacuum-Schmelze, Hanau, Germany) using a whole head CTF 275-Channel MEG system (VSM Med-Tech Systems Inc., Coquitlam, BC, Canada) in the MEG Center at CCHMC. The sampling rate of the MEG recordings was 6,000 Hz. An acquisition window was set to 3,000 milliseconds (ms) per trial, with a 2,000 ms pre-trigger baseline window. Data were recorded with a noise cancellation of third-order gradients. Subjects were asked to remain still, but if head movement during a recording was beyond 5 mm, that dataset was not included in analysis, and an additional dataset was recorded.

All subjects were familiarized with the MEG facilities, including the magnetically shielded room, MEG system, and the button box, and then provided the opportunity to opt out of participation. Once subjects agreed to participate in the study, it was reconfirmed that they were free from all possible metals. After that, the subjects laid on a specially designed MEG bed while a researcher attached three fiducial coils to the nasion, left, and right pre-auricular points. These three coils were subsequently activated at different frequencies for measuring participants' head positions relative to the MEG sensors. Just before the MEG recordings, subjects' heads were positioned in the MEG dewar (or helmet) and their head position was localized.

Magnetic resonance imaging (MRI) scan

Three-dimensional (3D) MRI was obtained using a 3T Philips Achieva scanner (Philips Healthcare, 3000 Minuteman Road, Andover, MA). Three fiducial marks were placed in identical locations to the positions of the three coils used in the MEG recordings, to allow for an accurate co-registration of the two data sets. Subsequently, all anatomical landmarks were made identifiable in the MRIs.

Time-frequency decomposition

MEG waveforms were transformed into spectrograms, the time-frequency representations of MEG data [17, 31], using MEG Processor, a customer-designed program for MEG data analyses [32, 33]. The spectral characteristics of MEG data were analyzed with spectrograms computed with the Morlet continuous wavelet algorithm [32–34]. Since frequency-temporal resolution changes with the "sigma value" (the number of wave cycles completed within a time window), the time-frequency analysis method was improved for this study by dynamically changing the sigma value according to frequency ranges [17, 31]. We analyzed neuromagnetic signals in three frequency ranges, which included 5–100 Hz, 100–1000 Hz and 1000–2884 Hz. We did not include neuromagnetic signals below 5 Hz, as the computation of such low-frequency components requires an extremely high number of data points. Moreover, activity below 5 Hz may include *pre-motor* activation, such as the readiness magnetic fields, which we took care to exclude from our analyses of the motor responses of patients with migraine. For each frequency range, we used 600 frequency bins. Consequently, the frequency resolution was 6.315 ((100–5 Hz)/600); 0.667 ((1000–100 Hz)/600); and 0.318 ((2884–1000 Hz)/600) data points per Hz for the three frequency ranges, respectively. To measure magnetic spectral power elicited by finger movements, accumulated spectrograms from 100 trials for the left finger and 100 trials for the right finger were computed separately. The magnetic polarity of the activity was part of the color-coding scheme of the "polarity spectrogram" (Figs. 1, 2, 3 and 4).

Sensor level analysis

The polarity spectrograms, which depict the positive and negative directions of the magnetic fields for each MEG sensor, were overlaid onto contour maps of the entire brain for visualizing the spatial distribution of the movement-elicited brain activation [13, 32]. These contour maps were used to demonstrate the source patterns. A global spectrogram (a summation of all sensors) for each condition (for left or for right finger movement) was computed for assessing the spectral components of the entire cortex. To quantify total brain activation that was elicited by movement, the absolute spectral power across sensors was computed using the root-mean-square (RMS) value excluding polarity information. To facilitate the measurements, we developed a toolbox, which could automatically measure the mean value for each frequency bin of all MEG sensors. The automatic measurements of the mean values of spectrograms from all MEG sensors showed less inter-individual variation among controls. The time window for quantifying spectral power at sensor levels was 10–270 ms for all the three frequency ranges. This time window was selected to capture typical movement-related magnetic fields without including the prior readiness fields [13, 14].

Source level analysis

Wavelet-based beamformer was used in the source analysis [32–34]. That is, in order to capture the dynamic spatiotemporal activity in the brain, we applied a sliding window in the source estimation process. Multiple local spheres were used for magnetic forward computing of the sources of activity. MEG Processor was used to compute and visualize magnetic sources [31, 35]. As described above in the sensor-level analysis, the time window for source estimation was also 10–270 ms for signals in the frequency ranges of 5–100 Hz, 100–1000 Hz and 1000–2,884 Hz. The whole brain was scanned with a 3-millimeter resolution grid. In comparison with our previous reports [31, 35], one methodological improvement in the present study was that the source power and goodness-of-fit (GOF) were computed

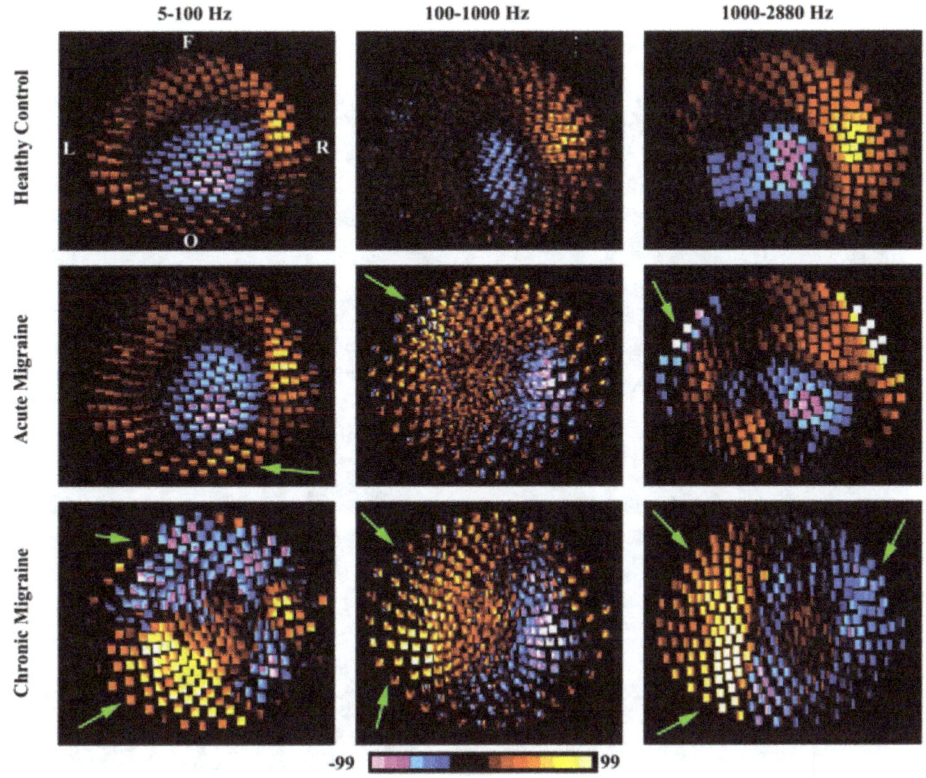

Fig. 1 Polarity contour maps of MEG data recorded from a representative chronic migraine subject, acute migraine subject, and control subject during left finger movements. The control subject shows activation predominantly around the primary motor area in all three-frequency bands. The acute migraine subject shows activation around the primary motor cortex as well as other areas (*green arrows*), including the left frontal region and the right occipital area. The chronic migraine subject shows activation out of the primary motor area, which appear to be stronger than the activation from the primary motor areas (*green arrow*). Neuromagnetic in 1000–2884 Hz shows the most disorganized pattern in the chronic migraine subject as compared with the control including activity distributed over the left frontal, left occipital, and right frontal regions. All contour maps are in the same orientation. "L" indicates left; "R" indicates right; "F" indicates frontal; "O" indicates occipital

for each grid position. The details of the methodology has been described in previous reports [32, 34].

Statistical analysis

The effects of chronic migraine on latency and spectral power were analyzed with Analyses of Variance (ANOVA). The fixed factor was the groups of migraine subjects versus controls. The dependent variables were latency and spectral power. The comparisons of chronic vs. control group, chronic vs. acute group, and acute vs. control group for left and right finger movements were performed with *Student* T-tests. The odds ratios of activity in brain areas other than the primary motor cortex among the chronic, acute, and control groups were analyzed with Fisher's exact tests. Since subjects performed left and right finger movements, the aforementioned statistical analyses were performed twice, one for each finger. $p < 0.05$ was considered significant for each paired comparison. Bonferroni correction was applied for multiple comparisons (i.e. since three frequency ranges were analyzed, $0.05/3 = 0.016$, only $p < 0.01$ was very conservatively considered to be significant).

Results

Clinical characteristics

The clinical characteristics are shown in Table 1. Control group participants were recruited to match the chronic migraine group in age, gender, and handedness. There was no headache in the control group. In the chronic migraine group, 15 of the 27 subjects were female, which was identical to the control group demographic, but different from the acute migraine group. The chronic migraine group has significantly higher frequency of headaches per month as compared with the acute migraine group ($p < 0.01$). T-tests show no significant differences between chronic and acute migraine groups in terms of the other parameters, including years of suffering from migraine, duration of headache, and severity of headache ($p > 0.05$). This suggests that differences in neural responses between groups may be associated with

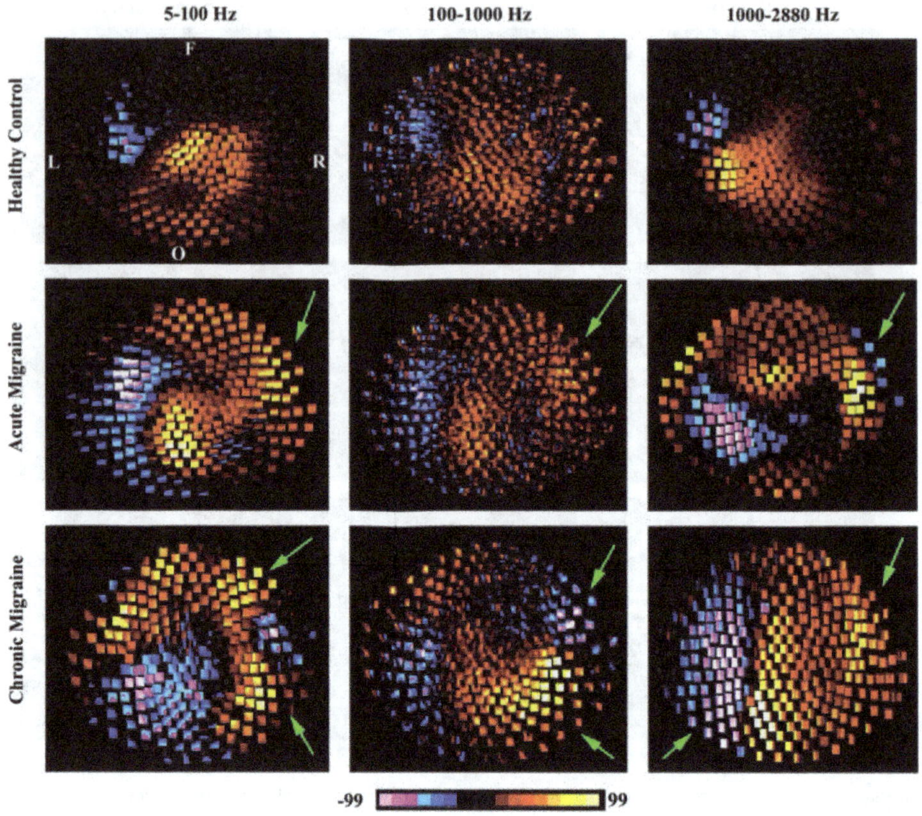

Fig. 2 Polarity contour maps of MEG data recorded from a representative chronic migraine subject, an acute migraine subject and a control during right finger movements. The control subject shows activation predominantly around the primary motor area. The acute migraine subject show activation around the primary motor cortex as well as other areas (*green arrows*). The chronic migraine subject shows activation out of the primary motor area, which appear to be overshadow the activation around the primary motor areas (*green arrow*). Neuromagnetic in 1000–2884 Hz shows the most disorganized pattern in the chronic migraine subject as compared with the control. All contour maps are in the same orientation. "L" indicates left; "R" indicates right; "F" indicates frontal; "O" indicates occipital

headache frequency as opposed to another feature distinguishing groups.

Behavioral data

The mean and standard deviation of the button-press response time after hearing the sound cue are shown in Table 2. There was a significant difference between the chronic migraine and control groups in terms of the response time for left finger movement ($p < 0.05$), but not for right finger movement. There was no statistical difference between the chronic migraine and acute migraine groups in terms of the response time for either left or right finger movement.

Sensor-level contour map

Low-frequency activation (5–100 Hz)

As shown in Figs. 1 (left hand) and 2 (right hand), as expected, the most consistent neuromagnetic activation in 5–100 Hz was identified around the primary motor region in the hemisphere contralateral to the finger pressing the button in the control, chronic and acute migraine groups (i.e. left hemisphere activation in response to right-hand button press, and right hemisphere activation in response to left-hand button press). However, the patient groups, with chronic and acute migraine, also show dispersed neuromagnetic activation outside of the typical primary motor activation (Green arrows in Figs. 1–2). Not only is this additional activity found in migraine groups and not controls, but the intensity of this activity appears to be stronger for chronic migraine subjects as compared to acute migraine subjects.

High-frequency activation (100–1000 Hz)

Contour maps revealed that the most consistent neuromagnetic activation in 100–1000 Hz was identified in the primary motor area in the contralateral hemisphere in all three groups of subjects (Figs. 1–2). We noted both chronic and acute migraine subjects showed dispersed neuromagnetic activation around the primary

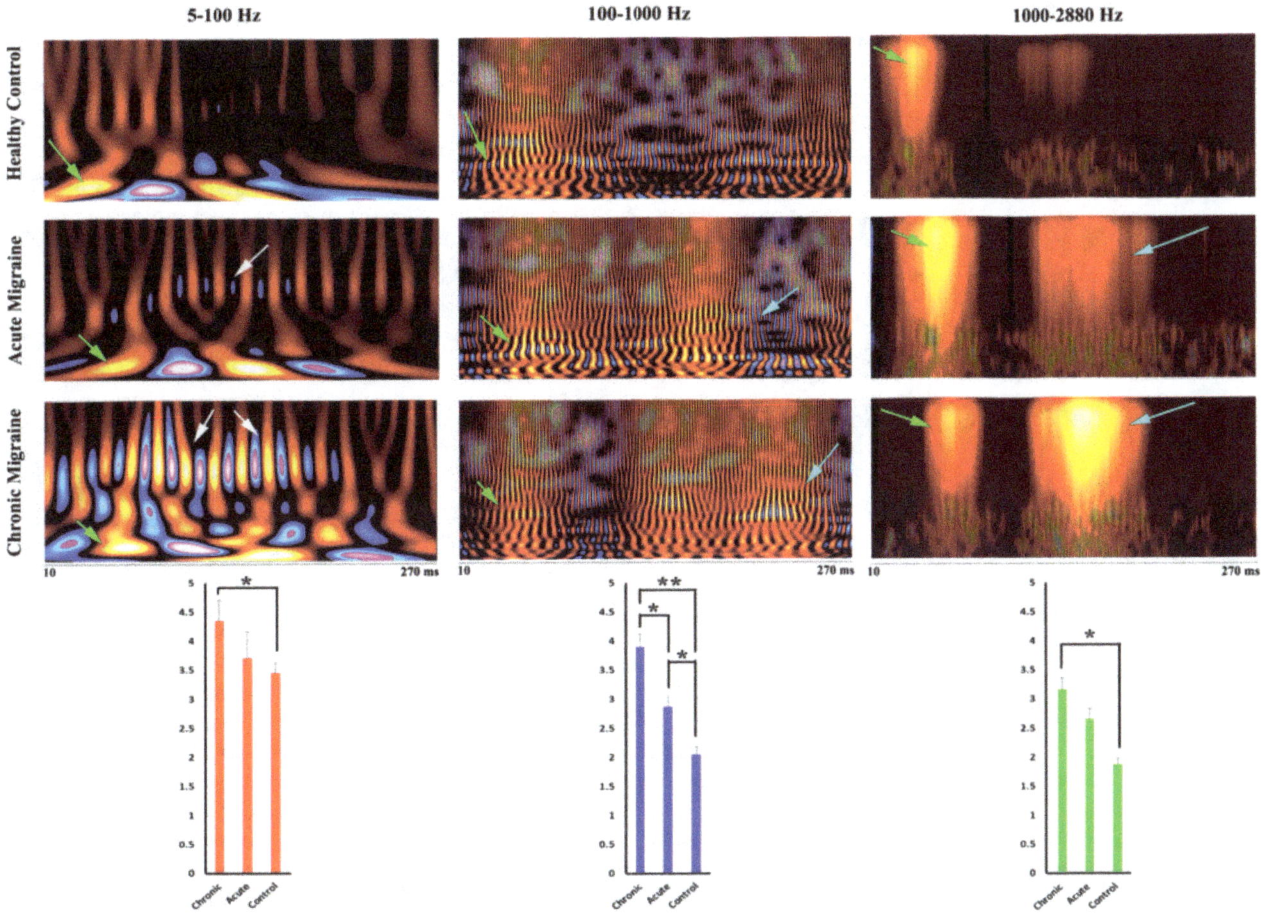

Fig. 3 Global spectrograms of MEG data recorded from a representative chronic migraine subject, an acute migraine subject, and a control during left finger movements. The spectrograms in 5–100 Hz show delayed spectral components in acute and chronic migraines (*light green arrows* indicate component 1, *dark green arrows* indicate component 2) as compared with controls. Spectral components around 70–80 Hz (*white arrows*) appear to be strong in chronic migraine, to be weak in acute migraine, and are not identifiable in the control. The spectrograms in 100–1000 Hz and 1000–2880 Hz reveal later components (*cyan arrows*) in chronic and acute migraine, but not in the controls. The vertical axis contains the frequency range (i.e., the minimum frequency at the bottom; maximum on the top). The horizontal axis contains the time window (from 10 ms to 270 ms). Below the spectrograms are bar graphs showing the spectral power of neuromagnetic activation elicited by left finger movements in chronic migraine subjects, acute migraine subjects and healthy controls. The bars show the mean and standard error of the spectral power of each group of subjects. "**" indicates $p < 0.001$; "*" indicates $p < 0.01$

motor region as compared with controls (Green arrows in Figs. 1–2).

Very high-frequency activation (1000–2884 Hz)

As in the lower frequency bands, contour maps revealed that the most consistent neuromagnetic activation in 1000–2884 Hz was identified in the primary motor area in the hemisphere contralateral to the finger pressing the button in the control groups (Figs. 1–2). The contour maps in the chronic migraine group were different from that of control and acute migraine groups (Green arrows in Figs. 1–2). The dipolar pattern around the primary motor region, which was consistently presented in control group, was not clearly identifiable in the chronic migraine group (Figs. 1–2).

Global spectrograms

Low-frequency activation (5–100 Hz)

As shown in Fig. 3 (responses to left-hand button press) and Fig. 4 (responses to right-hand button press), global spectrograms in 5–100 Hz revealed movement-elicited oscillatory activation (green arrows) in all three groups. We noted abnormal focal oscillatory increases (cyan arrows in Figs. 3–4) for acute and for chronic migraine subjects, that do not appear for controls. Bar graphs in Figs. 3 and 4 under each frequency band show quantitative measurements of the spectral power of neuromagnetic activation across the whole time window represented in the spectrogram. For both the right and left hand, in this frequency range, chronic migraine patients show significantly higher spectral power than controls (Figs. 3–4).

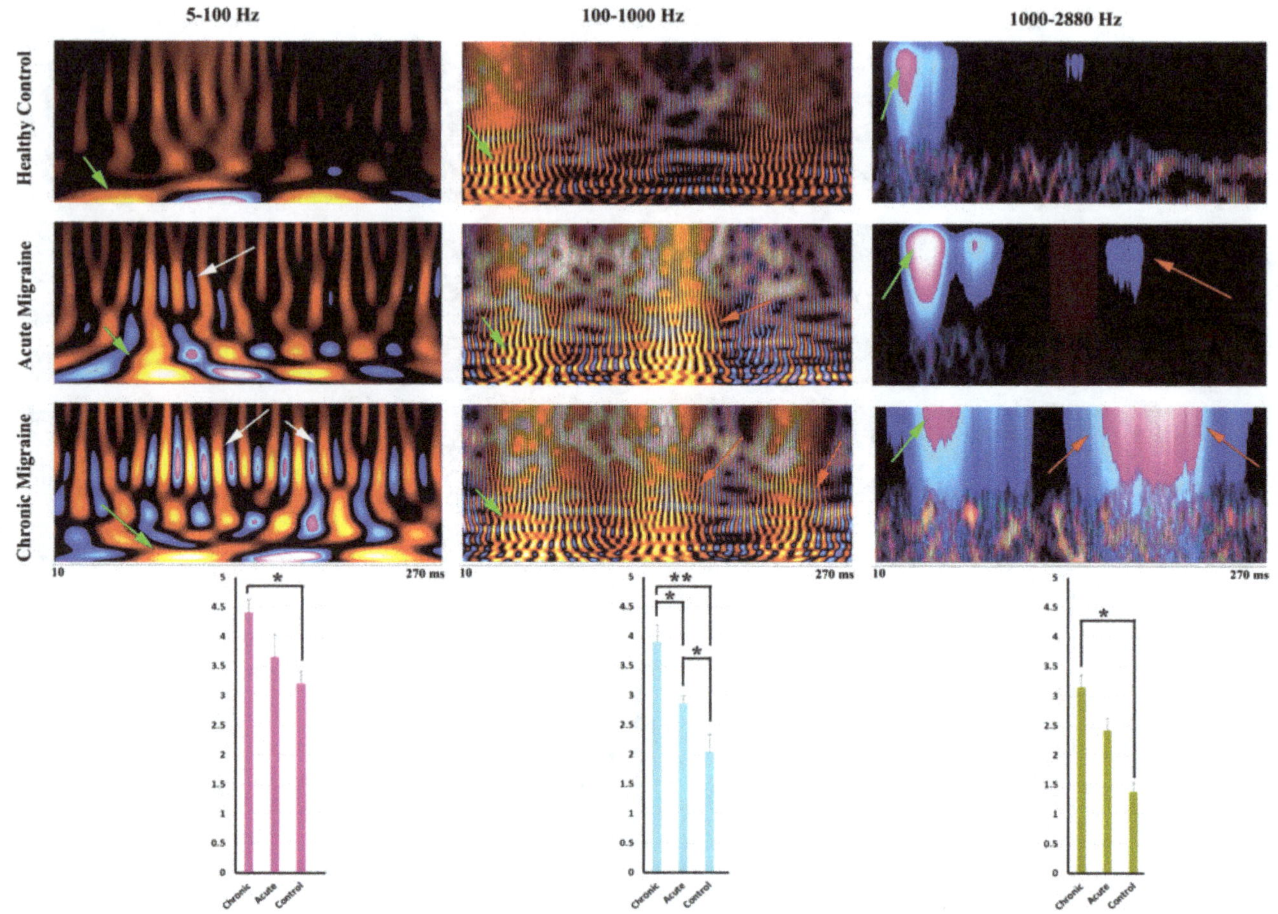

Fig. 4 Global spectrograms of MEG data recorded from a representative chronic migraine subject, an acute migraine subject and a control during left finger movements. The spectrograms in 5–100 Hz show delayed spectral components in acute and chronic migraines (*light green arrows* indicate component 1, *dark green arrows* indicate component 2) as compared with controls. Spectral components around 70–80 Hz (*white arrows*) appear to be strong in chronic migraine, to be weak in acute migraine, and are not identifiable in the control. The spectrograms in 100–1000 Hz and 1000–2880 Hz reveal later components (*cyan arrows*) in chronic and acute migraine, but not in the controls. The vertical axis contains the frequency range (i.e., the minimum frequency at the bottom; maximum on the top). The horizontal axis contains the time window (from 10 ms to 270 ms). Below the spectrograms are bar graphs showing the spectral power of neuromagnetic activation elicited by right finger movements in chronic migraine subjects, acute migraine subjects and healthy controls. The bars show the mean and standard error of the spectral power of each group of subjects. "**" indicates $p < 0.001$; "*" indicates $p < 0.01$

While all three groups show 2 early neuromagnetic increases (as indicated by green arrows in the first column of Figs. 3–4), acute and chronic migraines show delays in these responses. Figure 5 shows the exact latencies for each of these early increases in this frequency band. The first response increase, "Component 1", and the second response increase "Component 2" in the chronic migraine group are significantly slower than controls for both right and left hands, whereas acute migraines only show significant delays compared to controls for both hands in Component 1. Chronic migraines only show significantly delayed responses compared with acute migraines for Component 1 in the left hand. A 3-way ANOVA was run on the total sample of 81 participants to examine the effect of gender, age, and headache frequency on spectral power, and no significant interaction was found in this conventional frequency range.

High-frequency activation (100–1000 Hz)

Global spectrograms in 100–1000 Hz revealed movement-elicited high-frequency oscillatory activation (green arrows in Figs. 3–4) in all three groups. Abnormal focal oscillatory increases were also revealed for migraine groups but not for controls (Cyan arrows in Figs. 3–4). Due to the rapid oscillatory activity in this frequency range, latency differences could not be measured. Therefore, in these frequency ranges, differences between groups were detected in terms of spectral power only. The bar graph for the 100–1000 Hz range is shown below the spectrograms for each group in Figs. 3–4. As in the low frequency range,

Table 1 Demographic and Clinical Characteristics of Subjects

Parameters		Measurements		
		Chronic	Acute	Control
Gender (female/male)		15/12	19/8	15/12
Age (years) (mean ± SD)[a]		13.5 ± 3.1	14.2 ± 2.4	13.4 ± 3.2
Handedness (right/left)		24/3	24/3	24/3
Frequency of headache per month (mean ± SD)		20.3 ± 7.3	7.5 ± 3.6	0
Years of suffering from migraine (mean ± SD)		5.9 ± 4.1	3.8 ± 2.7	0
Duration of headache (hours) (mean ± SD)		9.1 ± 12.3	9.0 ± 4.6	0
Severity of headache (on scale: 0 ~ 10) (mean ± SD)		6.0 ± 1.9	6.5 ± 2.6	0
Pain type (Number of subjects; Multiple descriptions were allowed)	Throbbing	21	17	0
	Pressure	16	13	0
	Constant	12	6	0
	Sharp	6	6	0
	Squeezing	9	3	0
	Stabbing	6	2	0
	Others	1	2	0

[a] *SD* standard deviation

chronic migraines show significantly higher spectral power than controls for both hands. However, in addition to this finding, bar graphs indicate that acute migraines also show significantly higher spectral power than controls, as well as significantly lower spectral power than chronic migraines, for both hands. This suggests that the abnormal motor responses underlying acute migraines are only detectable in higher frequency ranges, whereas as chronic migraine abnormalities are more distributed across the frequency bands. A 3-way ANOVA was run on the total sample of 81 participants to examine the effect of age, gender, and headache frequency on spectral power. A significant effect of migraine frequency (and not age or gender) on spectral power was revealed (F (1, 26) = 13.21, $p = 0.003$). This finding suggests that higher frequencies such as these are crucial for detecting oscillatory differences underlying neurological disorders.

Table 2 Movement Response Time (milliseconds) after Hearing the Sound Cue

	Chronic (Mean ± SD) [b]	Acute (Mean ± SD)	Control (Mean ± SD)
Left-hand	425.3 ± 183.4[a]	413.8 ± 193.4	364.5 ± 142.6
Right hand	392.4 ± 157.9	387.4 ± 161.6	358.4 ± 146.2

[a] $P < 0.05$ (Chronic vs. control)
[b] *SD* standard deviation

Very high frequency activation (1000–2884 Hz)

Global spectrograms in the 1000–2884 Hz range revealed movement-elicited very high-frequency oscillatory activation (green arrows in Figs. 3–4) in all three groups. Due to the extreme speed of fluctuations, the individual very high frequency oscillations merged as clusters (See arrows in Figs. 3–4). We therefore measured the spectral power, but not latency. Compared to healthy controls, acute migraine subjects only showed slightly increased late activation. However, chronic migraine subjects showed much stronger late activation as compared to healthy controls and acute migraine subjects (cyan Arrows in Figs. 3–4). A 3-way ANOVA was run on the total sample of 81 participants to examine the effect of gender, age, and headache frequency on spectral power, and no significant interaction was found in this frequency range.

Magnetic Source Imaging

Low-frequency activation (5–100 Hz)

The most consistent location of neuromagnetic activation was the primary motor area (M1) in all three groups of subjects (Figs. 6–7). We also noted activation in the ipsilateral motor area (IMA), the premotor area (PMA), the supplementary motor area (SMA), the occipital area (OCA) and the deep brain area (DBA). The odds ratio of the activation in the aforementioned areas are quantified and summarized in bar graphs below each frequency band. For 5–100 Hz, chronic migraines showed significantly higher activation than controls in all of the above listed regions, for both hands. Acute migraines showed significantly higher activation than controls in all regions except for the deep brain area, for both hands. Interestingly, this is also the only region that showed significantly higher activation for chronic migraines as compared with acute migraines, for both hands (as indicated by a red asterisk as opposed to blue). This suggests that the deep brain area in this frequency band may be a biomarker distinguishing the chronification of migraines from acute migraines.

High-frequency activation (100–1000 Hz)

The most consistent location of neuromagnetic activation was the M1 in all three groups of subjects (Figs. 6–7). We also noted activation in the IMA, the PMA, the SMA, the OCA, and the DBA. Bar graphs below the MSI images show that in this frequency, chronic migraines have significantly higher activation in each of these regions than controls, for both hands. As in the lower frequencies, this range shows significant activation increases for acute migraines compared with controls in all of the above listed regions except for DBA, in both hands. Of note, in this frequency band this DBA region also shows significant increases for chronic over acute migraine activation, in both

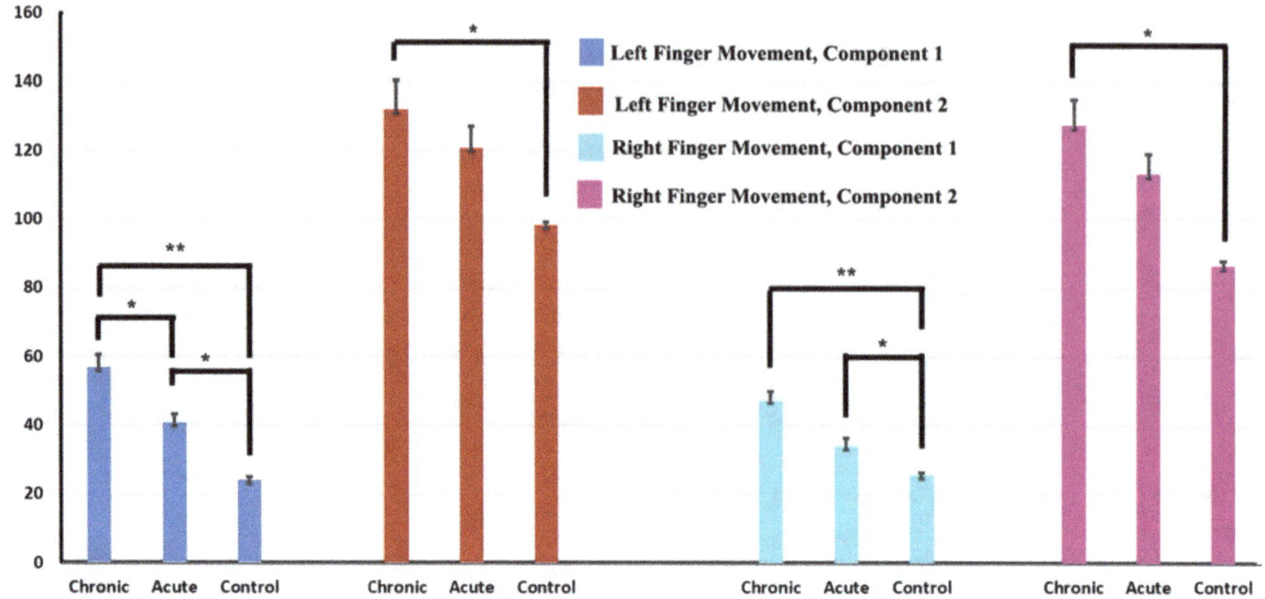

Fig. 5 The latencies of the first and second spectral components in 5–100 Hz in chronic migraine subjects, acute migraine subjects, and healthy control subjects. The x-axis measures time in milliseconds. The bars show the mean and standard error of latencies of spectral components in each group of subjects. The double asterisk indicates $p < 0.001$; and a single asterisk indicates $p < 0.01$

hands. Furthermore, the left hand shows significant increases for chronic versus acute in the IMA region.

Very High-frequency activation (1000–2884 Hz)

The most consistent location of neuromagnetic activation was the M1 in all three groups of subjects (Figs. 6–7). We also noted activation in the IMA, the PMA, the SMA, the OCA, and the DBA. Bar graphs beneath the MSI figure show significant increases in all of these regions for chronic migraines compared with controls, for both hands. Just as in the lower frequency bands, acute migraines show increases in all areas compared with controls, except in the DBA, where chronic migraines show a significant increase in activation compared with acute migraines, for both hands. There is also a significant increase for chronic versus acute migraines in the IMA for the right hand.

Frequency signature

A comparison of the contour maps and global spectrograms in three frequency ranges (5–100 Hz, 100–1000 Hz, and 1000–2884 Hz) revealed that there were frequency-dependent neuromagnetic abnormalities in chronic and acute migraine (Figs. 1–4). Very high-frequency signals, 1000–2884 Hz, revealed the most significant abnormalities underlying chronic migraine in terms of in the contour map patterns and the aberrant regions of activation revealed by magnetic source imaging. The 100–1000 Hz range also revealed the most significant spectral power abnormalities of chronic migraine in the global spectrograms. These findings suggest that investigations in frequency bands above 100 Hz are crucial for identifying the brain dysfunction underlying childhood neurological disorders, such as migraine, which is necessary for improved diagnosis and treatment.

Discussion

MEG data from the three groups of pediatric migraine subjects have demonstrated that there were spatial, temporal, and spectral neuromagnetic differences between pediatric migraine groups versus pediatric control subjects ($\mu = 13.4$ years), as well as between chronic migraine ($\mu = 13.5$ years) and acute migraine ($\mu = 14.2$ years) subjects during a button-press paradigm. We noted that clinical assessment of pediatric acute migraine has been well characterized in previous reports [13, 14, 36, 37]. However, assessment of pediatric chronic migraine seems relatively scarce. While typical diagnoses of chronic migraine require at least 15 headaches per month, the present study found that the average frequency tended to be even higher in the pediatric population investigated here (approximately 20/month).

The analyses of neuromagnetic signals in 5–100 Hz show that in the chronic migraine group the latency of early responses, labeled "Component 1" and "Component 2" here, was significantly delayed as compared with the control group during left and right finger movements. This latency finding is consistent with previous reports using conventional measurements of

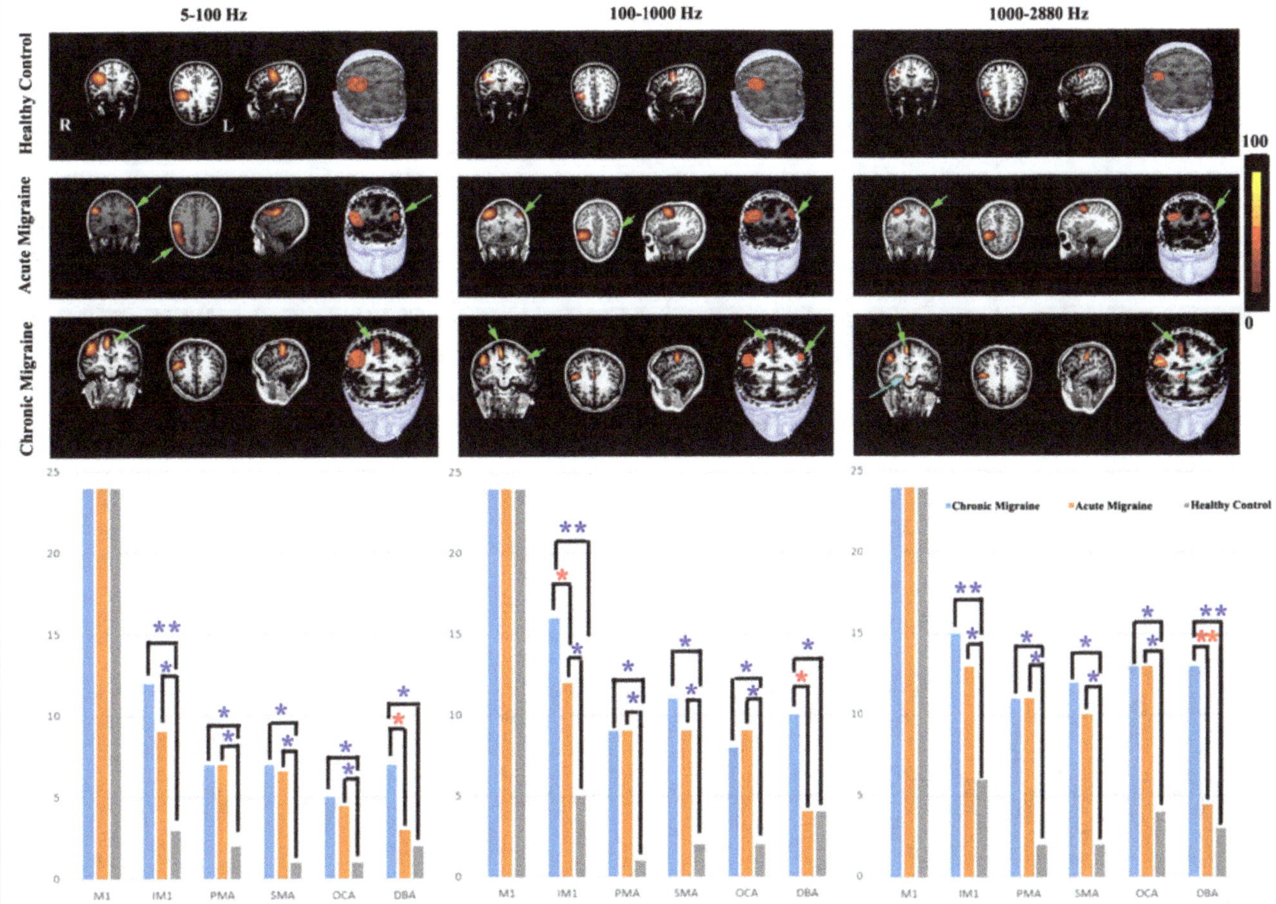

Fig. 6 Magnetic source imaging (MSI) showing the locations of neuromagnetic activation in response to left-finger movement in a representative chronic migraine subject, acute migraine subject, and control subject. The primary motor cortex in the hemisphere contralateral to the finger pressing the button is activated in all the three subjects (*no arrows*). The ipsilateral sensorimotor area, supplementary motor area, and the pre-motor areas are activated only in chronic and acute migraine subjects (*green arrows*). The deep brain area is activated only in the chronic migraine subject (*cyan arrows*). In all coronal and axial views, "R" indicates right and "L" indicates left. Below the MSI images are bar graphs indicating the sources of neuromagnetic activation elicited by left finger movements in three groups of subjects. The bars show the number of subjects having activation in each location in each group. M1 indicates primary motor area; IMA indicates ipsilateral motor area; PMA indicates pre-motor area; SMA indicates supplementary motor area; OCA incites occipital area and DBA indicates deep brain area. The odds ratio was statistically analyzed by comparing each group. The double asterisk indicates $p < 0.001$; and a single asterisk indicates $p < 0.01$. A red asterisk indicates a difference between acute and chronic migraines and blue asterisks represent the other group differences

waveform responses [18]. In addition to confirming prior waveform findings, the spectrograms of the present study provide novel frequency descriptions of neuromagnetic components.

The latency of the first spectral component in the chronic migraine group was also significantly delayed as compared with the acute migraine group, but only in left-finger movements. This phenomenon has not been revealed in any previous report. We expect that this finding results from the fact that the subjects in the migraine groups were predominately right-handed. Consequently, motor cortical dysfunction in chronic migraine during right finger movement may be more easily compensated for in right-handers, but as the left-hand is already weaker in these subjects, the addition of cortical dysfunction perhaps becomes more apparent during left-handed tasks; in this case in terms of latency.

In addition to timing differences, the present study also revealed significant differences between groups in terms of spectral power. Specifically, the neuromagnetic spectral power in 5–100 Hz in chronic migraine subjects was significantly increased compared to controls during left and right finger movements. Similar to previous reports on acute migraine [13, 14], a significant increase of brain activation suggests that the cortical excitability is elevated in migraine. This finding is consistent with previous MEG studies [16, 18]

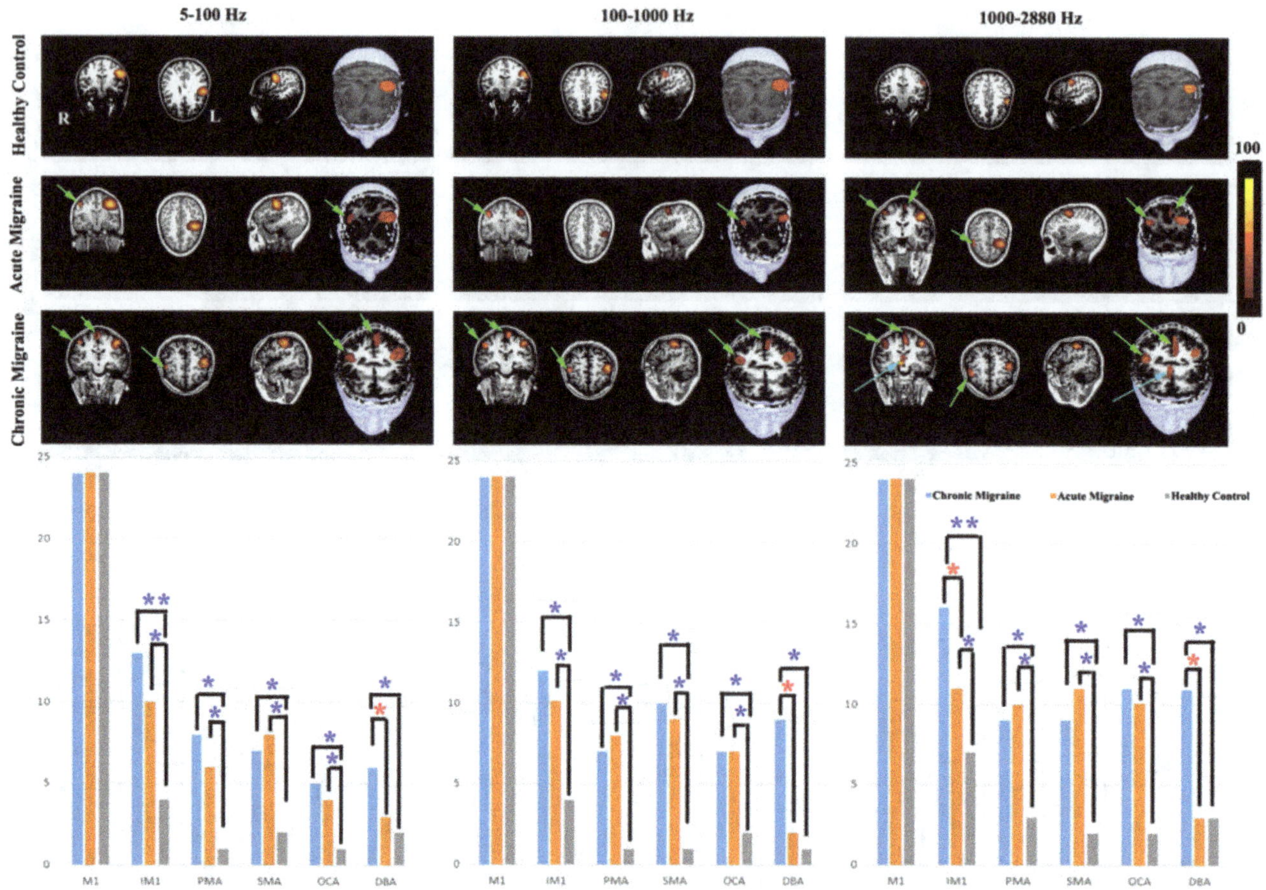

Fig. 7 Magnetic source imaging (MSI) showing the locations of neuromagnetic activation in response to right-finger movement in a representative chronic migraine subject, acute migraine subject, and control subject. The primary motor cortex in the hemisphere contralateral to the finger pressing the button is activated in all the three subjects (*no arrows*). The ipsilateral sensorimotor area and the supplementary motor area are activated in chronic and acute migraine subjects (*green arrows*). The deep brain area is activated only in the chronic migraine subject (*cyan arrows*). In all coronal and axial views, "R" indicates right and "L" indicates left. Below the MSI images are bar graphs indicating the sources of neuromagnetic activation elicited by right finger movements in three groups of subjects. The bars show the number of subjects having activation in each location in each group. M1 indicates primary motor area; IMA indicates ipsilateral motor area; PMA indicates pre-motor area; SMA indicates supplementary motor area; OCA incites occipital area and DBA indicates deep brain area. The odds ratio was statistically analyzed by comparing each group. The double asterisk indicates $p < 0.001$; and a single asterisk indicates $p < 0.01$. A red asterisk indicates a difference between acute and chronic migraines and blue asterisks represent the other group differences

and fMRI studies showing that migraine subjects have greater activation in the primary motor cortex compared to controls [38].

The data of the present study have also revealed that the spectral power of brain activation in 100–1,000 Hz in chronic migraine was significantly higher than that of the acute migraine. Though the exact cerebral mechanism remains unknown, the increase of high-frequency oscillations in 100–1,000 Hz may reflect the activation of the cortical-subcortical networks during the onset of discrete movements, or may signal the direct modulation of outputs from the subthalamic nucleus to the basal ganglia, thereby facilitating movement execution [39]. In fact, the present study and previous publications [13, 14, 40] support the notion of increased cortical excitability in the brain with chronic and acute migraine during headache attacks. Further, these findings suggest that the abnormality in chronic migraine is more severe than that of the acute migraine.

Source analyses revealed that both chronic and acute migraine subjects had distributed brain activation outside of the primary motor area. In comparison to controls, chronic migraine subjects had a significantly higher likelihood of activation in the ipsilateral sensorimotor area, the supplementary motor area, the premotor area, the occipital region, and the deep brain area. This observation is similar to many previous reports [41, 42]. The distinct spatial patterns suggest that the dysfunction associated with migraine recruits an abnormally large neural network for a basic motor task.

Analyses of magnetic sources also revealed that chronic migraine had significantly higher odds of having activation in the deep brain area in comparison with acute migraine and controls. Though the cerebral mechanisms underlying aberrant chronic activation remain unclear, we postulate that involvement of the deep brain area may indicate that brain dysfunction in chronic migraine goes beyond the cerebral cortex. From a clinical point of view, aberrant neuromagnetic signals from the deep brain areas may be unique to chronic migraine patients.

MEG signals in the 5–100 Hz, 100–1000 Hz, and 1000–2884 Hz appear to reveal different aspects of migraine-related abnormalities in both chronic and acute migraine, such as response latency, spectral power, and brain regions, respectively. Though previous reports have shown that the brain generates signals around 2632 Hz in the somatosensory cortex [43] and 2500 Hz in the epileptogenic regions [44], those previous reports are based on invasive intracranial recordings, and are limited to patients with intractable epilepsy who are surgical candidates [43, 44]. Therefore, this is the first report showing neuromagnetic signals in this frequency range (>100 Hz) in migraine subjects using *noninvasive* MEG. The results of the present study showed that, neuromagnetic signals can not only differentiate chronic migraine subjects from healthy controls, but also can also reveal differences between chronic migraine patients and acute migraine patients. The difference between chronic migraine and acute migraine may enable us to investigate the chronification of migraine attacks and develop new strategies to prevent acute migraine from developing into chronic migraine.

Conclusions

In summary, this study has demonstrated that chronic migraine subjects show aberrant neural activation in both low- and high-frequency ranges as compared with controls. The primary novel findings of the present study were (1) the identification of very high-frequency brain activation in chronic migraine subjects using MEG; (2) the determination of increased ictal cortical activation beyond the primary motor cortex in chronic migraine subjects during a button-press task; and (3) the observation of spatiotemporal and spectral differences between chronic and acute migraine. These findings support the notion that chronic migraine is a neurological disorder caused by cortical dysfunction and the evolution from acute migraine is manifested in further increases and delays in cortical and deep brain activation [45, 46].

Competing interests
All authors declared that there was no conflict of interest during the study.

Authors' contributions
KL carried out the recruitment, data acquisition, and manuscript preparation and submission. JX conceived of the study and its design, as well as carrying out the data acquisition and analysis, and drafting the manuscript. EC, HF, and DR participated in data acquisition. JA, JK, HO, and MK participated in recruitment and eligibility screening. SP and AH participated in study design, recruitment, and eligibility screening. All authors were given the opportunity to read and approve the final manuscript.

Acknowledgements
We thank Ms. Antoinette Green, Ms. Susan LeCates, Ms. Polly Vaughan, Ms. Shannon Cherney, Ms. Judy Bush, Ms. Paula Manning, Ms. Ann Segers and Ms. Janelle Allen for recruiting participants. We thank Prof. Paul Horn for helping with statistical analyses. The project described was supported by Grant Number 1R21NS081420 and R21NS072817 from the National Institute of Neurological Disorders and Stroke (NINDS), the National Institutes of Health.

Author details
[1]Division of Neurology, Cincinnati Children's Hospital Medical Center, 3333 Burnet Avenue, MLC 2015, Cincinnati, OH 45220, USA. [2]Department of Pediatrics, University of Cincinnati, College of Medicine, Cincinnati, OH, USA. [3]Division of Behavioral Medicine and Clinical Psychology, Cincinnati Children's Hospital Medical Center, Cincinnati, OH, USA.

References

1. Stovner LJ, Andree C (2010) Prevalence of headache in Europe: a review for the Eurolight project. J Headache Pain 11(4):289–299. doi:10.1007/s10194-010-0217-0
2. Lipton RB (2009) Tracing transformation: chronic migraine classification, progression, and epidemiology. Neurology 72(5 Suppl):S3–7. doi:10.1212/WNL.0b013e3181974b19
3. Bigal ME, Sheftell FD, Rapoport AM, Lipton RB, Tepper SJ (2002) Chronic daily headache in a tertiary care population: correlation between the International Headache Society diagnostic criteria and proposed revisions of criteria for chronic daily headache. Cephalalgia 22(6):432–438
4. Koenig MA, Gladstein J, McCarter RJ, Hershey AD, Wasiewski W (2002) Chronic daily headache in children and adolescents presenting to tertiary headache clinics. Headache 42(6):491–500
5. Seshia SS, Wang SJ, Abu-Arafeh I, Hershey AD, Guidetti V, Winner P, Wober-Bingol C (2010) Chronic daily headache in children and adolescents: a multi-faceted syndrome. Can J Neurol Sci 37(6):769–778
6. Bigal ME, Tepper SJ, Sheftell FD, Rapoport AM, Lipton RB (2004) Chronic daily headache: correlation between the 2004 and the 1988 International Headache Society diagnostic criteria. Headache 44(7):684–691. doi:10.1111/j.1526-4610.2004.04128.x
7. Bigal ME, Sheftell FD, Rapoport AM, Tepper SJ, Lipton RB (2002) Chronic daily headache: identification of factors associated with induction and transformation. Headache 42(7):575–581
8. Wheeler AH (1999) Chronic Daily Headache: Theory to Therapy. Curr Rev Pain 3(6):481–488
9. Saper JR (2008) Chronic daily headache: transformational migraine, chronic migraine, and related disorders. Curr Neurol Neurosci Rep 8(2):100–107
10. Hershey AD (2003) Chronic daily headaches in children. Expert Opin Pharmacother 4(4):485–491. doi:10.1517/14656566.4.4.485
11. Hershey AD, Kabbouche MA, Powers SW (2006) Chronic daily headaches in children. Curr Pain Headache Rep 10(5):370–376
12. Coppola G, Bracaglia M, Di Lenola D, Di Lorenzo C, Serrao M, Parisi V, Di Renzo A, Martelli F, Fadda A, Schoenen J, Pierelli F (2015) Visual evoked potentials in subgroups of migraine with aura patients. J Headache Pain 16:92. doi:10.1186/s10194-015-0577-6
13. Xiang J, deGrauw X, Korostenskaja M, Korman AM, O'Brien HL, Kabbouche MA, Powers SW, Hershey AD (2013) Altered cortical activation in adolescents with acute migraine: a magnetoencephalography study. J Pain 14(12):1553–1563. doi:10.1016/j.jpain.2013.04.009

14. Xiang J, Degrauw X, Korman AM, Allen JR, O'Brien HL, Kabbouche MA, Powers SW, Hershey AD (2013) Neuromagnetic abnormality of motor cortical activation and phases of headache attacks in childhood migraine. PLoS One 8(12):e83669. doi:10.1371/journal.pone.0083669
15. Bowyer SM, Shvarts V, Moran JE, Mason KM, Barkley GL, Tepley N (2012) Slow brain activity (ISA/DC) detected by MEG. J Clin Neurophysiol 29(4): 320–326. doi:10.1097/WNP.0b013e3182624342
16. Bowyer SM, Mason KM, Moran JE, Tepley N, Mitsias PD (2005) Cortical hyperexcitability in migraine patients before and after sodium valproate treatment. J Clin Neurophysiol 22(1):65–67
17. Huo X, Wang Y, Kotecha R, Kirtman EG, Fujiwara H, Hemasilpin N, Degrauw T, Rose DF, Xiang J (2011) High gamma oscillations of sensorimotor cortex during unilateral movement in the developing brain: a MEG study. Brain Topogr 23(4):375–384. doi:10.1007/s10548-010-0151-0
18. Wang X, Xiang J, Wang Y, Pardos M, Meng L, Huo X, Korostenskaja M, Powers SW, Kabbouche MA, Hershey AD (2010) Identification of abnormal neuromagnetic signatures in the motor cortex of adolescent migraine. Headache 50(6):1005–1016. doi:10.1111/j.1526-4610.2010.01674.x
19. Liu H, Ge H, Xiang J, Miao A, Tang L, Wu T, Chen Q, Yang L, Wang X (2015) Resting state brain activity in patients with migraine: a magnetoencephalography study. J Headache Pain 16:525. doi:10.1186/s10194-015-0525-5
20. Xiang J, Wang Y, Chen Y, Liu Y, Kotecha R, Huo X, Rose DF, Fujiwara H, Hemasilpin N, Lee K, Mangano FT, Jones B, DeGrauw T (2010) Noninvasive localization of epileptogenic zones with ictal high-frequency neuromagnetic signals. J Neurosurg Pediatr 5(1):113–122. doi:10.3171/2009.8.PEDS09345
21. Xiang J, Liu Y, Wang Y, Kirtman EG, Kotecha R, Chen Y, Huo X, Fujiwara H, Hemasilpin N, Lee K, Mangano FT, Leach J, Jones B, DeGrauw T, Rose D (2009) Frequency and spatial characteristics of high-frequency neuromagnetic signals in childhood epilepsy. Epileptic Disord 11(2):113–125. doi:10.1684/epd.2009.0253
22. Leahy RM, Mosher JC, Spencer ME, Huang MX, Lewine JD (1998) A study of dipole localization accuracy for MEG and EEG using a human skull phantom. Electroencephalogr Clin Neurophysiol 107(2):159–173
23. Siniatchkin M, Sendacki M, Moeller F, Wolff S, Jansen O, Siebner H, Stephani U (2012) Abnormal changes of synaptic excitability in migraine with aura. Cereb Cortex 22(10):2207–2216. doi:10.1093/cercor/bhr248
24. Antal A, Kriener N, Lang N, Boros K, Paulus W (2011) Cathodal transcranial direct current stimulation of the visual cortex in the prophylactic treatment of migraine. Cephalalgia 31(7):820–828. doi:10.1177/0333102411399349
25. Ward TN (2010) Transcranial magnetic stimulation. Headache 50(10):1629. doi:10.1111/j.1526-4610.2010.01786.x
26. Teepker M, Hotzel J, Timmesfeld N, Reis J, Mylius V, Haag A, Oertel WH, Rosenow F, Schepelmann K (2010) Low-frequency rTMS of the vertex in the prophylactic treatment of migraine. Cephalalgia 30(2):137–144. doi:10.1111/j.1468-2982.2009.01911.x
27. Lo YL (2010) Headache: migraine, magnetic stimulation and cortical excitability. Nat Rev Neurol 6(8):425–427. doi:10.1038/nrneurol.2010.109
28. Headache Classification Committee of the International Headache Society (1988) Classification and diagnostic criteria for headache disorders, cranial neuralgias and facial pain. Cephalalgia 8(Suppl 7):1–96
29. Hershey AD, Winner P, Kabbouche MA, Gladstein J, Yonker M, Lewis D, Pearlman E, Linder SL, Rothner AD, Powers SW (2005) Use of the ICHD-II criteria in the diagnosis of pediatric migraine. Headache 45(10):1288–1297. doi:10.1111/j.1526-4610.2005.00260.x
30. Hershey AD, Powers SW, Vockell AL, LeCates SL, Segers A, Kabbouche MA (2004) Development of a patient-based grading scale for PedMIDAS. Cephalalgia 24(10):844–849. doi:10.1111/j.1468-2982.2004.00757.x
31. Kotecha R, Xiang J, Wang Y, Huo X, Hemasilpin N, Fujiwara H, Rose D, deGrauw T (2009) Time, frequency and volumetric differences of high-frequency neuromagnetic oscillation between left and right somatosensory cortices. Int J Psychophysiol 72(2):102–110. doi:10.1016/j.ijpsycho.2008.10.009
32. Xiang J, Korman A, Samarasinghe KM, Wang X, Zhang F, Qiao H, Sun B, Wang F, Fan HH, Thompson EA (2015) Volumetric imaging of brain activity with spatial-frequency decoding of neuromagnetic signals. J Neurosci Methods 239:114–128. doi:10.1016/j.jneumeth.2014.10.007
33. Xiang J, Luo Q, Kotecha R, Korman A, Zhang F, Luo H, Fujiwara H, Hemasilpin N, Rose DF (2014) Accumulated source imaging of brain activity with both low and high-frequency neuromagnetic signals. Frontiers Neuroinformatics 8(57):57. doi:10.3389/fninf.2014.00057
34. Thompson EA, Xiang J, Wang YY (2015) Frequency-spatial beamformer for MEG source localization. Biomed Signal Process Contr 18:263–273. doi:10.1016/j.bspc.2015.01.004
35. Huo X, Xiang J, Wang Y, Kirtman EG, Kotecha R, Fujiwara H, Hemasilpin N, Rose DF, Degrauw T (2010) Gamma oscillations in the primary motor cortex studied with MEG. Brain Dev 32(8):619–624. doi:10.1016/j.braindev.2009.09.021
36. Hershey AD (2010) Current approaches to the diagnosis and management of paediatric migraine. Lancet Neurol 9(2):190–204. doi:10.1016/S1474-4422(09)70303-5
37. Guo X, Xiang J, Wang Y, O'Brien H, Kabbouche M, Horn P, Powers SW, Hershey AD (2012) Aberrant neuromagnetic activation in the motor cortex in children with acute migraine: a magnetoencephalography study. PLoS One 7(11):e50095. doi:10.1371/journal.pone.0050095
38. Rocca MA, Colombo B, Pagani E, Falini A, Codella M, Scotti G, Comi G, Filippi M (2003) Evidence for cortical functional changes in patients with migraine and white matter abnormalities on conventional and diffusion tensor magnetic resonance imaging. Stroke 34(3):665–670. doi:10.1161/01.STR.0000057977.06681.11
39. Cheyne D, Bells S, Ferrari P, Gaetz W, Bostan AC (2008) Self-paced movements induce high-frequency gamma oscillations in primary motor cortex. NeuroImage 42(1):332–342. doi:10.1016/j.neuroimage.2008.04.178
40. Ge HT, Liu HX, Xiang J, Miao AL, Tang L, Guan QS, Wu T, Chen QQ, Yang L, Wang XS (2015) Abnormal cortical activation in females with acute migraine: a magnetoencephalography study. Clin Neurophysiol 126(1):170–179. doi:10.1016/j.clinph.2014.03.033
41. Bowyer SM, Fleming T, Greenwald ML, Moran JE, Mason KM, Weiland BJ, Smith BJ, Barkley GL, Tepley N (2005) Magnetoencephalographic localization of the basal temporal language area. Epilepsy Behav 6(2):229–234. doi:10.1016/j.yebeh.2004.12.003
42. Gummadavelli A, Wang Y, Guo X, Pardos M, Chu H, Liu Y, Horn P, Zhang F, Xiang J (2013) Spatiotemporal and frequency signatures of word recognition in the developing brain: a magnetoencephalographic study. Brain Res 1498:20–32. doi:10.1016/j.brainres.2013.01.001
43. Sakura Y, Terada K, Usui K, Baba K, Usui N, Umeoka S, Yamaguchi M, Matsuda K, Tottori T, Mihara T, Nakamura F, Inoue Y (2009) Very high-frequency oscillations (over 1000 Hz) of somatosensory-evoked potentials directly recorded from the human brain. J Clin Neurophysiol 26(6):414–421. doi:10.1097/WNP.0b013e3181c298c9
44. Usui N, Terada K, Baba K, Matsuda K, Nakamura F, Usui K, Tottori T, Umeoka S, Fujitani S, Mihara T, Inoue Y (2010) Very high frequency oscillations (over 1000 Hz) in human epilepsy. Clin Neurophysiol 121(11):1825–1831. doi:10.1016/j.clinph.2010.04.018
45. Conforto AB, Moraes MS, Amaro E Jr, Young WB, Lois LA, Goncalves AL, Peres MF (2012) Increased variability of motor cortical excitability to transcranial magnetic stimulation in migraine: a new clue to an old enigma. J Headache Pain 13(1):29–37. doi:10.1007/s10194-011-0379-4
46. Rapoport A (2011) New frontiers in headache therapy. Neurol Sci 32(Suppl 1): S105–109. doi:10.1007/s10072-011-0542-3

4

Excessive daytime sleepiness is associated with an exacerbation of migraine

Jiyoung Kim[1], Soo-Jin Cho[2], Won-Joo Kim[3], Kwang Ik Yang[4], Chang-Ho Yun[5] and Min Kyung Chu[6*]

Abstract

Background: Previous studies have shown that migraine and sleep disturbances are closely associated. Excessive daytime sleepiness (EDS) is a common symptom of various types of sleep disturbance. Findings from clinic-based studies suggest that a high percentage of migraineurs experience EDS. However, the prevalence and clinical impact of EDS among migraineurs at the population level have rarely been reported. The objective of this study was to investigate the prevalence and impact of EDS among migraineurs using a population-based sample in Korea.

Methods: We selected a stratified random sample of Koreans aged 19 to 69 years and evaluated them using a semi-structured interview designed to identify EDS, headache type, and the clinical characteristics of migraine. If the score on the Epworth Sleepiness Scale (ESS) was more than or equal to 11, the participant was classified as having EDS.

Results: Of the 2,695 participants that completed the interview, 143 (5.3 %) and 313 (11.6 %) were classified as having migraine and EDS, respectively. The prevalence of EDS was significantly higher in participants with migraine (19.6 %) and non-migraine headache (13.4 %) compared to non-headache controls (9.4 %). Migraineurs with EDS had higher scores on the Visual Analogue Scale (VAS) for headache intensity (6.9 ± 1.8 vs. 6.0 ± 1.9, $p = 0.014$) and Headache Impact Test-6 (59.8 ± 10.2 vs. 52.5 ± 8.2, $p < 0.001$) compared to migraineurs without EDS.

Conclusions: Approximately 20 % of migraineurs had EDS in this population-based sample. Excessive daytime sleepiness was associated with an exacerbation of some migraine symptoms.

Keywords: Epidemiology, Excessive daytime sleepiness, Headache, Migraine, Sleep, Sleepiness

Background

Migraine and sleep disturbances are common neurological problems in the general population [1–3]. The close association between the two conditions has been reported in numerous clinic- and population-based studies. Both excessive sleep and sleep deprivation are common triggering factors of migraine and sleep may terminate an attack of migraine [4, 5]. Insomnia is a common comorbidity of migraine in cross-sectional and longitudinal studies [6, 7]. Habitual snoring and sleep bruxism are associated with an exacerbation of migraine [8, 9]. Morning headache in obstructive sleep apnea (OSA) patients may exhibit migraine-like headache [10]. Restless legs syndrome has been reported to be associated with migraine in case-controlled and population-based studies [11, 12].

Excessive daytime sleepiness (EDS) is defined as 'sleepiness in a situation when an individual would be expected to be awake and alert' [13]. EDS is not a disorder in and of itself, but represents symptoms of several broad conditions including poor sleep quality, depression, anxiety, sleep-disordered breathing, and obesity metabolic syndrome [14]. Besides impairing quality of life, EDS may lead to potentially problematic conditions such as attention deficits and sleep attacks [15]. The prevalence of EDS has ranged between 10 % and 20 % in the general population [16, 17].

For psychiatric conditions, anxiety and depression has been reported to be associated with EDS. Individuals with depression have frequently EDS (57.1 %) and a

* Correspondence: chumk@hallym.ac.kr
[6]Department of Neurology, Kangnam Sacred Heart Hospital, Hallym University College of Medicine, 1 Singil-ro, Yeongdeungpo-gu, Seoul 07441, South Korea
Full list of author information is available at the end of the article

quarter of individuals with EDS have moderate-to-severe depression in survey using Beck Depression Inventory [18, 19]. Anxiety was associated with an increased occurrence of EDS in a 20-year prospective community-based study from Switzerland [17].

The association between EDS and several common neurological diseases such as Parkinson's disease, epilepsy, and migraine has been previously reported. A case-controlled study from Italy noted that subjects with episodic migraine (EM) showed an increased odds ratio [14 % vs. 5 %; odds ratio (OR) = 3.1; 95 % confidence interval (CI) 1.1–8.9] for EDS compared to age- and sex-matched healthy controls [15]. Another case-controlled study showed a positive association between EDS and chronic migraine (CM) [20]. A case-series study in the United States showed that a significant proportion of participants with migraine also had EDS [21]. A community-based study in Norway showed increased ORs (OR = 3.3, 95 % CI 1.0–10.2) for EDS among migraineurs compared to headache-free individuals [22]. However, previous reports regarding the association between EDS and migraine were predominantly clinic-based studies and the association between them has seldom been examined in the general population. In addition, the clinical characteristics of migraine associated with EDS have not yet been reported.

The Korean Headache-Sleep Study (KHSS) is a nationwide population-based interview survey regarding headache and sleep disturbance [12]. It provides an opportunity to assess comorbidity between EDS and migraine as well as elucidate the clinical characteristics of migraine relative to the presence of comorbid EDS. The present study investigated 1) the prevalence of migraine and/or EDS in a general population-based sample; 2) the comorbidity between migraine and EDS in association with potential covariates such as anxiety, depression and poor sleep quality; and 3) the clinical characteristics of migraine comorbid with EDS using the data available from the KHSS.

Methods

Study population and survey process

The study was a nationwide, cross-sectional survey of headache and sleep in the Korean population in adults aged 19–69 years. The study design and methods have been previously described in detail [12]. Briefly, we adopted a two-stage systematic random sampling method in all Korean territories except Jeju-do, proportional to the distribution of the population, which resulted in a sample of 2,695 individuals. Subjects were stratified according to age, gender, size of residential area and educational level. To minimize bias, we informed participants that the topic of the survey was social health issues rather than headache. Trained interviewers conducted structured interviews using a questionnaire to diagnose headache type, sleep duration, sleepiness, anxiety, and depression door-to-door using a face-to-face interview. The interview included questions on headache symptoms and sleep status. All interviewers were employed by Gallup Korea and had previous social survey interviewing experience. The study was conducted from November 2011 to January 2012. It was approved by the institutional review board/ethics committee of Hallym University Sacred Heart Hospital and was performed in accordance with the ethical standards described in the 1964 Declaration of Helsinki and its subsequent amendments [23]. Written informed consent was obtained from all participants.

Migraine assessment

We diagnosed migraine using a questionnaire. The questionnaire established a headache profile which was designed to align with the second edition of the International Classification of Headache Disorders (ICHD-2) [24]. We investigated the severity of headache based on its effects on daily activity (mild, moderate, or severe) and using a visual analogue scale (VAS). Furthermore, we surveyed the headache frequency as following question. "How many days do you experience the headache every month?" Migraine was diagnosed based on the ICHD-2 criteria for migraine without aura (code 1.1) [24]. We did not attempt to separately diagnose migraine with and without aura. As such, both were included in the present study. The questions used to diagnose migraine have 75.0 % sensitivity and 88.2 % specificity, verified by comparing the diagnoses from the survey with those of doctors obtained from an additional telephone interview. This validation process has been previously described in detail [25].

Non-migraine headache assessment

If a participant responded positively to the question 'In the past year, have you had at least 1 headache lasting more than 1 min?' and was not diagnosed as having migraine, she or he was diagnosed as having non-migraine headaches.

Excessive daytime sleepiness, sleep duration and poor sleep quality assessment

We used the Epworth Sleepiness Scale (ESS) for assessing participants' daytime sleepiness. The total ESS score ranged from 0 to 24. If a participant scored more than or equal to 11 on the ESS, they were classified as having EDS. The ESS has been previously validated in the Korean language [26]. The Korean version of the ESS has been reported to have good internal consistency (Cronbach's $\alpha = 0.90$) and test-retest reliability ($r = 0.78$ to 0.93)

We assessed the weekday and weekend sleep durations of participants. Average sleep duration was defined as [(weekday sleep duration × 5) + (weekend sleep duration × 2)]/7. Short sleep duration was defined as average sleep duration of less than 6 h and poor sleep quality was defined as a Pittsburgh Sleep Quality Index score (PSQI) of more than 5.

Anxiety and depression assessment

We used the Goldberg Anxiety Scale (GAS) for measuring self-reported anxiety symptomology. If a participant provides a positive response for two or more of the first four screening questions and five or more of all GAS questions, they were characterized as having anxiety [27]. The Korean version of the GAS has been reported to have 82.0 % sensitivity and 94.4 % specificity [28].

The Patient Health Questionnaire-9 (PHQ-9) was used for diagnosing depression [29]. If a participant's PHQ-9 score was 10 or more, they were categorized as having depression. The Korean PHQ-9 has been found to have 81.1 % sensitivity and 89.9 % specificity [30].

Statistical analysis

We compared EDS prevalence among non-headache controls, and participants with non-migraine headache and migraine, using the chi-square test. We conducted a multivariable logistic regression analysis, adjusting for anxiety, depression, short sleep duration (average sleep duration less than 6 h), and poor sleep quality (a PSQI score of more than 5). We used logistic regression to evaluate the association between migraine and EDS according to headache frequency and calculated odds ratios (ORs) and their 95 % confidence intervals (CIs). We compared the clinical characteristics of participants with migraine with and without EDS using Student's *t*-test for continuous variables and the chi-square test for categorical variables. *p*-values of <0.05 were considered statistically significant. The results were analysed using the statistical software SPSS 22.0 (IBM, Armonk, NY, USA).

As with most survey studies, missing data from a lack of responding occurred on several items. The data reported are the available data and therefore some variables deviate from the overall sample size of $n = 2{,}695$. Imputation techniques were not employed to minimize non-response effects [31].

Results

Survey

Our interviewers approached 7,430 individuals and 3,114 of them agreed to take the survey. Of them, 2,695 subjects completed the survey (Fig. 1). The distribution of age, gender, size of residential area, and educational level were not significantly different from those of the Korean general population (Table 1).

Prevalence of migraine and non-migraine headache

Of the 2,695 respondents, 143 (5.3 %) met the ICHD-2 criteria for migraine and 1,130 (41.9 %) were classified as having non-migraine headache. Finally, 1,422 participants (52.8 %) were classified as non-headache controls.

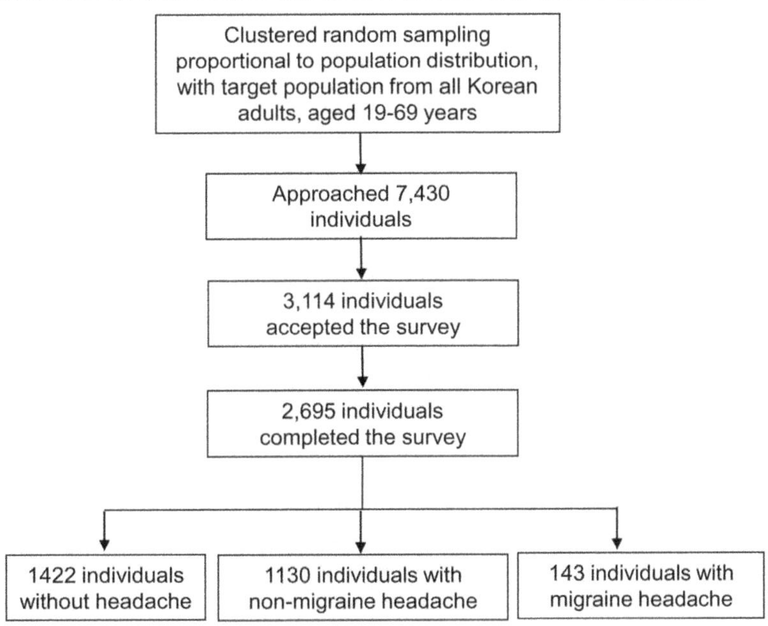

Fig. 1 Flow chart depicting participation in the Korean Headache-Sleep Study

Table 1 Sociodemographic distribution of all survey participants including migraine, non-migraine headache, and excessive daytime sleepiness

	Sample number	Total population	*p*-value	Migraine	Non-migraine headache	Excessive daytime sleepiness
	N (%)	N (%)		N, % (95 % CI)	N, % (95 % CI)	N, % (95 % CI)
Gender						
Men	1345 (49.3[a])	17,584,365 (50.6)	0.854[b]	36, 2.7 (1.8–3.5)	471, 35.0 (32.4–37.6)	161, 12.0 (10.2–13.7)
Women	1350 (50.7 [a])	17,198,350 (49.4)		107, 7.9 (6.5–9.4)	659, 49.0 (46.2–51.5)	152, 11.3 (9.6–12.9)
Age						
19–29	542 (20.5 [a])	7,717,947 (22.2)	0.917[b]	25, 4.5 (2.7–6.2)	231, 42.6 (38.4–46.8)	52, 9.6 (7.1–12.1)
30–39	604 (21.9 [a])	8,349,487 (24.0)		42, 7.0 (4.9–9.1)	269, 44.5 (40.6–48.5)	71, 11.8 (9.2–14.3)
40–49	611 (23.1 [a])	8,613,110 (24.8)		39, 6.5 (4.5–8.4)	277, 45.3 (41.4–49.3)	62, 10.1 (7.7–12.5)
50–59	529 (18.9 [a])	6,167,505 (17.7)		22, 4.1 (2.4-5.9)	204, 38.6 (34.4-42.7)	66, 12.5 (9.7-15.3)
60–69	409 (15.6 [a])	3,934,666 (11.3)		15, 3.9 (2.0–5.7)	149, 36.4 (31.7–41.1)	62, 15.2 (11.7–18.6)
Size of residential area						
Large city	1248 (46.3 [a])	16,776,771 (48.2)	0.921[b]	76, 6.1 (4.8–7.5)	525, 42.1 (39.3–44.8)	150, 12.0 (10.2–13.8)
Medium-to-small city	1186 (44.0 [a])	15,164,345 (43.6)		48, 4.0 (2.9–5.2)	488, 41.1 (38.3–43.9)	134, 11.3 (9.5–13.1)
Rural area	261 (9.7 [a])	2,841,599 (8.2)		19, 7.4 (4.2–10.6)	117, 44.8 (38.8–50.9)	29, 11.1 (7.3–14.9)
Educational level						
Middle school or less	393 (14.9 [a])	6,608,716 (19.0)	0.752[b]	22, 5.5 (4.2–7.7)	165, 42.0 (37.1–46.9)	58, 14.8 (11.2–18.3)
High school	1208 (44.5 [a])	15,234,829 (43.8)		50, 5.0 (3.8–6.3)	502, 41.6 (38.8–44.3)	135, 11.2 (9.4–13.0)
College or more	1068 (39.6 [a])	12,939,170 (37.2)		60, 5.6 (4.3–7.0)	457, 42.7 (39.8–45.8)	119, 11.1 (9.3–13.0)
Not responded				1, 3.8 (0.0–11.8)	6, 5.3 (0.3–9.6)	1, 3.8 (0.0–11.8)
Total	2695 (100.0 [a])	34,782,715 (100.0)		143, 5.3 (4.5–6.2)	1130, 41.9 (40.0–43.8)	313, 11.6 (10.4–12.8)

CI Confidence Interval
[a]Adjusted after age, gender, size of residential area and educational level
[b]Compared gender, age group, size of residential area, and educational level distributions between the sample of the present study and total population of Korea

Excessive daytime sleepiness and migraine

Three hundred and thirteen (11.6 %) subjects reported ESS scores in an excess of 11 and were therefore classified as having EDS (Table 1). Among the 143 participants with migraine, 28 (19.6 %) were classified as also having EDS. Of the 1,130 participants with non-migraine headache and the 1,422 classified as non-headache controls, 151 (13.4 %) and 134 (9.4 %) were classified as having EDS, respectively. The prevalence of EDS was significantly higher among participants with migraine (OR = 2.3, 95 % CI = 1.5–3.7, $p < 0.000$) and non-migraine headache (OR = 1.5, 95 % CI = 1.2–1.9, $p = 0.002$) compared to non-headache controls. However, the prevalence of EDS was not significantly different between participants with migraine and those with non-migraine headache (OR = 1.6, 95 % CI = 1.0–2.5, $p = 0.055$) (Fig. 2).

Univariable logistic regression revealed that EDS prevalence among participants with migraine (OR = 2.3, 95 % CI = 1.5–3.7, $p < 0.001$) and non-migraine headache (OR = 1.5, 95 % CI = 1.2–1.9, $p = 0.002$) had increased ORs for EDS compared to non-headache controls. Anxiety (OR = 2.4, 95 % CI = 1.7–3.2, $p < 0.001$), depression (OR = 6.2, 95 % CI = 4.2–9.1, $p < 0.001$), short sleep duration (OR = 1.4, 95 % CI = 0.9–1.9, $p = 0.122$), and poor sleep quality (OR = 3.3, 95 % CI = 2.6–4.3) also had increased ORs for EDS. In the multivariable logistic regression for EDS adjusting for anxiety and depression (Model 1), migraine was not associated with increased ORs for EDS. After adjusting for short sleep duration (<6 h) and poor sleep quality (PSQI score > 5) (Model 2), however, non-migraine headache and migraine were revealed to have statistically significant ORs for EDS. The final model adjusting for anxiety, depression, short sleep duration, and poor sleep quality (Model 3), indicated that those with non-migraine headache and migraine did not have statistically significant ORs for EDS relative to non-headache controls (Table 2).

Excessive daytime sleepiness according to the headache frequency of migraine

Although not statistically significant, there was a tendency towards increased prevalence of EDS in migraineurs with at least 10 attacks per month (OR = 1.5, 95 % CI = 0.4–5.8, $p = 0.557$) compared to those with less than one attack a month. The ESS scores were not significantly different among migraineurs with less than

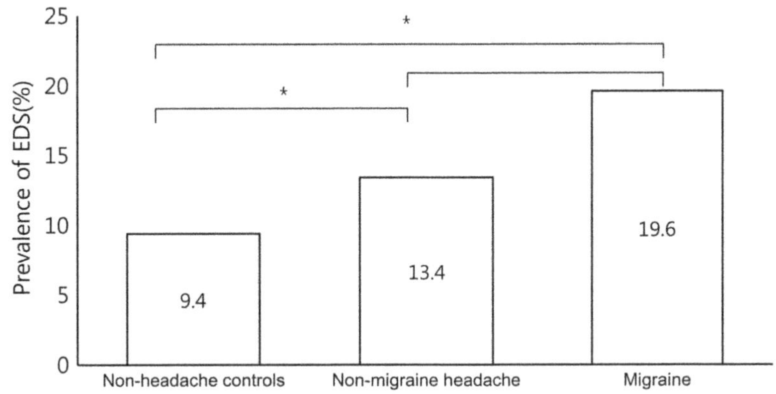

Fig. 2 Comparison of the prevalence of EDS among participants *$p < 0.05$

one attack per month (6.2 ± 3.8), 1–9 attacks per month (7.4 ± 4.6), or at least 10 attacks per month (7.2 ± 4.9, $p = 0.330$).

Clinical characteristics of subjects having migraine with and without EDS

We investigated the headache characteristics, headache frequency, VAS score for pain intensity, HIT-6 scores, psychiatric comorbidities such as anxiety and depression of participants with migraine grouped according the presence of EDS. Unilateral pain (39.3 % vs. 60.9 %, $p = 0.039$) was less prevalent and moderate-to-severe pain intensity (96.4 % vs. 76.5 %, p = 0.017) was more prevalent among migraineurs with EDS compared to migraineurs without EDS. Additionally, VAS scores for pain intensity (6.9 ± 1.8 vs. 6.0 ± 1.9, p = 0.014), HIT-6 scores (59.8 ± 10.2 vs. 52.5 ± 8.2, p < 0.001) and the prevalence of depression (42.9 % vs. 10.4 %, p < 0.001) was higher in migraineurs with EDS than those without EDS. The other measures did not significantly differ with the presence of EDS (Table 3).

Discussion

The key findings in the present study were: (1) the prevalence of migraine and EDS in the Korean general population were 5.3 % and 11.6 %, respectively; (2) the prevalence of EDS was significantly higher among participants with migraine (19.6 %) and non-migraine headache (13.4 %) compared to non-headache controls (9.4 %); and (3) some clinical characteristics of migraine were more profound among migraineurs with EDS compared to migraineurs without EDS.

The 1-year prevalence of migraine in the present study was 5.3 % (2.7 % for men and 7.9 % for women). The 1-year prevalence of migraine in Asian countries has been found to range between 4.7 % and 9.1 % in most previous studies [32]. Our findings are similar to those reported in previous studies from Asian countries. The prevalence of migraine in Asia is relatively lower than that of western countries.

We found that the prevalence of EDS was 11.6 % in the Korean general population. Previous population-based studies have reported EDS using ESS mostly ranging from 10 % to 20 %. Three Australian studies among adults reported that EDS prevalence ranged from 11.7 %

Table 2 Logistic regression to examine excessive daytime sleepiness by headache condition

	Univariable analysis for EDS		Multivariable analysis, adjusted for anxiety and depression (Model 1)		Multivariable analysis, adjusted for sleep duration and PSQI Score (Model 2)		Multivariable analysis, adjusted for anxiety, depression, sleep duration and PSQI score (Model 3)	
	OR	*P*-value	OR	*P*-value	OR	*P*-value	OR	*P*-value
Non-migraine headache	1.5 (1.2–1.9)	0.002	1.3 (1.0–1.7)	0.042	1.3 (1.0–1.7)	0.037	1.2 (0.9–1.5)	0.175
Migraine	2.3 (1.5–3.7)	<0.001	1.6 (1.0–2.6)	0.069	1.8 (1.2–2.9)	0.010	1.4 (0.8–2.2)	0.206
Anxiety	2.4 (1.7–3.2)	<0.001	1.3 (0.9–1.9)	0.135			1.2 (0.8–1.7)	0.504
Depression	6.2 (4.2–9.1)	<0.001	4.8 (3.1–7.4)	<0.001			3.7 (2.4–5.8)	<0.001
Short sleep duration (<6 h)	1.4 (0.9–1.9)	0.122			0.8 (0.5–1.2)	0.790	0.8 (0.5–1.1)	0.143
PSQI (PSQI score >5)	3.3 (2.6–4.3)	<0.001			3.3 (2.5–4.3)	<0.001	3.0 (2.2–3.8)	<0.001

EDS Excessive daytime sleepiness, *PSQI* Pittsburgh Sleep Quality Index

Table 3 Clinical characteristics and impact of migraine according to excessive daytime sleepiness

	Migraine with EDS, *N* = 28	Migraine without EDS, *N* = 115	*P*-value
Headache characteristics			
Unilateral pain, N (%)	11 (39.3)	70 (60.9)	0.039
Pulsating quality, N (%)	18 (64.3)	90 (78.3)	0.123
Moderate-to-severe pain intensity, N (%)	27 (96.4)	88 (76.5)	0.017
Aggravation by movement, N (%)	23 (82.1)	77 (67.0)	0.116
Nausea, N (%)	23 (82.1)	102 (88.7)	0.349
Vomiting, N (%)	11 (39.3)	44 (38.3)	0.920
Photophobia, N (%)	16 (57.1)	68 (59.1)	0.848
Phonophobia, N (%)	23 (82.1)	78 (67.8)	0.136
Osmophobia, N (%)	14 (50.0)	54 (47.0)	0.722
Headache frequency, mean ± SD	5.1 ± 7.2	3.5 ± 5.9	0.178
VAS for pain intensity, mean ± SD	6.9 ± 1.8	6.0 ± 1.9	0.014
HIT-6 score, mean ± SD	59.8 ± 10.2	52.5 ± 8.2	<0.001
Anxiety, N (%)	11 (39.3)	32 (27.8)	0.236
Depression, N (%)	12 (42.9)	12 (10.4)	<0.001

EDS Excessive daytime sleepiness, *VAS* Visual Analogue Scale, *HIT-6* Headache Impact Test-6

to 15.3 % [33–35]. A study in Singapore revealed an EDS prevalence of 9.0 % [36]. A previous study using data from the Korean Genome Epidemiology Study found that the prevalence of EDS was 12.2 % [37]. Our study showed a similar EDS prevalence to that from previous studies and therefore verified the reliability of the sampling and EDS diagnosis in our study.

Excessive daytime sleepiness has been reported to be associated with poor sleep quality and psychiatric conditions [38, 39]. Poor sleep quality is reported to be associated psychiatric conditions [40–42]. Furthermore, migraineurs were reported to have poor sleep quality and higher psychiatric comorbid conditions compared to non-headache controls [43–45]. In the present study, participants with migraine had an increased OR for EDS compared to non-headache controls in the univariable regression analysis. After adjusting for anxiety, depression, short sleep duration, and poor sleep quality, migraine was no longer a significant predictor of EDS while poor sleep quality and depression maintained significant associations with EDS (Table 3). Previous case-controlled studies have demonstrated similar findings. EM and CM had increased ORs for EDS in a univariate analysis [15, 20]. However, after adjusting for poor sleep quality, drugs, and gender, EM and CM were no longer statistically significant. These findings suggest that a significant association between migraine and EDS in a univariable analysis may be attributable to poor sleep quality and/or depression among migraineurs rather than the migraine itself.

In the present study, migraineurs with EDS experienced more severe headache intensity, reported a higher impact of the headache, and more depressive symptomology than those without EDS. These findings suggest that migraineurs with EDS have more severe clinical burden than migraineurs without EDS. Considering findings in the present study, physicians should carefully investigate the level of EDS and factors that exacerbate it, such as poor sleep quality and depressive symptomology when caring for patients with migraine.

This study had some limitations. First, although our research is a large population-based study with low sampling error, its statistical power for executing a subgroup analysis was limited. Some results might not have reached statistical significance because of the limited sample size. Second, this study is cross-sectional and the directionality of the association is uncertain. It cannot be determined whether migraine causes EDS or vice versa. Third, we surveyed the sleep habits of participants based solely on self-report. Further, we did not use any tool to evaluate characteristics of sleep such as polysomnography, which could further explore the sleep architecture, total sleep time, sleep efficiency, or other relevant sleep variables among participants with EDS.

Our study has several strengths. First, this study has a large sample size in a population-based setting and the estimated sampling error was low. Second, we investigated risk factors for EDS after adjusting for sleep duration. Third, we assessed the clinical features of migraine in participants with EDS compared with those without EDS.

Conclusions

In summary, migraineurs had a higher prevalence of EDS relative to non-headache controls. Further, migraineurs with EDS experienced a more severe headache, depressive mood, and higher impact of headache. The presence of EDS should be carefully evaluated in migraineurs, in order to relieve the headache as well as reduce the impact of headache.

Abbreviations

EDS, excessive daytime sleepiness; ESS, epworth Sleepiness Scale; VAS visual Analogue Scale; OSA, obstructive sleep apnea; EM, episodic migraine; CI, confidence interval; CM, chronic migraine; ICHD, International Classification of Headache Disorders; KHSS, Korean Headache-Sleep Study; PSQI, Pittsburgh Sleep Quality Index score; GAS, Goldberg Anxiety Scale; PHQ-9 Patient Health Questionnaire-9; HIT-6 Headache Impact Test-6; OR odds ratio

Competing interests

The authors declare that they have no conflicting interests.

Authors' contributions

JYK conceptualized and designed the study, analyzed the data, and wrote the manuscript. SJC conceptualized and designed the study, and wrote the manuscript. JMK conceptualized and collected the data. KIY conceptualized and collected the data. CHY conceptualized and collected the data. MKC conceptualized and designed the study, collected and analyzed the data, and wrote the manuscript. All authors read and approved the final manuscript.

Acknowledgements

The authors would like to thank Gallup Korea for providing technical support for the Korean Headache-Sleep Study.

Funding

This Study was Supported by a 2011-Grant from Korean Academy of Medical Sciences.

Author details

[1]Department of Neurology, Bio Medical Research Institute, Pusan National University Hospital, Pusan National University School of Medicine, Busan, South Korea. [2]Department of Neurology, Dongtan Sacred Heart Hospital, Hallym University College of Medicine, Hwaseong, South Korea. [3]Department of Neurology, Gangnam Severance Hospital, Yonsei University College of Medicine, Seoul, South Korea. [4]Sleep Disorders Center, Department of Neurology, Soonchunhyang University College of Medicine, Cheonan Hospital, Cheonan, South Korea. [5]Clinical Neuroscience Center, Department of Neurology, Seoul National University Bundang Hospital, Seongnam, South Korea. [6]Department of Neurology, Kangnam Sacred Heart Hospital, Hallym University College of Medicine, 1 Singil-ro, Yeongdeungpo-gu, Seoul 07441, South Korea.

References

1. Rains JC, Poceta JS, Penzien DB (2008) Sleep and headaches. Curr Neurol Neurosci Rep 8(2):167–175
2. Aguggia M, Cavallini M, Divito N, Ferrero M, Lentini A, Montano V et al (2011) Sleep and primary headaches. Neurol Sci 32(Suppl 1):S51–54
3. Freedom T, Evans RW (2013) Headache and sleep. Headache 53(8): 1358–1366
4. Kelman L, Rains JC (2005) Headache and sleep: examination of sleep patterns and complaints in a large clinical sample of migraineurs. Headache 45(7):904–910
5. Inamorato E, Minatti-Hannuch SN, Zukerman E (1993) The role of sleep in migraine attacks. Arq Neuropsiquiatr 51(4):429–432
6. Sancisi E, Cevoli S, Vignatelli L, Nicodemo M, Pierangeli G, Zanigni S et al (2010) Increased prevalence of sleep disorders in chronic headache: a case-control study. Headache 50(9):1464–1472
7. Odegard SS, Sand T, Engstrom M, Stovner LJ, Zwart JA, Hagen K (2011) The long-term effect of insomnia on primary headaches: a prospective population-based cohort study (HUNT-2 and HUNT-3). Headache 51(4):570–580
8. Scher AI, Lipton RB, Stewart WF (2003) Habitual snoring as a risk factor for chronic daily headache. Neurology 60(8):1366–1368
9. Fernandes G, Franco AL, Goncalves DA, Speciali JG, Bigal ME, Camparis CM (2013) Temporomandibular disorders, sleep bruxism, and primary headaches are mutually associated. J Orofac Pain 27(1):14–20
10. Suzuki K, Miyamoto M, Miyamoto T, Numao A, Suzuki S, Sakuta H et al (2015) Sleep apnoea headache in obstructive sleep apnoea syndrome patients presenting with morning headache: comparison of the ICHD-2 and ICHD-3 beta criteria. J Headache Pain 16:56
11. Schurks M, Winter AC, Berger K, Buring JE, Kurth T (2012) Migraine and restless legs syndrome in women. Cephalalgia 32(5):382–389. doi:10.1177/0333102412439355
12. Cho SJ, Chung YK, Kim JM, Chu MK (2015) Migraine and restless legs syndrome are associated in adults under age fifty but not in adults over fifty: a population-based study. J Headache Pain 16:554
13. Arand D, Bonnet M, Hurwitz T, Mitler M, Rosa R, Sangal RB (2005) The clinical use of the MSLT and MWT. Sleep 28(1):123–144
14. Bixler EO, Vgontzas AN, Lin HM, Calhoun SL, Vela-Bueno A, Kales A (2005) Excessive daytime sleepiness in a general population sample: the role of sleep apnea, age, obesity, diabetes, and depression. J Clin Endocrinol Metab 90(8):4510–4515
15. Barbanti P, Fabbrini G, Aurilia C, Vanacore N, Cruccu G (2007) A case-control study on excessive daytime sleepiness in episodic migraine. Cephalalgia 27(10):1115–1119
16. Carskadon MA (1993) Evaluation of excessive daytime sleepiness. Neurophysiol Clin 23(1):91–100
17. Hasler G, Buysse DJ, Gamma A, Ajdacic V, Eich D, Rossler W et al (2005) Excessive daytime sleepiness in young adults: a 20-year prospective community study. J Clin Psychiatry 66(4):521–529
18. Chellappa SL, Araujo JF (2006) Excessive daytime sleepiness in patients with depressive disorder. Rev Bras Psiquiatr 28(2):126–129
19. Hublin C, Kaprio J, Partinen M, Heikkila K, Koskenvuo M (1996) Daytime sleepiness in an adult, Finnish population. J Intern Med 239(5):417–423
20. Barbanti P, Aurilia C, Egeo G, Fofi L, Vanacore N (2013) A case-control study on excessive daytime sleepiness in chronic migraine. Sleep Med 14(3):278–281
21. Peres MF, Stiles MA, Siow HC, Silberstein SD (2005) Excessive daytime sleepiness in migraine patients. J Neurol Neurosurg Psychiatry 76(10):1467–1468
22. Odegard SS, Engstrom M, Sand T, Stovner LJ, Zwart JA, Hagen K (2010) Associations between sleep disturbance and primary headaches: the third Nord-Trondelag Health Study. J Headache Pain 11(3):197–206
23. World Medical A (2001) Ethical principles for medical research involving human subjects. Eur J Emerg Med 8(3):221–223
24. Headache Classification Subcommittee of the International Headache S (2004) The international classification of headache disorders: 2nd edition. Cephalalgia 24(Suppl 1):9–160
25. Kim BK, Chu MK, Lee TG, Kim JM, Chung CS, Lee KS (2012) Prevalence and impact of migraine and tension-type headache in Korea. J Clin Neurol 8(3):204–211
26. Cho YW, Lee JH, Son HK, Lee SH, Shin C, Johns MW (2011) The reliability and validity of the Korean version of the Epworth sleepiness scale. Sleep Breath 15(3):377–384
27. Goldberg D, Bridges K, Duncan-Jones P, Grayson D (1988) Detecting anxiety and depression in general medical settings. BMJ 297(6653):897–899
28. Lim JY, Lee SH, Cha YS, Park HS, Sunwoo S (2001) Reliability and validity of anxiety screening scale. J Korean Acad Fam Med 22(8):1224–1232
29. Pignone MP, Gaynes BN, Rushton JL, Burchell CM, Orleans CT, Mulrow CD et al (2002) Screening for depression in adults: a summary of the evidence for the U.S. Preventive services task force. Ann Intern Med 136(10):765–776
30. Choi HS, Choi JH, Park KH, Joo KJ, Ga H, Ko HJ et al (2007) Standardization of the Korean version of Patient Health Questionnaire-9 as a screening instrument for major depressive disorder. J Korean Acad Fam Med 28(2):114–119
31. Little RJ, Rubin DB (2014) Statistical analysis with missing data. New York: John Wiley & Sons

32. Peng KP, Wang SJ (2014) Epidemiology of headache disorders in the Asia-pacific region. Headache 54(4):610–618
33. Hayley AC, Williams LJ, Kennedy GA, Berk M, Brennan SL, Pasco JA (2014) Prevalence of excessive daytime sleepiness in a sample of the Australian adult population. Sleep Med 15(3):348–354
34. Vashum KP, McEvoy MA, Hancock SJ, Islam MR, Peel R, Attia JR et al (2015) Prevalence of and associations with excessive daytime sleepiness in an Australian older population. Asia Pac J Public Health 27(2):NP2275–2284
35. Bartlett DJ, Marshall NS, Williams A, Grunstein RR (2008) Sleep health New South Wales: chronic sleep restriction and daytime sleepiness. Intern Med J 38(1):24–31
36. Ng TP, Tan WC (2005) Prevalence and determinants of excessive daytime sleepiness in an Asian multi-ethnic population. Sleep Med 6(6):523–529
37. Joo S, Baik I, Yi H, Jung K, Kim J, Shin C (2009) Prevalence of excessive daytime sleepiness and associated factors in the adult population of Korea. Sleep Med 10(2):182–188
38. Guilleminault C, Brooks SN (2001) Excessive daytime sleepiness: a challenge for the practising neurologist. Brain 124(Pt 8):1482–1491
39. Pagel JF (2009) Excessive daytime sleepiness. Am Fam Physician 79(5):391–396
40. Buysse DJ, Reynolds CF 3rd, Monk TH, Berman SR, Kupfer DJ (1989) The Pittsburgh Sleep Quality Index: a new instrument for psychiatric practice and research. Psychiatry Res 28(2):193–213
41. Perlis ML, Giles DE, Buysse DJ, Tu X, Kupfer DJ (1997) Self-reported sleep disturbance as a prodromal symptom in recurrent depression. J Affect Disord 42(2–3):209–212
42. Ford DE, Kamerow DB (1989) Epidemiologic study of sleep disturbances and psychiatric disorders. An opportunity for prevention? JAMA 262(11): 1479–1484
43. Wang Y, Xie J, Yang F, Wu S, Wang H, Zhang X et al (2015) Comorbidity of poor sleep and primary headaches among nursing staff in north China. J Headache Pain 16:88
44. Morgan I, Eguia F, Gelaye B, Peterlin BL, Tadesse MG, Lemma S et al (2015) Sleep disturbances and quality of life in Sub-Saharan African migraineurs. J Headache Pain 16:18
45. Breslau N, Schultz LR, Stewart WF, Lipton RB, Lucia VC, Welch KM (2000) Headache and major depression: is the association specific to migraine? Neurology 54(2):308–313

5

Field testing of the ICHD-3β and expert opinion criteria for chronic migraine

Huahua Jiang[1], Yong Deng[1], Yixin Zhang[1], Jieli Jin[1], Xueying Kong[1], Qiuwen Zhu[1], Kuiyun Wang[2] and Jiying Zhou[1*]

Abstract

Background: Chronic headache (CrH) occurs commonly in the population, and chronic migraine (CM) accounts for much of the CrH. Diagnostic criteria for CM remain controversial, and this could lead to undertreatment of CM. The purpose of this study was to analyze the clinical profiles of CM and to field test the International Classification of Headache Disorders-3β criteria (ICHD-3β) and Expert Opinion criteria (EO) for CM application.

Methods: We retrospectively reviewed the medical records of CrH patients in our headache clinic during the period. Eligible patients were selected from CrH population based on Silberstein and Lipton criteria (S-L) for CM, and meanwhile fulfilled with migraine days at least 8 days/month. Then we evaluated the characteristics of clinic profiles and outcomes between patients diagnosed CM using ICHD-3β and EO criteria. Field tested the CM criteria Of ICHD-3β and EO.

Results: In a total of 710 CrH patients , 261 (36.8 %) were recruited with CM based on both S-L criteria and fulfilled at least 8 migraine days/month. Be understandable, all the 261 patients met the EO criteria, and only 185 (70.9 %) met ICHD-3β for CM. For the 76 patients who met EO but not ICHD-3β, 70 had atypical migraine attacks (probable migraine, PM), and another 6 had typical migraine attacks but less than a total history of 5 attacks. Although 173 (66.3 %) were concurrent with medication overuse, just one patient overused triptans and none used ergot agents. Clinical features were not significantly different between the ICHD-3β and EO criteria groups ($P > 0.05$), and neither were outcomes of prophylaxis ($P = 0.966$). Total migraine prophylaxis effectiveness was 73 %.

Conclusion: Migraine-specific analgesics are rarely used in China, permitting patients with PM to avail themselves of "migraine days" is a reasonable accommodation for this difficult condition. In our hands, use of the new EO criteria for diagnosis of CM increases the sensitivity and maintains the specificity of decision making, and therefore should be adopted in CM management practice.

Keywords: Chronic disease, Humans, International classification of diseases, Migraine disorders/classifications, Migraine disorders/diagnosis

Background

Chronic headache (CrH) refers to a group of headache disorders occurring at least 15 days/month exceeding 3 months, including those associated with medication overuse [1, 2]. Approximately 3 to 5 % of the adult population worldwide have CrH [2]. In practice, the most common form of CrH in patients presenting to headache clinics is CM [2–6]. However, the diagnostic criteria for CM remain controversial.

Transformed migraine (now called chronic migraine, CM) was first proposed by Silberstein and Lipton (S-L) in 1994 [6]. It was classified as CM with or without medication overuse (CM+ and CM-, respectively) [6]. CM criteria were standardized in the Second Edition of the International Classification of Headache Disorders (ICHD-2) in 2004, which required migraine symptoms to be present at least 15 days/month and excluded medication overuse headache (MOH) [7]. Revised criteria (ICHD-2R) published in 2006 modified this, requiring

* Correspondence: zheadache@163.com
[1]Department of Neurology, The First Affiliated Hospital of Chongqing Medical University, 1st You Yi Road, Yu Zhong District, Chongqing 400016, China
Full list of author information is available at the end of the article

headache at least 15 days/month but also migraine symptoms on at least 8 days. It was still difficult to apply these ICHD-2R criteria in patients with MOH [8].

The International Classification of Headache Disorders, 3rd edition, beta version (ICHD-3β) was published in 2013 [9]. The ICHD-3β criteria for CM require headache at least 15 days/month for least 3 months; it includes migraine with or without aura and believed migraine day relieved by a triptan or ergot derivative, on at least 8 days/month. It also allows CM with and without MOH [9]. However, CrH with probable migraine (PM) are not considered while diagnoses CM by ICHD-3β criteria, not mention the situation that migraine-specific analgesics are still not available worldwide. Thankfully, a paper describing Expert Opinion on diagnostic criteria for CM was published in 2014 [10]. The criteria address PM for treatment of headache with triptans and ergot derivatives [10]. Thus, the purpose of this study was to perform field testing of the ICHD-3β and Expert Opinion criteria (EO) for CM in our patient population.

Methods

Study population

A retrospective study was conducted in the headache clinic of the First Affiliated Hospital of Chongqing Medical University in China. Consecutive patient visits presenting with a principal complaint of headache from January 2013 to December 2015 were candidate for this study.

All headache patients with CrH were reviewed by two doctors independently (H.J., Y.D). The diagnosis of CrH was confirmed with at least 15 days/month over a period lasting more than 3 months, which had been defined in our previous study [11]. Eligible patients were selected from CrH if their signs and symptoms fulfilled the criteria for CM according to S-L criteria [6], and with migraine days at least 8 days/month [12]. Patients with other primary CrH (chronic tension-type headache (CTTH), new daily persistent headache (NDPH) and chronic cluster headache et al.) and secondary headaches were excluded [13]. MRI and/or CT scans were performed if clinically necessary. If the headache could not be accurately categorized as either primary or secondary, it was classified as headache not otherwise specified (headache NOS) [11].

The patients were treated empirically with flunarizine (5 mg/day), amitriptyline (25–50 mg/day), topiramate (75 mg/day), metoprolol (25–50 mg/day) or venlafaxine (75 mg/day), based on the specialist's judgements (JY Zhou) and patient's preferences. Additionally, overused analgesics were withdrawn in order to address MOH. Patients were informed to discontinue the overused analgesics and meanwhile started prophylactic treatment. Medication responses were classified as significant effectiveness (50 % reduction in headache days of moderate to severe headache), partial effectiveness, and no improvement or worsening symptoms.

Date collection

All individuals presenting with a principal complaint of headache were interviewed face-to-face by a headache specialist (JY Zhou). The medical history and a detailed structured self-administered questionnaire were completed by 7 doctors (H.J., Y.D,, Y. Z., J.J., X.K., Q.Z., K.W). The questionnaire was validated for headache diagnosis by previous study [5, 11, 14], and included the following components: demographic characteristics, clinical features of headache (onset age, course, location, duration, frequency, intensity, aggravation after physical activity and associated symptoms); history of head injury; past medical history and drug intake for headache; family history. Treatment follow up was then at a 3 to 6-month visit for face-to-face consult, or by telephone interviews, based on previous trials that the migraine prevention should reasonably last for 3–6 months for response and tolerability evaluation [15, 16].

Standard study protocol and patient consents

Our study protocol was approved by the hospital ethics board. All patients gave their informed consent before collecting headache information.

Statistical analysis

Statistical analysis was performed using SPSS software, version 20.0 (Chicago, IL, USA). The characteristics of the study population were analyzed using descriptive statistics. Quantitative variables were expressed as mean ± standard deviation (SD). Qualitative variables were expressed as frequency (proportion). The Student's t test and chi-squared test were used for comparison of clinical parameters between groups. $P < 0.05$ was considered to be statistically significant.

Results

During the study period (January 2013 to December 2015), 2733 patient visits with main complaint of headache were recorded (Fig. 1). A total of 710 (26.0 %) had CrH. Of the CrH patients, 261 (36.8 %) patients were diagnosed as CM based on the S-L criteria, 14.1 % (100/710) had CTTH, 2 % (14/710) had NDPH, 8.3 % (59/710) other primary headache, 28.2 % (200/710) secondary headache and 10.7 % (76/710) headache NOS. CM patients were female predominant (73.2 %) and the mean age was 49.5 years (range from 11 to 83 years).

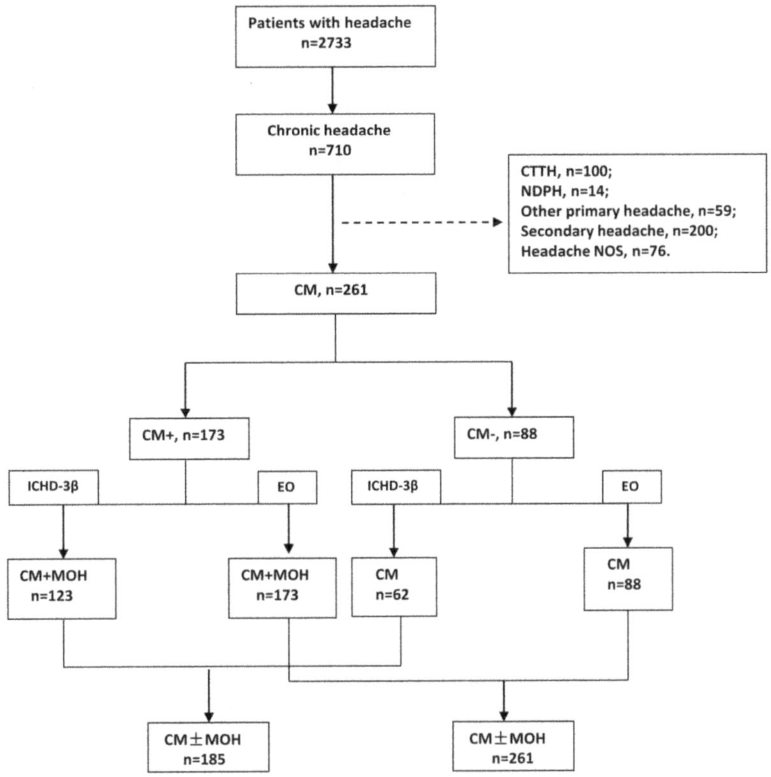

Fig. 1 Flow chart of the study. CTTH: chronic tension-type headache; NDPH: new daily persistent headache; Headache NOS: headache not otherwise specified; CM: chronic migraine ; CM- : chronic migraine without medication overuse; CM+: chronic migraine with medication overuse; ICHD-3β: International Classification of Headache Disorders,3rd edition beta version; EO: Expert Opinion criteria; MOH: medication overuse headache

The classification of CM using ICHD-3β and EO criteria

Among 261 CM patients, 66.3 % (173/261) overused medication. Of the 88 CM patients without medication overuse, 100 % met EO criteria for CM, but only 62 (70 %) fulfilled ICHD-3β criteria for this diagnosis, as 26 patients had PM being not included in ICHD-3β. Patients with medication overuse were classified as MOH according to ICHD-3β and EO criteria which allow both CM and MOH diagnoses. Of the 173 CM patients with documented medication overuse, 123 (71.1 %) patients fulfilled CM and MOH based on ICHD-3β, other 50 patients were diagnosed with PM. In contrast, all 173 (100 %) patients fulfilled CM and MOH based on EO (Table 1). In total, of 261 CM patients, 70.9 % (185) fulfilled ICHD-3β criteria for CM, and all 261 patients fulfilled EO criteria for CM.

Table 2 summarizes the subtypes of migraine in CM based on ICHD-3β and EO. The subtypes of migraine based on S-L criteria for CM include migraine without aura (MO), migraine with aura (MA), and PM. Among all 261 patients, there were 183 patients meeting the criteria for MO, 8 patients with MA and 70 patients meeting the criteria for PM. Of the 183 MO patients, 177 (96.7 %) patients fulfilled MO based on ICHD-3β criteria for CM, other 6 patients just had less than 5 migraine episodes. 8 (100 %) MA patients fulfilled MA subtypes. The migraine subtypes in EO were in accordance with those in S-L criteria.

Table 1 Classification of patients with CM based on S-L, using ICHD-3β and EO

S-L	ICHD-3β	*n* (%)	EO	*n* (%)
261		185 (70.9 %)		261 (100 %)
CM-, *n* = 88	CM	62 (70.5 %)	CM	88 (100 %)
CM+, *n* = 173	CM + MOH	123 (71.1 %)	CM + MOH	173 (100 %)

Abbreviations: *S-L* silberstein and lipton criteria, *CM* chronic migraine without medication overuse, *CM+* chronic migraine with medication overuse, *ICHD-3β* international classification of headache disorders,3rd edition beta version, *EO* expert opinion criteria, *CM* chronic migraine, *CM + MOH* chronic migraine with medication overuse headache

Table 2 Subtypes of migraine in CM based on ICHD-3β and EO

S-L	ICHD-3β	*n* (%)	EO	*n* (%)
n = 261		185 (70.9 %)		261 (100 %)
MO, *n* = 183	MO	177 (96.7 %)	MO	183 (100 %)
MA, *n* = 8	MA	8 (100 %)	MA	8 (100 %)
PM, *n* = 70	–	–	PM	70 (100 %)

Abbreviations: *S-L* silberstein and lipton criteria, *MO* migraine without aura, *MA* migraine with aura, *PM* probable migraine, *ICHD-3β* international classification of headache disorders, 3rd edition beta version, *EO* expert opinion criteria

The clinical features of CM by ICHD-3β and EO criteria

The clinical features of CM patients based on ICHD-3β and EO criteria are shown in Table 3. Demographic profiles showed no significant differences. Mean age was from 48.5 to 49.5 years, and females predominated (73.2–74.1 %). The body mass index averaged from 22.9 to 23.2, within the normal range. The majority of patients (77.8–78.9 %) had not completed high school.

Table 3 Clinical features of CM based on ICHD-3β and EO criteria

	ICHD-3β *n* = 185	EO *n* = 261	*P*-value
Age (years), mean (SD)	48.5 ± 11.4	49.54 ± 11.5	0.364
Gender, *n* (%)			0.837
Female	137 (74.1 %)	191 (73.2 %)	
Male	48 (24.9 %)	70 (26.8 %)	
BMI, mean (SD)	23.2 ± 3.7	22.9 ± 3.6	0.418
Educational level, *n* (%)			0.783
< high school	149 (77.8 %)	206 (78.9 %)	
≥ high school	42 (22.2 %)	55 (21.1 %)	
Frequency of headache days, mean (SD)	23.5 ± 6.4	23.7 ± 6.4	0.750
Frequency of migraine days, mean (SD)	19.9 ± 7.9	20.4 ± 7.9	0.519
Age of onset of migraine, mean (SD)	31.7 ± 12.1	32.1 ± 12.4	0.727
Courses of migraine, mean (SD)	16.8 ± 10.9	17.4 ± 11.7	0.588
Age of onset of CM, mean (SD)	42.3 ± 12.0	42.9 ± 12.1	0.624
Courses of CM, mean (SD)	6.2 ± 8.2	6.8 ± 8.4	0.503
Currently used acute analgesics, *n* (%)			0.811
Yes	154 (83.2 %)	215 (82.5 %)	
No	31 (16.8 %)	46 (17.6 %)	
Category of used analgesics, *n* (%)			0.773
Single analgesics	9 (5.8 %)	14 (6.5 %)	
Combination analgesics	81 (52.6 %)	105 (48.8 %)	
Multiple analgesics	64 (41.6 %)	96 (44.7 %)	
Ergots	0	0	
Triptans	1 (0.6 %)	1 (0.5 %)	0.813
Medication overuse, *n* (%)			0.964
Yes	123 (66.5 %)	173 (66.3 %)	
No	62 (33.5 %)	88 (33.7 %)	
Family headache history, *n* (%)			0.995
Yes	100 (54.1 %)	141 (54.0 %)	
No	85 (45.9 %)	120 (46.0 %)	

Abbreviations: *CM* chronic migraine, *BMI* body mass index, *ICHD-3β* international classification of headache disorders,3rd edition beta version, *EO* expert opinion criteria

No headache characteristics were significantly different between the ICHD-3β and EO groups. Frequency of headache was almost identical (23.5–23.7 days per month) by either standard. The courses of migraine were 16.8–17.4 years and the courses of CM were 6.2–6.8 years. The mean age of onset of migraine was 31.7–32.1 years and the mean onset age of CM was 42.3–42.9 years. Most patients (82.5–82.7 %) took analgesic medications. About half (48.8–52.6 %) used combination analgesics, and 41.6–44.7 % of patients were taking multiple analgesics. Just 5.8–6.5 % of patients used simple analgesics. No patients ever used ergots, and only one patient tried triptans. About 54 % of patients had family headache history.

Treatment outcomes

A total of 250 patients received migraine prophylaxis (flunarizine, $n = 141$; amitriptyline, $n = 58$; topiramate, $n = 20$; metoprolol, $n = 25$; and venlafaxine, $n = 6$). Of these, 62 patients (25 %) were lost to follow-up (flunarizine, $n = 38$; amitriptyline, $n = 14$; topiramate, $n = 4$; and metoprolol, $n = 5$). The causes of lost were of incorrect telephone numbers ($n = 54$), or refusal to follow-up ($n = 7$). One patient discontinued venlafaxine due to nausea.

Figure 2 summarizes the treatment response of CM. There was no difference between groups in ICHD-3β and EO ($P = 0.966$). A total of 71.6–72.9 % of the patients had significant reduction of headaches, 15.4–16.4 % of patients had a partial response and the balance (11–12 %) had no improvement which meant these patients had no response to migraine prophylaxis.

Discussion

This was the first study to evaluate clinical applicability of ICHD-3β and EO criteria for CM. CM is a disabling disorder that is underdiagnosed and undertreated [17]. The prevalence rate of CM is variable. A systematic review in 2003 summarized 12 population-based studies using several definitions for frequent migraine and determined that the global prevalence of CM varied from 0.0 to 5.1 %, with most estimates in the range of 1.4 to 2.2 % [18]. In our study, among 2733 headache patients, a total of 710 patients had CrH. Of the CrH patients, 26.1 % (185/710) patients fulfilled ICHD-3β criteria for CM, but 36.8 % (261/710) patients were diagnosed CM based on EO, and the benefit outcomes who received migraine prophylaxis were identical between the two groups.

In a large US population-based sample, CM accounted for 7.68 % of all migraine cases based on ICHD-2 [19]. Another study, at the Danish Headache Centre, showed that CM accounted for 4.3 % of migraine or tension-type headache based on ICHD-2R [13]. It appears that the proportion of CM varied because of different population sampling techniques or diagnostic criteria.

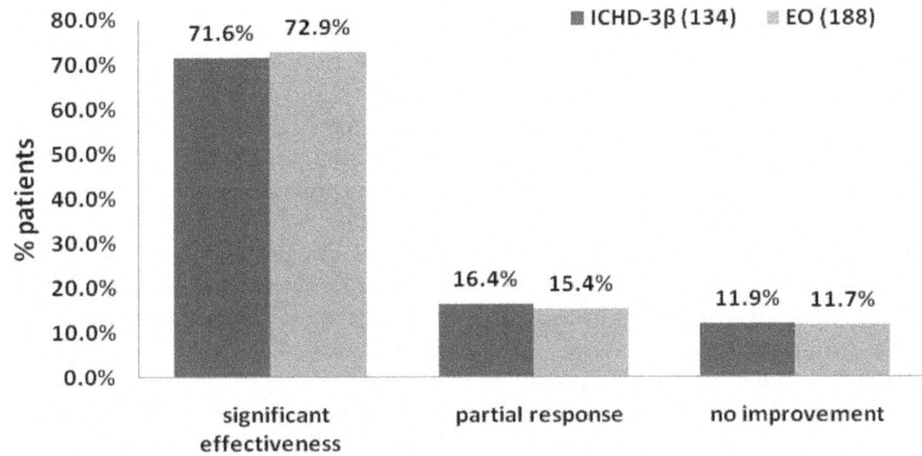

Fig. 2 Treatment response of chronic migraine. ICHD-3β: International Classification of Headache Disorders,3rd edition beta version; EO: Expert Opinion criteria

At present, there is no "gold standard" for diagnosis of CM in clinical practice. ICHD-3β is still considered to be a testing version, and the revised criteria (EO) were proposed in 2014. Table 4 showed the diagnostic criteria of CM.

The three systems of criteria recognize CM with medication overuse. The S-L criteria have been used widely in clinical practice. The criteria required a history of migraine or increasing headache frequency with decreasing severity of migrainous features over at least 3 months, and required a history of transformation. In current opinion, CM is not considered to be a complication of migraine, so the transformation process form episodic attack to continuous pain is not essential condition. Previous study showed that CM can be the initial subtype [20].

The criteria of ICHD-3β require presence of headache on at least 15 days/month for at least 3 months, and establish a diagnostic treatment link to migraine day. It requires migraine with/without an aura or relieved by a triptan or ergot derivative on ≥ 8 days/month. However, it might be too restrictive for application. Firstly, patients with CM often have difficulty recalling their prior migraine attacks as required by item B. Secondly, when analgesic agents are used, migraine features are often not typical or characteristic. Moreover, even migraine-

Table 4 Diagnostic criteria for CM according to S-L, ICHD-3β and EO criteria

S-L	ICHD-3β	EO
A. Daily or almost daily (>15 days a month) head pain for >1 month	A. Headache on ≥15 days per month for at least 3 months	A. Headache on ≥15 days per month for at least 3 months
B. Average headache duration of >4 h a day (if untreated)	B. Occurring in a patient who has had at least 5 attacks fulfilling criteria for 1.1 Migraine without aura and/or 1.2 migraine with aura	B. On ≥8 days per month on average ≥4 hours/day for at least 3 months, 1 or more of the following criteria were fulfilled 1. Criteria C and D for 1.1 migraine without aura 2. Criteria B and C for 1.2 migraine with aura 3. Criteria A and B for 1.5 probable migraine
C. At least one of the following: 1. History of episodic migraine meeting any HIS criteria 1.1-1.6 2. History of increasing headache frequency with deceasing severity of migrainous features over at least 3 months 3. Headache at some time meets HIS criteria for migraine 1.1-1.6 other than duration	C. On ≥8 days per month for at least 3 months, one or more of the following criteria were fulfilled 1. Criteria C and D for 1.1 migraine without aura 2. Criteria B and C for 1.2 migraine with aura 3. Believed by the patient to be migraine at onset and relieved by a triptan or ergot derivative	C. Not better accounted for by another ICHD-3 diagnosis
D. Dose not meet criteria for new daily persistent headache (4.7) or hemicrania compounds continua (4.8)	D. Not better accounted for by another ICHD-3 diagnosis.	D. Does not meet criteria for new daily persistent headache (4.7) or hemicrania continua (4.8)

Abbreviations: *S-L* silberstein and lipton criteria, *ICHD-3β* international classification of headache disorders, 3rd edition beta version, *EO* expert opinion criteria, *CM* chronic migraine

specific analgesics can be effective against other primary headaches, such as cluster headaches, as well as other secondary headaches.

ICHD-3β requires migraine-specific medication as one of the criteria, as patients in some countries took triptans prescribed by their headache clinics, and this could increase the sensitivity of the criteria [21]. A survey in Italy showed that triptans were used by 46.4 % of patients with a previous diagnosis of migraine [17]. Another survey in Latin American showed that 70 % of MOH overused ergotamine, and most of them were migraine sufferers prior to MOH [22]. However, in our population in China, very few patients used triptans or ergot derivatives for treatment of migraine episodes [5, 11, 23]. This may be because that other types of analgesics were not only effective and cheaper than tripans. In this study, just one patient tried triptans, and triptans worked in this patient. The patient had consulted to stop triptans out of overuse. Although PM is considered a migraine subtype by the ICHD-3β, PM days are not counted as migraine days in the CM criteria. Thus some CrH with PM cannot be classified and had no specific diagnosis.

Headache experts proposed revised criteria (EO) in 2014 [10]. The new criteria (1) removed the criterion B that requires CM to occur in a patient with ≥ 5 prior migraine episodes; (2) added PM to C3 regarding treatment and relief of headache by a triptan or ergot agent, and (3) added a requirement that the headache does not meet criteria for NDPH or hemicrania continua. In our study, 70 (26.8 %) patients had atypical migraine episodes, fulfilled the PM [9]. Analyze the 70 PM patients according to the PM criteria, the most criteria not satisfied with was criterion D (associated symptoms), which were up to 70 % (49/70); and criterion B (typical headache duration) was not satisfied in 11.4 % (8/70); criterion C (typical headache features) in 18.6 % (13/70). Migraine attacks might resolve quickly if treated early in the course and before the full symptom complex develops. Additionally, a study in Turkish had reported that migraine characteristics, especially associated symptoms, were less prominent in the CM population, and the phenotype of CM may be associated with the course of classification [24]. So, allowing probable migraines to be a justification for the patient taking a "migraine day", also serves to include less developed attacks without relying on a migraine-specific treatment response [25].

Among 261 CM patients fulfilling EO criteria, female patients (191, 73.2 %) predominated. This was similar to previous results [5, 26]. The average of age of our patients was 49.5 years, consistent with earlier studies [5, 27]. Most of our patients reported a relatively low level of formal education, which was consistent with our previous study [5]. These patients with CM had an average duration of migraine attacks of 17.4 years, although this is shorter than in another recent study [28]. We note that 82.5 % of our patients took acute analgesics, and 67.6 % had MOH, which was similar to other studies [16, 29, 30]. Finally, the proportion of patients with a positive family headache history was similar to our previous study [5].

Our study was not designed to investigate therapeutic strategies or agents for the treatment of CM, but it did suggest that most patients with CM benefited from 3 to 6-months of treatment with medications for migraine prophylaxis.

Conclusion

This study was designed to field-test the new EO criteria for CM, beside the ICHD-3β criteria. Migraine-specific analgesics are rarely used in China, accounting for 0.4 % of the agents overused. Given that the ICHD-3β criteria utilize treatment with migraine-specific medication as one of the key data points, it makes this clinical tool less applicable in our clinical setting, and argues for use of the EO criteria. Our results indicate that CrH with PM should be classified into CM based on EO, which will allow more CM sufferers to receive correct diagnosis and adequate treatment. The EO criteria appear to increase the diagnostic sensitivity without lowering specificity, and should be adopted in CM management practice in our setting. Also in our setting, permitting patients with PM to avail themselves of "migraine days" is a reasonable accommodation for treatment of this difficult condition.

Limitation

This was a retrospective study and selection bias was inevitable. In addition, we treated these patients using medications for migraine prophylaxis. Therefore, further study is needed to establish the efficacy and safety of migraine-specific medications, including different agents, dosage forms, and routes of administration. Moreover, we did not evaluate the disability of these patients, and the factor should be taken into consideration when evaluating the impact of headache. And given that our data were based on patients referred to a specialty clinic for neurological disease, it necessarily will not represent profiles of migraine sufferers in the general population.

Clinical implication

This study was of major importance for neurologists because chronic migraine (CM) is a disabling disorder that is underdiagnosed and undertreated, and diagnostic criteria for CM remain controversial. In addition, this study analyzed the clinical profiles of CM and to field test the ICHD-3β and Expert Opinion criteria for CM. Migraine-specific analgesics are rarely used in China, permitting patients with probable migraine to avail themselves of "migraine days" is a reasonable accommodation for this difficult condition. The Expert Opinion criteria appear to increase the diagnostic sensitivity without lowering specificity, and should be adopted in CM management practice in our setting.

Abbreviations

CM: Chronic migraine; CrH: Chronic headache; EO: Expert opinion criteria; ICHD-2: Second Edition of the International Classification of Headache Disorders; ICHD-2R: Revised ICHD-2; ICHD-3β: International Classification of Headache Disorders, 3rd edition, beta version; MA: Migraine with aura; MOH: Medication overuse headache; PM: Probable migraine

Acknowledgments

Appreciation is extended to the members who helped to complete headache questionnaires at the neurology outpatient clinic of the First Affiliated Hospital of Chongqing Medical University in China. We also thank all participants.

Funding

This study was supported by the Natural Science Foundation Project of Chongqing Science and Technology Commission [NO. cstc2013jjB10009].

Authors' contribution

HJ, YZ, JZ conceived the idea for this study. Questionnaire survey data was completed by HJ,YD, YZ, JJ, XK, QZ, KW and interviewed face-to-face by JZ. Initial sample was analysed by HJ,YD. The paper was drafted by HJ. All authors reviewed and approved the final manuscript.

Competing interests

The authors declare that they have no competing interests.

Author details

[1]Department of Neurology, The First Affiliated Hospital of Chongqing Medical University, 1st You Yi Road, Yu Zhong District, Chongqing 400016, China. [2]Department of Neurology, The first people's Hospital of Jintang County, Sichuan, China.

References

1. Zwart JA, Dyb G, Hagen K, Svebak S, Holmen J (2003) Analgesic use: A predictor of chronic pain and medication overuse headache The Head–HUNT Study. Neurology 61(2):160–164
2. Sancisi E, Cevoli S, Vignatelli L, Nicodemo M, Pierangeli G, Zanigni S, Montagna P (2010) Increased prevalence of sleep disorders in chronic headache: a case-control study. Headache 50(9):1464–1472
3. Pascual J, Colás R, Castillo J (2001) Epidemiology of chronic daily headache. Curr Pain Headache Rep 5(6):529–536
4. Sanin LC, Mathew NT, Bellmeyer LR, Ali S (1994) The International Headache Society (IHS) headache classification as applied to a headache clinic population. Cephalalgia 14(6):443–446
5. Huang Q, Li W, Li N, Wang J, Tan G, Chen L, Zhou J (2013) Elevated blood pressure and analgesic overuse in chronic daily headache: an outpatient clinic-based study from China. J Headache Pain 14(1):1
6. Silberstein SD, Lipton RB, Sliwinski M (1996) Classification of daily and near-daily headaches field trial of revised IHS criteria. Neurology 47(4):871–875
7. Headache Classification Subcommittee of the International Headache Society (2004) The International Classification of Headache Disorders: 2nd edition. Cephalalgia 24 Suppl 1:9–160
8. Olesen J, Bousser MG, Diener HC, Dodick D, First M, Goadsby PJ, Nappi G (2006) New appendix criteria open for a broader concept of chronic migraine. Cephalalgia 26(6):742–746
9. Headache Classification Committee of the International Headache Society (IHS (2013) The international classification of headache disorders, (beta version). Cephalalgia 33(9):629–808
10. Silberstein SD, Lipton RB, Dodick DW (2014) Operational diagnostic criteria for chronic migraine: expert opinion. Headache 54(7):1258–1266
11. Wang Y, Zhou J, Fan X, Li X, Ran L, Tan G, Liu B (2011) Classification and clinical features of headache patients: an outpatient clinic study from China. J Headache Pain 12(5):561–567
12. Zeeberg P, Olesen J, Jensen R (2009) Medication overuse headache and chronic migraine in a specialized headache centre: field-testing proposed new appendix criteria. Cephalalgia 29(2):214–220
13. Schwedt (2014) Chronic migraine. BMJ 348:g1416
14. Li N, Wang J, Huang Q, Tan G, Chen L, Zhou J (2012) Clinical features of new daily persistent headache in a tertiary outpatient population. Headache 52(10):1546–1552
15. Silberstein SD, US Headache Consortium (2000) Practice parameter: Evidence-based guidelines for migraine headache (an evidence-based review) Report of the Quality Standards Subcommittee of the American Academy of Neurology. Neurology 55(6):754–762
16. Pascual J, El Berdei Y, Gómez-Sánchez JC (2007) How many migraine patients need prolonged (>1 year) preventive treatment? Experience with topiramate. J Headache Pain 8(2):90–93
17. Cevoli S, D'Amico D, Martelletti P, Valguarnera F, Del Bene E, De Simone R, Bussone G (2009) Underdiagnosis and undertreatment of migraine in Italy: a survey of patients attending for the first time 10 headache centres. Cephalalgia 29(12):1285–1293
18. Natoli JL, Manack A, Dean B, Butler Q, Turkel CC, Stovner L, Lipton RB (2010) Global prevalence of chronic migraine: a systematic review. Cephalalgia 30(5):599–609
19. Buse DC, Manack AN, Fanning KM, Serrano D, Reed ML, Turkel CC, Lipton RB (2012) Chronic migraine prevalence, disability, and sociodemographic factors: results from the American Migraine Prevalence and Prevention Study. Headache 52(10):1456–1470
20 Zhang Y, Kong Q, Chen J, Li L, Wang D, Zhou J (2016) International Classification of Headache Disorders 3rd edition beta-based field testing of vestibular migraine in China: Demographic, clinical characteristics, audiometric findings and diagnosis statues. Cephalalgia 36(3):240–248
21 Bigal ME, Rapoport AM, Sheftell FD, Tepper SJ, Lipton RB (2007) The International Classification of Headache Disorders revised criteria for chronic migraine—field testing in a headache specialty clinic. Cephalalgia 27(3):230–234
22 Shand B, Goicochea MT, Valenzuela R, Fadic R, Jensen R, Tassorelli C, Nappi G (2015) Clinical and demographical characteristics of patients with medication overuse headache in Argentina and Chile: analysis of the Latin American Section of COMOESTAS Project. J Headache Pain 16(1):1
23 Dong Z, Chen X, Steiner TJ, Hou L, Di H, He M, Yu S (2015) Medication-overuse headache in China: Clinical profile, and an evaluation of the ICHD-3 beta diagnostic criteria. Cephalalgia 35(8):644–651
24 Yalın OÖ, Uluduz D, Özge A, Sungur MA, Selekler M, Siva A (2016) Phenotypic features of chronic migraine. J Headache Pain 17(1):1
25 Lipton RB, Silberstein SD (2015) Episodic and chronic migraine headache: breaking down barriers to optimal treatment and prevention. Headache 55(S2):103–122
26 Ferrari A, Leone S, Vergoni AV, Bertolini A, Sances G, Coccia CPR, Sternieri E (2007) Similarities and differences between chronic migraine and episodic migraine. Headache 47(1):65–72
27 Katsarava Z, Schneeweiss S, Kurth T, Kroener U, Fritsche G, Eikermann A, Limmroth V (2004) Incidence and predictors for chronicity of headache in patients with episodic migraine. Neurology 62(5):788–790
28 Cho SJ, Song TJ, Chu MK (2016) Outcome of Chronic Daily Headache or Chronic Migraine. Curr Pain Headache Rep 20(1):1–10
29 Bigal ME, Serrano D, Buse D, Scher A, Stewart WF, Lipton RB (2008) Acute migraine medications and evolution from episodic to chronic migraine: a longitudinal population-based study. Headache 48(8):1157–1168
30 Negro A, Martelletti P (2011) Chronic migraine plus medication overuse headache: two entities or not? J Headache Pain 12(6):593–601

6

Insomnia in probable migraine: a population-based study

Jiyoung Kim[1], Soo-Jin Cho[2], Won-Joo Kim[3], Kwang Ik Yang[4], Chang-Ho Yun[5] and Min Kyung Chu[6*]

Abstract

Background: Insomnia is a common complaint among individuals with migraine. The close association between insomnia and migraine has been reported in clinic-based and population-based studies. Probable migraine (PM) is a migrainous headache which fulfills all but one criterion in the migraine diagnostic criteria. However, an association between insomnia and PM has rarely been reported. This study is to investigate the association between insomnia and PM in comparison with migraine using data from the Korean Headache-Sleep Study.

Methods: The Korean Headache-Sleep Study is a nation-wide cross-sectional survey for all Korean adults aged 19–69 years. The survey was performed via face-to-face interview using a questionnaire on sleep and headache. If an individual's Insomnia Severity Index score was ≥15.5, she/he was diagnosed as having insomnia.

Results: Of 2695 participants, the prevalence of migraine, PM and insomnia was 5.3, 14.1 and 3.6 %, respectively. The prevalence of insomnia among subjects with PM was not significantly different compared to those with migraine (8.2 % vs. 9.1 %, $p = 0.860$). However, insomnia prevalence in subjects with PM was significantly higher than in non-headache controls (8.2 % vs. 1.8 %, $p < 0.001$). Insomnia Severity Index score was significantly higher in subjects with migraine compared to those with PM (6.8 ± 5.8 vs. 5.5 ± 5.8, $p = 0.012$). Headache frequency and Headache Impact Test-6 score were significantly higher in subjects with migraine and PM with insomnia compared to those without insomnia. Multivariable linear analyses showed that anxiety, depression, headache frequency and headache intensity were independent variables for contributing the ISI score among subjects with PM.

Conclusions: The prevalence of insomnia among subjects with PM was not significantly different compared to those with migraine. Anxiety, depression, headache frequency and headache intensity were related with ISI score in subjects with PM.

Keywords: Insomnia, Headache, Migraine, Probable migraine, Epidemiology

Background

Insomnia and migraine are common complaints among the general population, affecting 10–30 % and 5–15 % of the general population, respectively [1–3]. Both individuals with insomnia and individuals with migraine experience a limitation of functions and a decrease in quality of life(QOL) due to their symptoms [4–6]. Recent studies have revealed that both conditions imposed a huge amount of personal and social burdens [4, 7].

* Correspondence: chumk@hallym.ac.kr
[6]Department of Neurology, Kangnam Sacred Heart Hospital, Hallym University College of Medicine, Seoul, Republic of Korea
Full list of author information is available at the end of the article

A close association between insomnia and migraine has been described in previous population-based studies [8–16]. In cross-sectional studies, individuals with migraine had an increased risk of having insomnia [odds ratio (OR) = 1.4–2.6] compared to non-migraineurs and individuals with insomnia had a higher risk of having migraine (OR = 1.5–1.7) compared to individuals without insomnia [8, 11–16]. Longitudinal studies also showed an increase risk [relative risk (RR) = 1.7] for having insomnia among individuals with migraine after 11 years [9]. The association was stronger for those with high frequency migraine. Conversely, individuals with insomnia showed an increased risk of having migraine at 11-year follow-up (RR = 1.7) [10].

Probable migraine (PM) is a migrainous headache fulfilling all but one of the criteria for migraine [17]. Probable migraine was reported to be a common subtype of migraine, with a 1-year prevalence rate ranging from 4.3 to 14.6 % according to the previous population-based studies [18–20]. PM is a common headache type for visiting doctors in neurology department [21]. Individuals with PM often experienced headache-related disability and decreased QOL like migraine [18, 19]. Therefore, PM is an important type of headache in clinical practice.

Although insomnia appears to be closely associated with migraine, the association between insomnia and PM has rarely been reported. The Korean Headache-Sleep Study (KHSS) was a population-based survey regarding headache type and sleep and provided an opportunity to evaluate the association between insomnia and PM. In the present study, we 1) described the prevalence of insomnia, migraine and PM across a general population-based sample; 2) compared the prevalence of insomnia between migraine and PM; and 3) assessed the impact of insomnia in clinical characteristics of migraine and PM using the data from KHSS.

Methods

Survey

We used data from the KHSS in the present study. The KHSS was a nationwide, cross-sectional survey regarding headache types, symptoms of anxiety and depression, and sleep status among the adult population aged 19–69 years. The study design and methods of KHSS have been previously described in detail [22]. Briefly, we used a 2-stage clustered random sampling method for all Korean territories except Jeju-do, proportional to the population distribution. All interviewers were employees of Gallup Korea and had previously experience with social survey interviewing. The survey was conducted by door-to-door visits and face-to-face interviews from November 2011 to January 2012. The study was approved by the institutional review board/ethics committee of Hallym University Sacred Heart Hospital and was performed in accordance with the ethical standards laid out in the 1964 Declaration of Helsinki and its subsequent amendments [23]. Informed consent was obtained from all participants before each interview.

Assessment of migraine and PM

Diagnoses of migraine and PM were based on criteria A to D for migraine without aura (code 1.1) in the second edition of the International Classification of Headache Disorders (ICHD-2) [A, at least five attacks; B, attack duration of 4–72 h; C, any 2 of the 4 typical headache characteristics (i.e., unilateral location, pulsating quality, moderate-to-severe pain intensity, and aggravation by or caused by routine physical activity); and D, attacks associated with at least one of the following: nausea, vomiting, or both photophobia and phonophobia] [17]. Subjects who met all of these criteria were considered to have migraine, whereas subjects who met all criteria except one were considered to have PM. Cases with headaches that met the criteria for both PM and tension-type headaches did not receive a PM diagnosis, as per ICHD-2. Because migraine and PM with aura (codes 1.2.1 and 1.6.2, respectively) are difficult to document using the questionnaire method, we did not evaluate aura [24]. Accordingly, these conditions were classified as migraine and PM in the present study.

Assessment of insomnia

We used the Insomnia Severity Index (ISI) to diagnose and classify insomnia among subjects. The ISI is a brief self-reported questionnaire that measures the patient's perception of insomnia severity [25]. The ISI is composed of 7 items that evaluate various aspects of insomnia symptoms. Each ISI item was rated on a scale of 0–4. The total ISI score were divided into 4 categories: 0–7, no clinically significant insomnia; 8–14, subthreshold insomnia; 15–21: moderate insomnia; and 22–28: severe insomnia. If a participant's ISI score was 15.5 or more, she/he was diagnosed as having insomnia. The Korean version of ISI was previously validated with good sensitivity and specificity and showed a 15.5 cut-off score for discriminating patients with insomnia [26].

Assessment of anxiety and depression

We used the Goldberg Anxiety Scale (GAS) to diagnose anxiety among subjects. This scale comprises four screening items and five supplementary items [27, 28]. Subjects who answered positively for two or more screening items and five or more of all scale items were classified as having anxiety. The Korean version of the scale has an 82.0 % sensitivity and 94.4 % specificity for diagnosing anxiety [28].

The Patient Health Questionnaire-9(PHQ-9) was used to diagnose depression [29]. Subjects who had scores of 10 or more on this measure were considered to have depression. The Korean version of PHQ-9 has an 81.1 % sensitivity and 89.9 % specificity [30].

Analyses

The Kolmogorov–Smirnov test was used to evaluate the normality of the distribution; after the normality was confirmed, we utilized Student's t-test and Chi-square test for comparison of prevalence rates where appropriate. If the normality of the distribution was not confirmed, we used Mann–Whitney *U* test. Multiple linear regression analysis with stepwise selection was used to evaluate contributing factors for ISI score among patients with

PM. A significance level of $p < 0.05$ was set for all analyses. Statistical analyses were performed with the Statistical Package for the Social Sciences 22.0 (SPSS 22.0; IBM, Armonk, NY, USA).

As with most survey sampling designs, there were missing data (resulting from non-response) for several variables. All of the reported results are based on the available data; as such, the total numbers of some variables diverge from 2695 because of missing data for that particular variable. Imputation techniques were not used because we wanted to minimize non-response effects [31].

Results

Survey

Interviewers approached 7430 individuals. Although three thousand one hundred and fourteen agreed to participate in the survey (rejection rate 58.1 %), 419 individuals withdrew from participation in the interview. Overall, 2695 subjects completed the survey (cooperation rate 36.3 %; Fig. 1). We found no significant differences in the distributions of age, gender, size of residential area, and educational level from those of the general population of Korea (Table 1).

Prevalence of migraine, PM and insomnia

Of the 2695 subjects, 143 (5.3 %) were classified as having migraine and 379 (14.1 %) were classified as having PM during the previous year. Among participants, 333 (12.4 %) had subthreshold insomnia, 83 (3.1 %) had moderate insomnia and 26 (1.0 %) had severe insomnia. Ninety six (3.6 %) reported ≥ 15.5 ISI score and were classified as having insomnia (Table 1).

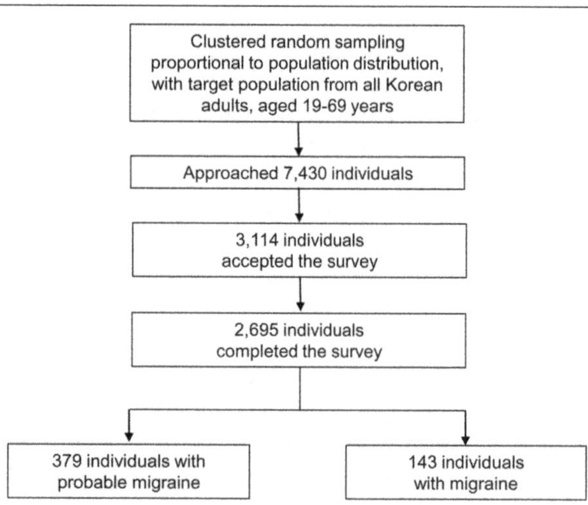

Fig. 1 Flow chart depicting the participation of subjects in the Korean Headache-Sleep Study

Prevalence and severity of insomnia among subjects with migraine and PM

Thirteen (9.1 %) subjects with migraine and 31 (8.2 %) subjects with PM were diagnosed as having insomnia. The prevalence of insomnia among subjects with PM was not significantly different compared to those with migraine ($p = 0.860$). Compared to non-headache controls (1.8 %), the prevalence of insomnia among subjects with migraine [OR = 5.6, 95 % confidence interval (CI) = 2.8–11.2, $p < 0.001$] and PM (OR = 5.0, 95 % CI = 2.9–8.5, $p < 0.001$) was significantly higher. Subjects with migraine had higher ISI score compared to subjects with PM (6.8 ± 5.8 vs. 5.5 ± 5.8, $p = 0.012$). The proportion of severe insomnia (2.8 % vs. 2.4 %, $p = 0.782$) and moderate insomnia (6.3 % vs. 7.1 %, $p = 0.739$) was not significantly different between migraine and PM. However, the proportion of subclinical insomnia was higher among subjects with migraine compared to those with PM (28.7 % vs. 16.4 %, $p = 0.002$) (Fig. 2).

Demographic and clinical characteristics of subjects with migraine and PM according to the presence of insomnia

Subjects with migraine and PM who had insomnia showed significantly higher GAS score and PHQ-9 score compared to those without insomnia. However, sociodemographic variables such as age, proportion of gender, size of residential and education level were not different according to the presence of insomnia (Table 2).

Headache characteristics of migraine and PM according to the presence of insomnia

The median and 25–75 % interquantile range values of the headache frequency, Visual Analog Scale (VAS) score for headache intensity and Headache Impact Test-6 (HIT-6) score were shown in Table 3. Subjects with migraine and PM who had insomnia showed significantly higher headache frequencies per month [migraine: 4.0, (2.0–11.0) vs. 1.0 (0.3–4.0), $p = 0.004$; PM: 2.0 (0.4–4.0) vs. 1.0 (0.3–2.0), $p = 0.004$] and HIT-6 scores [migraine: 65.0 (59.5–71.5) vs. 52.0 (47.0–60.0), $p < 0.001$; PM: 54.0 (48.0–62.0) vs. 45.5 (42.0–52.0), $p < 0.001$] compared to those without insomnia. Subjects with PM who had insomnia showed significantly higher VAS score for headache intensity [PM: 6.0 (5.0–7.0) vs. 5.0 (4.0–6.0), $p < 0.001$) compared to those without insomnia, but subjects with migraine who had insomnia [migraine: 7.0 (5.5–8.5) vs. 6.0 (5.0–7.0), $p = 0.076$] did not show significantly different VAS score compared to those without insomnia.

Multiple linear regression analyses for contributing factors for ISI score in subjects with PM

We performed the multiple linear regression analyses of clinical variables including sociodemographic variables

Table 1 Sociodemographic characteristics of survey participants; the total Korean population; and cases identified as having migraine, probable migraine, and insomnia

	Survey participants N (%)	Total population N (%)	*P-value*	Migraine N, % (95 % CI)	Probable migraine N, % (95 % CI)	Insomnia N, % (95 % CI)
Gender						
Men	1345 (49.3)	17,584,365 (50.6)	*0.854*[a]	36, 2.7 (1.8–3.5)	136, 10.1 (8.5–11.8)	33, 2.5 (1.6–3.3)
Women	1350 (50.7)	17,198,350 (49.4)		107, 7.9 (6.5–9.4)	243, 17.9 (15.8–19.9)	83, 4.7 (3.5–5.8)
Age						
19–29	542 (20.5)	7,717,947 (22.2)	*0.917*[a]	25, 4.5 (2.7–6.2)	69, 12.6 (9.8–15.4)	14, 2.6 (1.2–3.9)
30–39	604 (21.9)	8,349,487 (24.0)		42, 7.0 (4.9–9.1)	102, 16.8 (13.7–19.8)	19, 3.1 (1.7–4.5)
40–49	611 (23.1)	8,613,110 (24.8)		39, 6.5 (4.5–8.4)	102, 16.8 (13.9–19.8)	21, 3.4 (2.0–4.9)
50–59	529 (18.9)	6,167,505 (17.7)		22, 4.1 (2.4–5.9)	62, 11.6 (8.8–14.4)	23, 4.3 (2.6–6.1)
60–69	409 (15.6)	3,934,666 (11.3)		15, 3.9 (2.0–5.7)	44, 11.2 (8.1–14.2)	19, 4.6 (2.6–6.7)
Size of residential area						
Large city	1248 (46.3)	16,776,771 (48.2)	*0.921*[a]	76, 6.1 (4.8–7.5)	180, 14.4 (12.4–16.3)	47, 3.8 (2.7–4.8)
Medium-to-small city	1186 (44.0)	15,164,345 (43.6)		48, 4.0 (2.9–5.2)	174, 14.7 (12.7–16.7)	41, 3.8 (2.4–4.5)
Rural area	261 (9.7)	2,841,599 (8.2)		19, 7.4 (4.2–10.6)	25, 9.7 (6.1–13.3)	8, 3.1 (1.0–5.2)
Education level						
Middle school or less	393 (14.9)	6,608,716 (19.0)	*0.752*[a]	22, 5.5 (4.2–7.7)	44, 11.5 (8.4–14.7)	23, 5.9 (3.5–8.2)
High school	1208 (44.5)	15,234,829 (43.8)		60, 5.0 (3.8–6.3)	178, 14.7 (12.7–16.7)	40, 3.3 (2.3–4.3)
College or more	1068 (39.6)	12,939,170 (37.2)		60, 5.6 (4.3–7.0)	155, 14.4 (12.3–16.5)	32, 3.0 (2.0–4.0)
Not responded	26 (1.0)			1, 3.8 (0.0–11.8)	2, 7.7 (0.0–18.7)	1, 3.8 (0.0–11.8)
Total	2695 (100.0)	34,782,715 (100.0)		143, 5.3 (4.5–6.2)	379, 14.1 (12.7–15.4)	96, 3.6 (2.9–4.3)

CI Confidence Interval
[a]Comparison of gender, age group, size of residential area, and educational level distributions between the sample in the present study and the total population of Korea

(age, gender, size of residential area, educational level), GAS score, PHQ-9 score, headache frequency and VAS score to evaluate the contributing factors for ISI score (Table 4). The strongest contributing factor was PHQ-9 score ($\beta = 0.530$, $p < 0.001$), followed by GAS score ($\beta = 0.268$, $p < 0.001$), headache frequency ($\beta = 0.119$, $p < 0.001$) and VAS score ($\beta = 0.076$, $p = 0.026$) for headache intensity.

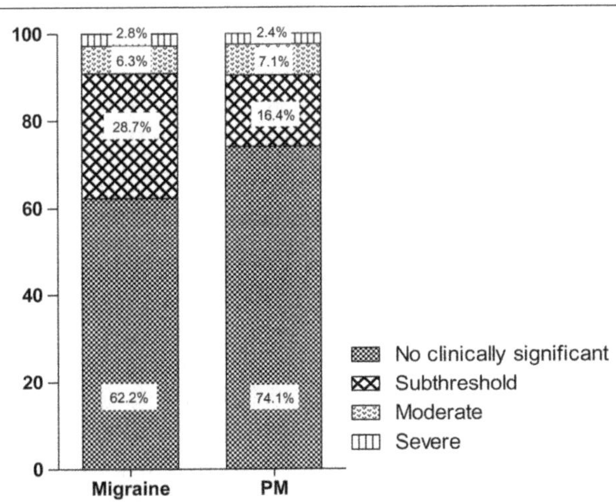

Fig. 2 Distribution of insomnia severity in subjects with migraine and probable migraine

Discussion

The main findings in the present study are as follows: 1) The prevalence of migraine, PM and insomnia in the Korea population was 5.3, 14.1 and 3.6 %, respectively; 2) The prevalence of insomnia among subjects with PM (8.2 %) was not significantly different compared to that among subjects with migraine (9.1 %); 3) Headache frequency and HIT-6 score of subjects were higher among migraine and PM subjects with insomnia compared to those without insomnia.

The 1-year prevalence of migraine (5.3 %) in the present study was lower than in previous studies from European (10–25 %) and North American (9–16 %) countries [1]. However, the 1-year prevalence of migraine in Asian countries was 4.7 to 9.1 %, which were lower compared to that in European and North American studies [32]. The migraine prevalence in our study was similar to previous studies in Asian countries.

The 1-year prevalence rate of PM was 14.1 % in the present study. Previous epidemiological studies have

Table 2 The difference of demographic and clinical variables in subjects with migraine and PM according to insomnia status

	Migraine			PM		
	Insomnia (+), $N = 13$	Insomnia (–), $N = 130$	*p*	Insomnia, $N = 31$	Insomnia, $N = 348$	*p*
Age, years	43.3 ± 16.3	41.0 ± 12.0	*0.653*[a]	45.0 ± 13.2	41.6 ± 12.5	*0.151*
Female, n (%)	10 (76.9 %)	97 (74.6 %)	*0.855*	21 (67.7 %)	222 (63.8 %)	*0.702*
Size of residential area			*0.857*			*0.382*
Large city, n (%)	7 (53.8 %)	69 (53.1 %)		14 (45.2 %)	166 (47.7 %)	
Medium-to-small city, n (%)	5 (38.5 %)	43 (33.1 %)		13 (41.9 %)	161 (46.3 %)	
Rural city, n (%)	1 (7.7 %)	18 (13.8 %)		4 (12.9 %)	21 (6.0 %)	
Education level			*0.081*			*0.886*
Middle school or less, n (%)	6 (46.2 %)	16 (12.3 %)		3 (9.7 %)	4 (11.8 %)	
High school, n (%)	3 (23.1 %)	57 (43.8 %)		16 (51.6 %)	162 (46.6 %)	
College or more, n (%)	4 (30.8)	56 (43.1 %)		12 (38.7 %)	143 (41.1 %)	
No answer, n (%)	0 (0.0 %)	1 (0.8 %)		0 (0.0 %)	2 (0.6 %)	
GAS score	6.4 ± 2.1	3.3 ± 2.3	*<0.001*[a]	6.6 ± 1.8	2.4 ± 2.1	*<0.001*
PHQ-9 score	12.3 ± 6.4	4.0 ± 4.2	*<0.001*[a]	12.3 ± 6.7	2.8 ± 3.1	*<0.001*

PM Probable migraine, *GAS* Goldberg Anxiety Scale, *PHQ-9* The Patient Health Questionnaire-9, *SD* Standard deviation
Values are expressed as mean ± SD, [a]Mann-Whitney *U* test

reported 1-year prevalence rates of PM ranging from 4.3 to 14.6 %. Thus, the prevalence rate of PM in the present study was similar to those in the previous studies [18, 20, 33–36].

The prevalence of insomnia (≥15.5 ISI score) in the present study was 3.6 %. Insomnia prevalence has been previously reported, ranging from 15.3 to 22.8 % in Asian countries including Korea [37–39]. These findings are inconsistent with the present study. This may reflect different insomnia diagnostic criteria. Most previous population-based studies about insomnia probed insomnia symptoms by asking whether subjects had difficult falling asleep, staying asleep and waking too early in the morning. A previous population-based study reported prevalence of insomnia symptoms at least three nights per week was 17.0 %, but insomnia disorder prevalence based on Diagnostic and Statistical Manual of Mental Disorders (DSM)-IV criteria was 5.0 % in this study [39].

Although the prevalence rate of insomnia was not significantly different between subjects with migraine and PM, the ISI score was significantly different between the two groups in the present study. The difference was associated with the higher prevalence of subthreshold insomnia (8 ≤ ISI score ≤ 14) among subjects with migraine compared to those with PM. The prevalence rate of insomnia in subjects with migraine and PM was higher compared to non-headache controls in the present study. The finding agrees with findings in previous studies concerning the association between headache and insomnia [3]. Cross-sectional studies showed that headache or migraine had increased ORs compared to non-headache controls and longitudinal studies showed bidirectional comorbidity of two conditions: subjects with insomnia showed an increased risk for headache at 11-year follow up and vice versa [10, 40].

A few studies have addressed the relationship between PM and insomnia among children. Children with adult-like migraine had a higher prevalence of sleep disorders compared to non-headache controls (disorders of initiating and maintaining sleep; migraine 37.1 % vs controls 9.2 %, disorders of arousals; migraine 59.3 % vs controls 10.2 %) [41]. Sleep disorders in infancy could be good predictors for the development of headache [42].

Table 3 Headache frequency, headache pain intensity (VAS score), and Headache Impact Test-6 score in subjects with migraine or PM according to insomnia status

	Migraine			PM		
	Insomnia (+), $N = 13$	Insomnia (–), $N = 130$	*p*	Insomnia (+), $N = 31$	Insomnia (–), $N = 348$	*p*
	Median (25–75 %)	Median (25–75 %)		Median (25–75 %)	Median (25–75 %)	
Headache frequency[a] (per 1 month)	4.0 (2.0–11.0)	1.0 (0.3–4.0)	*0.004*	2.0 (0.4–4.0)	1.0 (0.3–2.0)	*0.004*
VAS score for headache intensity[a]	7.0 (5.5–8.5)	6.0 (5.0–7.0)	*0.076*	6.0 (5.0–7.0)	5.0 (4.0–6.0)	*<0.001*
HIT-6 score[a]	65.0 (59.5–71.5)	52.0 (47.0–60.0)	*<0.001*	54.0 (48.0–62.0)	45.5 (42.0–52.0)	*<0.001*

PM Probable migraine, *VAS* Visual Analogue Scale, *HIT-6* Headache Impact Test-6
[a]Mann-Whitney *U* test

Table 4 Analysis of contributing factors related to the ISI score in subjects with PM

	Unstandardized coefficients		Standardized coefficients	t	P	Tolerance	VIF
	B	Standard error	Beta				
PHQ-9 score	0.695	0.054	0.530	12.876	<0.001	0.643	1.556
GAS score	0.654	0.103	0.268	6.316	<0.001	0.607	1.646
Headache frequency	0.124	0.035	0.119	3.537	<0.001	0.956	1.046
VAS score for headache intensity	0.249	0.111	0.076	2.240	0.026	0.940	1.063

ISI Insomnia severity index, *PM* Probable migraine, *GAS* Goldberg Anxiety Scale, *PHQ-9* The Patient Health Questionnaire-9, *VAS* Visual Analogue Scale
$R^2 = 0.592$, $R^2_{adj} = 0.588$

In the present study demonstrated that depression (PHQ-9 score), anxiety (GAD-7 score), headache frequency and headache intensity (VAS score) were independently associated with insomnia (ISI score) among individuals with PM (Table 4). This finding was similar to findings in the previous studies among migraineurs. A study including 78 migraineurs and 208 healthy controls revealed that sleep quality and headache frequency was significantly associated after adjusting anxiety and depression [43]. Another study demonstrated that migraineurs had more sleep problems than healthy controls even after adjusting lifetime anxiety and depression [44].

In the present study, headache frequency and HIT-6 score were higher in migraine and PM subjects with insomnia than in those without insomnia. Since a high headache frequency is one risk factor for chronification of headaches, our finding suggests that insomnia may be associated with the chronification of migraine and PM. We also noted that insomnia was associated with a higher HIT-6 score in subjects with migraine and PM. This finding may imply an increased burden of migraine and PM with the presence of insomnia [45]. Physicians should evaluate accompanying insomnia in subjects with migraine and PM. Careful investigation of the main causes of insomnia including psychiatric co-morbidity is also necessary.

This study has some limitations. First, although the questionnaire in this study was validated for migraine, it was not specifically validated for PM. However, the questionnaire itself was based on ICHD-2 and PM was classified based on the ICHD-2 diagnostic criteria. Second, although this study is population-based and had low sampling error, its statistical power was limited in terms of examining the subgroups. In other words, some results might not have reached statistical significance in subgroup analysis because of the limited sample size.

Despite these limitations, our study has several strengths. First, our study was based on clustered random sampling proportional to the Korean population distribution with low sampling error. This condition allowed us to accurately investigate the prevalence of insomnia, migraine, and PM among the Korean adult population. Second, this study explored the relation between PM and insomnia. This relation has been rarely studied. Third, we investigated both anxiety and depression, which are common comorbidities among subjects with insomnia and migraine, and assessed the effect of anxiety and depression in the association of insomnia with migraine and PM. Balancing the limitations and strengths, we believe that the present study accurately describes the association between insomnia and PM in comparison with migraine.

Conclusions

The prevalence rate of insomnia in individuals with PM is not significantly different compared to those with migraine. Insomnia aggravates headache symptoms among individuals with PM as well as among individuals with migraine.

Abbreviations

CI: Confidence interval; DSM-IV: Diagnostic and Statistical Manual of Mental Disorders-IV; HIT-6: Headache Impact Test-6; ICHD: International Classification of Headache Disorders; ISI: Insomnia severity index; KHSS: Korean Headache-Sleep Study; OR: Odds ratio; PHQ-9: Patient Health Questionnaire-9; PM: Probable migraine; QOL: Quality of life; GAS: Goldberg Anxiety Scale; RR: Relative risk; VAS: Visual Analogue Scale

Acknowledgements

The authors would like to thank Ms. Yejie Yun, Daewon Foreign Language High School, Seoul, Republic of Korea, for improving the use of English in the manuscript, and Gallup Korea for providing technical support for the Korean Headache-Sleep Study.

Funding

This Study was Supported by a 2011-Grant from Korean Academy of Medical Sciences.

Authors' contributions

JYK conceptualized and designed the study, analyzed the data, and wrote the manuscript. SJC conceptualized and collected the data. WJK conceptualized and collected the data. KIY conceptualized and collected the data. CHY conceptualized and collected the data. MKC conceptualized and designed the study, collected and analyzed the data, and wrote the manuscript. All authors read and approved the final manuscript.

Competing interests

The authors declare that they have no competing interests.

Author details
[1]Department of Neurology, Bio Medical Research Institute, Pusan National University Hospital, Pusan National University School of Medicine, Busan, Republic of Korea. [2]Department of Neurology, Dongtan Sacred Heart Hospital, Hallym University College of Medicine, Hwaseong, Republic of Korea. [3]Department of Neurology, Gangnam Severance Hospital, Yonsei University College of Medicine, Seoul, Republic of Korea. [4]Sleep Disorders Center, Department of Neurology, Cheonan Hospital, Soonchunhyang University College of Medicine, Cheonan, Republic of Korea. [5]Clinical Neuroscience Center, Department of Neurology, Seoul National University Bundang Hospital, Seongnam, Republic of Korea. [6]Department of Neurology, Kangnam Sacred Heart Hospital, Hallym University College of Medicine, Seoul, Republic of Korea.

References

1. Stovner L, Hagen K, Jensen R, Katsarava Z, Lipton R, Scher A, Steiner T, Zwart JA (2007) The global burden of headache: a documentation of headache prevalence and disability worldwide. Cephalalgia 27(3):193–210
2. Morin CM, LeBlanc M, Daley M, Gregoire JP, Merette C (2006) Epidemiology of insomnia: prevalence, self-help treatments, consultations, and determinants of help-seeking behaviors. Sleep Med 7(2):123–130
3. Uhlig BL, Engstrom M, Odegard SS, Hagen KK, Sand T (2014) Headache and insomnia in population-based epidemiological studies. Cephalalgia 34(10):745–751
4. Daley M, Morin CM, LeBlanc M, Gregoire JP, Savard J, Baillargeon L (2009) Insomnia and its relationship to health-care utilization, work absenteeism, productivity and accidents. Sleep Med 10(4):427–438
5. Bolge SC, Doan JF, Kannan H, Baran RW (2009) Association of insomnia with quality of life, work productivity, and activity impairment. Qual Life Res 18(4):415–422
6. Leonardi M, Steiner TJ, Scher AT, Lipton RB (2005) The global burden of migraine: measuring disability in headache disorders with WHO's Classification of Functioning, Disability and Health (ICF). J Headache Pain 6(6):429–440
7. Blumenfeld AM, Varon SF, Wilcox TK, Buse DC, Kawata AK, Manack A, Goadsby PJ, Lipton RB (2011) Disability, HRQoL and resource use among chronic and episodic migraineurs: results from the International Burden of Migraine Study (IBMS). Cephalalgia 31(3):301–315
8. Ødegård SS, Engstrøm M, Sand T, Stovner LJ, Zwart J-A, Hagen K (2010) Associations between sleep disturbance and primary headaches: the third Nord-Trøndelag Health Study. J Headache Pain 11(3):197–206
9. Ødegård SS, Sand T, Engstrøm M, Stovner LJ, Zwart JA, Hagen K (2011) The Long-Term Effect of Insomnia on Primary Headaches: A Prospective Population-Based Cohort Study (HUNT-2 and HUNT-3). Headache: J Head Face Pain 51(4):570–580
10. Ødegård SS, Sand T, Engstrøm M, Zwart J-A, Hagen K (2013) The impact of headache and chronic musculoskeletal complaints on the risk of insomnia: longitudinal data from the Nord-Trøndelag health study. J Headache Pain 14(1):1–10
11. Sutton DA, Moldofsky H, Badley EM (2001) Insomnia and health problems in Canadians. Sleep 24(6):665–670
12. Sivertsen B, Krokstad S, Overland S, Mykletun A (2009) The epidemiology of insomnia: associations with physical and mental health. The HUNT-2 study. J Psychosom Res 67(2):109–116
13. Lucchesi LM, Speciali JG, Santos-Silva R, Taddei JA, Tufik S, Bittencourt LR (2010) Nocturnal awakening with headache and its relationship with sleep disorders in a population-based sample of adult inhabitants of Sao Paulo City, Brazil. Cephalalgia 30(12):1477–1485
14. Budhiraja R, Roth T, Hudgel DW, Budhiraja P, Drake CL (2011) Prevalence and polysomnographic correlates of insomnia comorbid with medical disorders. Sleep 34(7):859–867
15. Huang GB, Yao LT, Hou JX, Zhang ZJ, Xin YT, Wu XY, Lu GY, Chen ZQ, Huang JP (2013) Epidemiology of migraine in the She ethnic minority group in Fujian province, China. Neurol Res 35(7):684–692
16. Lateef T, Swanson S, Cui L, Nelson K, Nakamura E, Merikangas K (2011) Headaches and sleep problems among adults in the United States: findings from the National Comorbidity Survey-Replication study. Cephalalgia 31(6):648–653
17. Headache Classification Subcommittee of the International Headache S (2004) The International Classification of Headache Disorders: 2nd edition. Cephalalgia 24(Suppl 1):9–160
18. Lanteri-Minet M, Valade D, Geraud G, Chautard MH, Lucas C (2005) Migraine and probable migraine–results of FRAMIG 3, a French nationwide survey carried out according to the 2004 IHS classification. Cephalalgia 25(12):1146–1158
19. Kim BK, Chung YK, Kim JM, Lee KS, Chu MK (2013) Prevalence, clinical characteristics and disability of migraine and probable migraine: a nationwide population-based survey in Korea. Cephalalgia 33(13):1106–1116
20. Silberstein S, Loder E, Diamond S, Reed ML, Bigal ME, Lipton RB, Group AA (2007) Probable migraine in the United States: results of the American Migraine Prevalence and Prevention (AMPP) study. Cephalalgia 27(3):220–229
21. Kim BK, Cho SJ, Kim BS, Sohn JH, Kim SK, Cha MJ, Song TJ, Kim JM, Park JW, Chu MK, Park KY, Moon HS (2016) Comprehensive Application of the International Classification of Headache Disorders Third Edition, Beta Version. J Korean Med Sci 31(1):106–113
22. Cho SJ, Chung YK, Kim JM, Chu MK (2015) Migraine and restless legs syndrome are associated in adults under age fifty but not in adults over fifty: a population-based study. J Headache Pain 16:554
23. World Medical A (2001) World Medical Association Declaration of Helsinki. Ethical principles for medical research involving human subjects. Bull World Health Organ 79(4):373–374
24. Stang PE, Osterhaus JT (1993) Impact of migraine in the United States: data from the National Health Interview Survey. Headache 33(1):29–35
25. Bastien CH, Vallieres A, Morin CM (2001) Validation of the Insomnia Severity Index as an outcome measure for insomnia research. Sleep Med 2(4):297–307
26. Cho YW, Song ML, Morin CM (2014) Validation of a Korean version of the insomnia severity index. J Clin Neurol 10(3):210–215
27. Goldberg D, Bridges K, Duncan-Jones P, Grayson D (1988) Detecting anxiety and depression in general medical settings. BMJ 297(6653):897–899
28. Lim JY, Lee SH, Cha YS, Park HS, Sunwoo S (2001) Reliability and validity of anxiety screening scale. J Korean Acad Fam Med 22(8):1224–1232
29. Pignone MP, Gaynes BN, Rushton JL, Burchell CM, Orleans CT, Mulrow CD, Lohr KN (2002) Screening for depression in adults: a summary of the evidence for the U.S. Preventive Services Task Force. Ann Intern Med 136(10):765–776
30. Choi HS, Choi JH, Park KH, Joo KJ, Ga H, Ko HJ, Kim SR (2007) Standardization of the Korean version of Patient Health Questionnaire-9 as a screening instrument for major depressive disorder. J Korean Acad Fam Med 28(2):114–119
31. Rubin DB, Little RJ (2002) Statistical analysis with missing data. J Wiley & Sons, Hoboken
32. Peng KP, Wang SJ (2014) Epidemiology of headache disorders in the Asia-pacific region. Headache 54(4):610–618
33. Rains JC, Penzien DB, Lipchik GL, Ramadan NM (2001) Diagnosis of migraine: empirical analysis of a large clinical sample of atypical migraine (IHS 1.7) patients and proposed revision of the IHS criteria. Cephalalgia 21(5):584–595
34. Bigal ME, Kolodner KB, Lafata JE, Leotta C, Lipton RB (2006) Patterns of medical diagnosis and treatment of migraine and probable migraine in a health plan. Cephalalgia 26(1):43–49
35. Patel NV, Bigal ME, Kolodner KB, Leotta C, Lafata JE, Lipton RB (2004) Prevalence and impact of migraine and probable migraine in a health plan. Neurology 63(8):1432–1438
36. Vukovic V, Plavec D, Pavelin S, Janculjak D, Ivankovic M, Demarin V (2010) Prevalence of migraine, probable migraine and tension-type headache in the Croatian population. Neuroepidemiology 35(1):59–65
37. Yeo BK, Perera IS, Kok LP, Tsoi WF (1996) Insomnia in the community. Singapore Med J 37(3):282–284
38. Kim K, Uchiyama M, Okawa M, Liu X, Ogihara R (2000) An epidemiological study of insomnia among the Japanese general population. Sleep 23(1):41–47
39. Ohayon MM, Hong SC (2002) Prevalence of insomnia and associated factors in South Korea. J Psychosom Res 53(1):593–600
40. Sivertsen B, Lallukka T, Salo P, Pallesen S, Hysing M, Krokstad S, Simon O (2014) Insomnia as a risk factor for ill health: results from the large population-based prospective HUNT Study in Norway. J Sleep Res 23(2):124–132
41. Esposito M, Roccella M, Parisi L, Gallai B, Carotenuto M (2013) Hypersomnia in children affected by migraine without aura: a questionnaire-based case-control study. Neuropsychiatr Dis Treat 9:289–294
42. Dosi C, Riccioni A, Della Corte M, Novelli L, Ferri R, Bruni O (2013) Comorbidities of sleep disorders in childhood and adolescence: focus on migraine. Nat Sci Sleep 5:77–85

43. Walters AB, Hamer JD, Smitherman TA (2014) Sleep disturbance and affective comorbidity among episodic migraineurs. Headache 54(1):116–124
44. Vgontzas A, Cui L, Merikangas KR (2008) Are sleep difficulties associated with migraine attributable to anxiety and depression? Headache 48(10):1451–1459
45. Sauro KM, Rose MS, Becker WJ, Christie SN, Giammarco R, Mackie GF, Eloff AG, Gawel MJ (2010) HIT-6 and MIDAS as measures of headache disability in a headache referral population. Headache 50(3):383–395

Nonspecific periaqueductal gray lesions on T2WI in episodic migraine

Zhiye Chen[1,2], Xiaoyan Chen[2], Mengqi Liu[1], Shuangfeng Liu[1], Lin Ma[1*] and Shengyuan Yu[2*]

Abstract

Background: The specific periaqueductal gray (PAG) lesions with migraine-like headache were easily identified on conventional MR images in clinical practice, and the aim of this study is to investigate the nonspecific periaqueductal gray (PAG) lesions in episodic migraine (EM) patients based on T2 weighted imaging (T2WI).

Methods: T2WI images were obtained from 18 EM patients and 18 normal controls (NC) on 3.0 T MR system. The images were observed by two experienced radiologists, and the lesions were identified on T2WI by consensus by 2 experienced neuroradiologists blinded to the patient identity. Chi-Square test was performed for the significance test.

Results: Ring-like hyperintensity lesions (HILs) around the PAG region were observed in 14 EM patients and in 5 NCs on T2WI. Four EM patients and 13 NCs were normal in PAG region. The significance was revealed by Chi-Square test ($P = 0.003$).

Conclusion: HIL of PAG may be the direct evidence of the EM genesis, and the further structural and functional study should be performed to elucidate the neuromechanism of migraine pathogenesis.

Keywords: Episodic migraine, Periaqueductal gray, Hyperintensity lesions, Magnetic resonance imaging

Background

Periaqueductal gray (PAG) was a center with powerful descending antinociceptive neuronal network, which include various layered neurons around the aquaeductus mesencephali [1, 2]. PAG dysfunction was recognized in migraine [3], and the PAG dysfunction may be associated with iron deposition and may be considered as a possible "generator" of migraine attacks [1, 4, 5].

The PAG lesions with migraine-like headache were mainly identified in multiple sclerosis [6–10] and infarction [11]. These lesions could be considered as specific lesions because of definite clinical diagnosis. Brain T2-visible hyperintensity lesions commonly presented in migraine patients [12, 13], and these T2 lesions may be seen in gray matter, and commonly located in white matter. However, T2-visible PAG lesions were not reported up to now. Compared with the previous reported specific lesions, the T2-visible lesions could be called as nonspecific lesions.

Above referred to specific PAG lesions could lead to migraine or migraine-like symptoms, herein, we hypothesize that non-specific PAG lesions on T2WI may present in the migraine and may be the direct evidence of migraine. To address this hypothesis, we prospectively obtained oblique axial T2WI data from 18 EM patients, and observed the signal and appearance of the T2-visible lesions on PAG region in EM patients, and the same observation was performed in NCs.

Methods

Subjects

Written informed consent was obtained from all participants according to the approval of the ethics committee of the local institutional review board. Eighteen EM patients were recruited from the International Headache Center, Department of Neurology, Chinese PLA General Hospital. All the following inclusion criteria should be fulfilled: 1) EM is defined as migraine attack days being less than 15 days per month. The definition of migraine refers to 1.1 Migraine without aura and 1.2 Migraine with aura in ICHD 3beta [14]; 2) no migraine preventive medication used in the past 3 months; 3) age between

* Correspondence: cjr.malin@vip.163.com; yusy1963@126.com
[1]Department of Radiology, Chinese PLA General Hospital, 28 Fuxing Road, Beijing 100853, China
[2]Department of Neurology, Chinese PLA General Hospital, 28 Fuxing Road, Beijing 100853, China

20 and 60 years; 4) right-handed; 5) absence of any chronic disorders, including hypertension, hypercholesterolemia, diabetes mellitus, cardiovascular diseases, cerebrovascular disorders, neoplastic diseases, infectious diseases, connective tissue diseases, other subtypes of headache, chronic pain other than headache, severe anxiety or depression preceding the onset of headache, psychiatric diseases, etc.; 6) absence of alcohol, nicotine, or other substance abuse; and 7) patient's willingness to engage in the study. Eighteen NCs were recruited from the hospital's staff and their relatives. Inclusion criteria were similar to those of patients, except for the first two items. NCs should never have had any primary headache disorders or other types of headache in the past year. General demographic and headache information were registered and evaluated in our headache database. Additionally, we evaluated anxiety, depression, and cognitive function of all the participants by using the Hamilton Anxiety Scale (HAMA) [15], the Hamilton Depression Scale (HAMD) [16], and the Montreal Cognitive Assessment (MoCA) Beijing Version (www.mocatest.org). The exclusion criteria were the following: cranium trauma, illness interfering with central nervous system function, psychotic disorder, and regular use of a psychoactive or hormone medication. The study protocol was approved by the Ethical Committee of Chinese PLA General Hospital and complied with the Declaration of Helsinki. Informed consent was obtained from all participants before the study. MRI scans were taken in the interictal stage at least three days after a migraine attack for EM patients. All the patients were given with the Visual Analogue Scale (VAS) and the Migraine Disability Assessment Scale (MIDAS). All the subjects were right-handed and underwent conventional MRI examination to exclude the subjects with cerebral infarction, malacia, or occupying lesions. Alcohol, nicotine, caffeine, and other substances were avoided for at least 12 h before MRI examination.

MRI acquisition

Images were acquired on a GE 3.0 T MR system (DISCOVERY MR750, GE Healthcare, Milwaukee, WI, USA) and a conventional eight-channel quadrature head coil was used. All subjects were instructed to lie in a supine position, and formed padding was used to limit head movement. Oblique axial T2-weighted imaging (T2WI)(TR = 5000 ms, TE = 113.4 ms, FOV = 24 cm × 24 cm, Matrix = 384 × 384, slice thickness = 6.0 mm, slice space = 1.0 mm) were obtained. Besides these, T1 fluid-attenuated inversion recovery (T1-FLAIR) and diffusion weighted imaging (DWI) were also acquired. The T1-FLAIR parameters included: TR/TE = 2040 ms/6.9 ms, FOV = 24 cm × 24 cm, Matrix = 384 × 256, slice thickness = 6.0 mm, slice space = 1.0 mm. DWI parameters included: TR/TE = 6000 ms/65.7 ms, FOV = 24 cm × 24 cm, matrix = 192 × 192, slice thickness = 6.0 mm, slice space = 1.0 mm) with b = 1000 s/mm2 applied in the x, y, and z directions and b = 0 s/mm2 without motion-probing gradients, followed by automatic generation of isotropic DWI. All the images had the same location, FOV, slice thickness and slice space.

MR image review

All the T2WI data were reviewed on the picture archiving and communication system (PACS) workstation. MR images were reviewed with the same film layout, magnification, and field of view, without the names of the subjects. The imaging findings were blindly reviewed in consensus by two experienced neuroradiologists without knowing the clinical information.

Definition of MR signs in PAG region on T2WI

Hyperintensity lesions (HIL) (Figs. 1 and 2) was defined as follows: (1) the lesion's signal was higher compared with normal brain tissue; (2) the lesion around the aquaeductus mesencephali; (3) the lesion with ring-like slight hyperintensity could be called as ring sign, and the lesion with irregular ring-like could be called as dot-ring sign with least three dots in the ring. (4) the lesion was not visible on T1WI and DWI; (5) no abnormal signal except PAG region. The exclusion criterion included: (1) acute infarction in the PAG region or peri-PAG region which would be visible on DWI; (2) mass lesion in the PAG region or peri-PAG region; (3) inflammatory demyelinating lesions in the PAG region or peri-PAG region; (4) multiple supratentorial abnormal signal on T2WI.

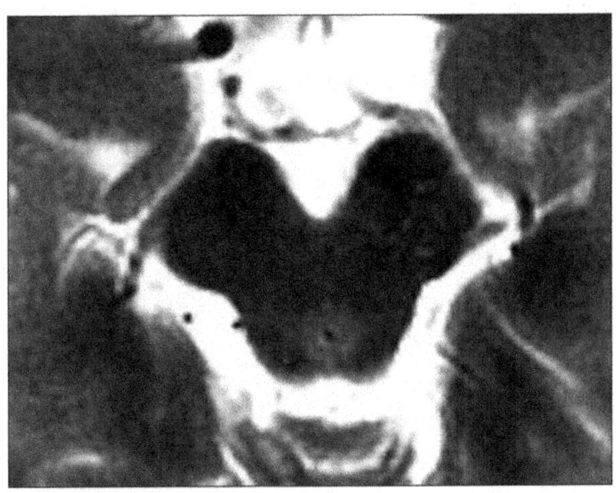

Fig. 1 Ring-like slight hyperintensity lesion (ring sign) around the aquaeductus mesencephali, and the flow void in the aquaeductus mesencephali could be seen

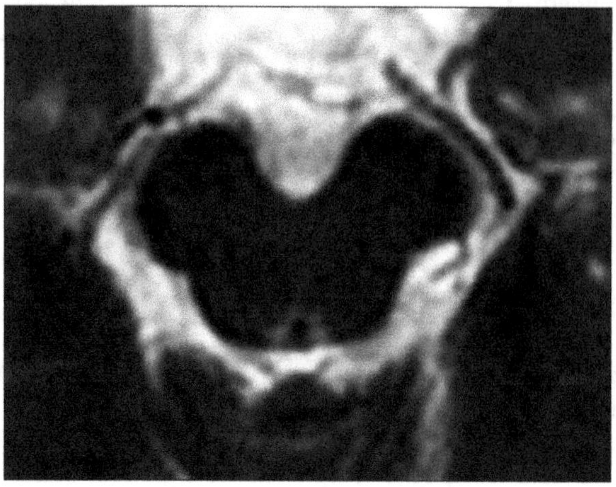

Fig. 2 Irregular ring-like hyperintensity (dot-ring sign) around the aquaeductus mesencephali

Statistical analysis

The statistical analysis was performed by using PASW Statistics 18.0. The significance differences of HIL between EM group and NC group were computed using Pearson Chi-Square test. The Spearman's correlation analysis was applied between migraine duration and positive PAG lesions on T2WI. Significant difference was set at a P value of < 0.05.

Results

Demography and neuropsychological test

Demographic and clinical data are summarized in Table 1. Eighteen EM patient (F/M = 14/4) and 18 age and sex-matched NCs (F/M = 14/4) were enrolled. There was no significant difference for age between EM (33.39 ± 10.69 years old) and NC (33.16 ± 10.77 years old). The scores of HAMA, HAMD and MoCA were 15.67 ± 9.85, 10.89 ± 7.26 and 29.17 ± 1.47, respectively. The disease duration was 12.44 ± 8.07 years, and the scores of VAS and MIDAS were 8.33 ± 1.50 and 16 ± 17.94, respectively.

Table 1 The clinical characteristics of EM patients and health cases (normal control, NC)

	EM	NC
Num (F/M)	18 (14/4)	18 (14/4)
Age*	33.39 ± 10.69	33.16 ± 10.77
HAMA*	15.67 ± 9.85	NA
HAMD*	10.89 ± 7.26	NA
MoCA*	29.17 ± 1.47	NA
DD (yrs)	12.44 ± 8.07	NA
VAS	8.33 ± 1.50	NA
MIDAS	16 ± 17.94	NA

NA Not available, *DD* disease duration
*There was no significant between EM and NC ($P > 0.05$)

Comparison of HIL between EM group and NC group

HIL was observed in 14 EM patients (14/18) and was observed in 5 NCs (5/18). The Chi-Square test demonstrated there was significant difference between EM and NC group ($P = 0.003$) (Table 2).

Correlation analysis between migraine duration and PAG lesion

Spearman's correlation analysis showed that there was no significant correlation between migraine duration and PAG lesion on T2WI ($P = 0.347$).

Discussion

Migraines are a common type of primary headaches with a reported prevalence of approximately 5.7 % in men and 17.0 % in women [17], and affect 12 % of the population worldwide [18]. In China, the prevalence of migraine is 9.3 % of the general population [19]. Migraines are also a major cause of chronic headaches, with approximately 2.5 % of EM transformed to new-onset chronic migraine [20]. Therefore, the neuromechanism of migraine has been the key focus of research [21].

The current MRI study about the role of PAG in migraine genesis mainly focused on the voxel-based morphometry [12], resting-state functional MRI [22, 23], diffusion kurtosis imaging [24], positron emission tomography [25], and ion deposition study [1]. Conventional MRI studies reported the specific T2 lesions in PAG region which lead to migraine or migraine-like symptoms, and non-specific T2 lesions in PAG region was still not revealed up to now. In this study, we prospectively observed the MR appearance of PAG on the T2WI. The findings were interesting, and the ring-like HILs were identified in most of the cases. Further statistical analysis demonstrated that there was significant difference between EM and NC group. Therefore, it was reasonable to assume that HIL might be the major feature of EM on conventional MR imaging.

A previous study [12] demonstrated that gray matter density in PAG was increased compared with normal controls, and these findings may be associated with the signal increased in T2WI, which reflect the hydrogen proton increasing. HILs of PAG region also indicated that axons in this region might undergo degeneration, which might be associated with migraine attack [12]. Besides, ion deposition load may aggravate the PAG burden, and then lead to the dysfunction of PAG [1].

Spearman's correlation analysis also demonstrated that there was no significant correlation between migraine

Table 2 Comparison of HIL of PAG between EM and NC

T2 lesion	EM	NC	Chi-Square Value	P value
Positive	14	5	9.028	0.003
Negative	4	13		

duration and PAG lesions, which was not consistent with the previous study [1]. In this study, positive correlation was found for duration of illness with R2' (transverse relaxation rates reflecting ion deposition extent) in the EM group. The R2' change may indicate PAG dysfunction, and it was not visible on T2WI. While HIL was visible on T2WI, and no correlation with migraine duration may suggest that nonspecific PAG lesion would be an intrinsic changes for EM. Besides, it may be associated with the small sample size.

In this study, HILs included ring sign and dot-ring sign, which may be have different pathophysiological mechanism. For the ring sign, it commonly was around the aqueductus mesencephali, and showed slight homogeneous hyperintensity. Based on the previous documents, it may be associated the ion deposition [1], frequent episodic activation [26], increased mean kurtosis and mean diffusivity value based on diffusion kurtosis imaging (DKI) [24] and altered functional connectivity [22], and this sign may be the direct imaging response for the intrinsic functional changes of PAG. While dot-ring sign always encircled the aqueductus mesencephali, and it may be associated with the ependyma [27], which would facilitates movement of iron, bound to ferritin, into brain and the neuron by the transferrin transporter [28–30]. Herein, the exact pathophysiology mechanism should further be investigated.

In the clinical practice, the specific lesions in PAG could easily be noticed while the non-specific lesion such as HILs commonly might be neglected. This study provided the direct imaging evidence for the change of PAG region in EM, and it was also easy to be identified on the T2WI, and could be applied with the routine MRI examination. The main limit of this study was that the sample of this study was relative small, and it would be necessary to increase the sample size in the future study.

Conclusion

In conclusion, HIL was a non-specific T2 lesion of PAG, and it might be the predominant MR hallmark and evidence for EM patients.

Abbreviations

EM: Episodic migraine; HIL: Hyperintensity lesion; NC: Normal controls; PAG: Periaqueductal gray; T2WI: T2 weighted imaging

Acknowledgements

This work was supported by the National Natural Sciences Foundation of China (81371514), Special Financial Grant from the China Postdoctoral Science Foundation (2014 T70960) and the Foundation for Medical and health Sci & Tech innovation Project of Sanya (2016YW37).

Authors' contributions

Category 1: (a) Conception and Design: LM; SYY. (b) Acquisition of Data: ZYC; MQL; SFL; XYC. (c) Analysis and Interpretation of Data: ZYC. Category 2: (a) Drafting the Article: ZYC. (b) Revising It for Intellectual Content: LM; SYY. All authors read and approved the final manuscript.

Competing interests

The authors declare that they have no competing interests.

References

1. Welch KM, Nagesh V, Aurora SK, Gelman N (2001) Periaqueductal gray matter dysfunction in migraine: cause or the burden of illness? Headache 41:629–637
2. Smith GST, Savery D, Marden C, López Costa JJ, Averill S, Priestley JV, Rattray M (1994) Distribution of messenger RNAs encoding enkephalin, substance P, somatostatin, galanin, vasoactive intestinal polypeptide, neuropeptide Y, and calcitonin gene-related peptide in the midbrain periaqueductal grey in the rat. J Comp Neurol 350:23–40.
3. Raskin NH, Yoshio H, Sharon L (1987) Headache may arise from perturbation of brain. Headache J Head Face Pain 27:416–420
4. Kruit MC, Launer LJ, Overbosch J, van Buchem MA, Ferrari MD (2009) Iron accumulation in deep brain nuclei in migraine: a population-based magnetic resonance imaging study. Cephalalgia 29:351–359
5. Tepper SJ, Lowe MJ, Beall E, Phillips MD, Liu K, Stillman MJ, Horvat M, Jones SE (2012) Iron deposition in pain-regulatory nuclei in episodic migraine and chronic daily headache by MRI. Headache 52:236–243
6. Gee JR, Chang J, Dublin AB, Vijayan N (2005) The association of brainstem lesions with migraine-like headache: an imaging study of multiple sclerosis. Headache 45:670–677
7. Haas DC, Kent PF, Friedman DI (1993) Headache caused by a single lesion of multiple sclerosis in the periaqueductal gray area. Headache 33:452–455
8. Lin GY, Wang CW, Chiang TT, Peng GS, Yang FC (2013) Multiple sclerosis presenting initially with a worsening of migraine symptoms. J Headache Pain 14:70
9. Tortorella P, Rocca MA, Colombo B, Annovazzi P, Comi G, Filippi M (2006) Assessment of MRI abnormalities of the brainstem from patients with migraine and multiple sclerosis. J Neurol Sci 244:137–141
10. Fragoso YD, Brooks JB (2007) Two cases of lesions in brainstem in multiple sclerosis and refractory migraine. Headache 47:852–854
11. Wang Y, Wang XS (2013) Migraine-like headache from an infarction in the periaqueductal gray area of the midbrain. Pain Med 14:948–949
12. Rocca MA, Ceccarelli A, Falini A, Colombo B, Tortorella P, Bernasconi L, Comi G, Scotti G, Filippi M (2006) Brain gray matter changes in migraine patients with T2-visible lesions: a 3-T MRI study. Stroke 37:1765–1770
13. Fazekas F, Koch M, Schmidt R, Offenbacher H, Payer F, Freidl W, Lechner H (1992) The prevalence of cerebral damage varies with migraine type: a MRI study. Headache 32:287–291
14. Headache Classification Committee of the International Headache Society (IHS) (2013) The International Classification of Headache Disorders, 3rd edition (beta version). Cephalalgia 33:629–808.
15. Maier W, Buller R, Philipp M, Heuser I (1988) The Hamilton Anxiety Scale: reliability, validity and sensitivity to change in anxiety and depressive disorders. J Affect Disord 14:61–68
16. Hamilton M (1967) Development of a rating scale for primary depressive illness. Br J Soc Clin Psychol 6:278–296
17. Scher AI, Gudmundsson LS, Sigurdsson S, Ghambaryan A, Aspelund T, Eiriksdottir G, van Buchem MA, Gudnason V, Launer LJ (2009) Migraine headache in middle age and late-life brain infarcts. JAMA 301:2563–2570
18. Gomez-Beldarrain M, Oroz I, Zapirain BG, Ruanova BF, Fernandez YG, Cabrera A, Anton-Ladislao A, Aguirre-Larracoechea U, Garcia-Monco JC (2015) Right fronto-insular white matter tracts link cognitive reserve and pain in migraine patients. J Headache Pain 17:4
19. Yu S, Liu R, Zhao G, Yang X, Qiao X, Feng J, Fang Y, Cao X, He M, Steiner T (2012) The prevalence and burden of primary headaches in China: a population-based door-to-door survey. Headache 52:582–591
20. Lipton RB (2009) Tracing transformation: chronic migraine classification, progression, and epidemiology. Neurology 72:S3–S7
21. Chen Z, Chen X, Liu M, Liu S, Shu S, Ma L, Yu S (2016) Altered functional connectivity of the marginal division in migraine: a resting-state fMRI study. J Headache Pain 17:89
22. Schwedt TJ, Larson-Prior L, Coalson RS, Nolan T, Mar S, Ances BM, Benzinger T, Schlaggar BL (2014) Allodynia and descending pain modulation in migraine: a resting state functional connectivity analysis. Pain Med 15:154–165
23. Schwedt TJ, Schlaggar BL, Mar S, Nolan T, Coalson RS, Nardos B, Benzinger T, Larson-Prior LJ (2013) Atypical resting-state functional connectivity of affective pain regions in chronic migraine. Headache 53:737–751

24. Ito K, Kudo M, Sasaki M, Saito A, Yamashita F, Harada T, Yokosawa S, Uwano I, Kameda H, Terayama Y (2016) Detection of changes in the periaqueductal gray matter of patients with episodic migraine using quantitative diffusion kurtosis imaging: preliminary findings. Neuroradiology 58:115–120
25. Maniyar FH, Sprenger T, Schankin C, Goadsby PJ (2014) The origin of nausea in migraine-a PET study. J Headache Pain 15:84
26. Welch KM, Cao Y, Aurora S, Wiggins G, Vikingstad EM (1998) MRI of the occipital cortex, red nucleus, and substantia nigra during visual aura of migraine. Neurology 51:1465–1469
27. Lisanti CJ, Asbach P, Bradley WG Jr (2005) The ependymal "Dot-Dash" sign: an MR imaging finding of early multiple sclerosis. AJNR Am J Neuroradiol 26:2033–2036
28. Benkovic SA, Connor JR (1993) Ferritin, transferrin, and iron in selected regions of the adult and aged rat brain. J Comp Neurol 338:97–113
29. Morris CM, Candy JM, Bloxham CA, Edwardson JA (1992) Distribution of transferrin receptors in relation to cytochrome oxidase activity in the human spinal cord, lower brainstem and cerebellum. J Neurol Sci 111:158–172
30. Morris CM, Candy JM, Omar S, Bloxham CA, Edwardson JA (1994) Transferrin receptors in the parkinsonian midbrain. Neuropathol Appl Neurobiol 20: 468–472

8

Resting-state EEG power and coherence vary between migraine phases

Zehong Cao[1,2,3], Chin-Teng Lin[1,3*], Chun-Hsiang Chuang[1,3], Kuan-Lin Lai[4,6], Albert C. Yang[5,6,7], Jong-Ling Fuh[4,6] and Shuu-Jiun Wang[4,6,8*]

Abstract

Background: Migraine is characterized by a series of phases (inter-ictal, pre-ictal, ictal, and post-ictal). It is of great interest whether resting-state electroencephalography (EEG) is differentiable between these phases.

Methods: We compared resting-state EEG energy intensity and effective connectivity in different migraine phases using EEG power and coherence analyses in patients with migraine without aura as compared with healthy controls (HCs). EEG power and isolated effective coherence of delta (1–3.5 Hz), theta (4–7.5 Hz), alpha (8–12.5 Hz), and beta (13–30 Hz) bands were calculated in the frontal, central, temporal, parietal, and occipital regions.

Results: Fifty patients with episodic migraine (1–5 headache days/month) and 20 HCs completed the study. Patients were classified into inter-ictal, pre-ictal, ictal, and post-ictal phases ($n = 22, 12, 8, 8$, respectively), using 36-h criteria. Compared to HCs, inter-ictal and ictal patients, but not pre- or post-ictal patients, had lower EEG power and coherence, except for a higher effective connectivity in fronto-occipital network in inter-ictal patients ($p < .05$). Compared to data obtained from the inter-ictal group, EEG power and coherence were increased in the pre-ictal group, with the exception of a lower effective connectivity in fronto-occipital network ($p < .05$). Inter-ictal and ictal patients had decreased EEG power and coherence relative to HCs, which were "normalized" in the pre-ictal or post-ictal groups.

Conclusion: Resting-state EEG power density and effective connectivity differ between migraine phases and provide an insight into the complex neurophysiology of migraine.

Keywords: Migraine without aura, Resting-state, EEG, Power, Isolated effective coherence

Background

Migraine is a common and potentially disabling neurological disorder that affects about 11 % of people worldwide [1], including 9.1 % in Taiwan [2]. A minority of migraine patients (13–31 %) experience aura symptoms prior to headache onset [3, 4]. Although some patients with migraine without aura exhibit other prodromal symptoms [3], their migraine attacks are generally unpredictable [5]. Taking abortive medications during the early stages of a migraine attack increases medication efficacy and reduces recurrence [6]. Therefore, pre-emptive detection of migraine attacks may be clinically beneficial, especially for patients with migraine without aura.

* Correspondence: Chin-Teng.Lin@uts.edu.au; sjwang@vghtpe.gov.tw
[1]Faculty of Engineering and Information Technology, University of Technology Sydney, Sydney, Australia
[4]Neurological Institute, Taipei Veterans General Hospital, Taipei, Taiwan
Full list of author information is available at the end of the article

Although the underlying pathophysiology of migraine is still unclear, prior neurophysiological studies have shown abnormal cortical evoked potentials [7, 8] in different stimulus models of migraine, such as lacking habituation of visual and auditory cortex excitability [9] and reduced motor and visual cortical thresholds [10]. Specifically, compared to controls, migraine patients show increased phase synchronization after stimulation during the migraine-free inter-ictal phase (between post- and pre-ictal phases) [11, 12]. Furthermore, in the pre-ictal phase (before migraine attacks), migraine patients exhibit normal habituation of visually-evoked and auditory-evoked potentials [13], but decreased motor cortex activity [14]. However, resting-state cortical activities, such as EEG power density and effective connectivity, have not been studied much in relation to particular migraine phases [15, 16].

There has been growing interest in resting-state functional and effective connectivity in recent years [17]. Compared to stimulation-related tasks, resting-state experiments, in which additional cortical activations are not induced, are more convenient and comfortable for migraine patients. Previous resting-state studies have shown dynamic EEG power changes in migraine patients [15, 16, 18]. EEG coherence, which involves cross-correlation between signals in the frequency domain to reveal interrelationships of EEG signals, is a widely used measure of functional connectivity [19]. High-level coherence between two EEG signals reflects synchronized neuronal oscillations, whereas low-level coherence suggests desynchronized neural activity. Although EEG coherence analysis has been applied to study migraine-related neural abnormalities in stimulation tasks [11, 12], resting-state EEG coherence in different phases of migraine has not yet been examined. The notion of EEG-detected connectivity is supported by resting-state functional MRI studies showing significant network changes in migraine [20, 21]. Additionally, classical coherence analysis has disadvantages such as volume conduction and influences from common sources or indirect connections [17]. These are typical problems when bivariate approaches are used instead of multivariate approaches. To solve these inherent problems, new connectivity measurement, such as isolated effective coherence (iCoh) [22], has been proposed to render more accurate interactions among the cerebral regions. This study aimed to investigate dynamic changes in resting-state EEG power intensity and brain connectivity networks across different phases of migraine (inter-ictal, pre-ictal, ictal, and post-ictal). In particular, we focused on a subgroup of migraine patients with low frequency because prediction of migraine attacks in this group could have substantial clinical utilities.

Methods

Subjects

Patients with migraine without aura, who were diagnosed by board-certified neurologists at the Headache Clinic, Taipei Veterans General Hospital (VGH) as having low-frequency migraine (1–5 days per month) were invited to join this study. Diagnoses of migraine without aura were based on the ICHD-2 criteria [23]. Age-matched HCs were enrolled from hospital colleagues, their relatives, or friends who did not have past or family histories of migraine, nor any headache attack during the past year.

Each patient kept a headache diary and completed a structured questionnaire on demographics, headache profile, medical history, and medication use. The headache profiles included the duration of migraine history (years), the severity of migraine, headache frequency (days per month), and Migraine Disability Assessment (MIDAS). In addition, the Beck Depression Inventory (BDI) and Hospital Anxiety Depression Scale (HADS) were administered to screen for psychological disturbances. On EEG study days, patients' migraine phases were designated as inter-ictal, pre-ictal, ictal, or post-ictal based on the patients' headache diaries (Fig. 1a). Ictal phase was coded when patients had suffered a migraine attack on the day of EEG study. Pre-ictal and post-ictal phases were coded when patients were within

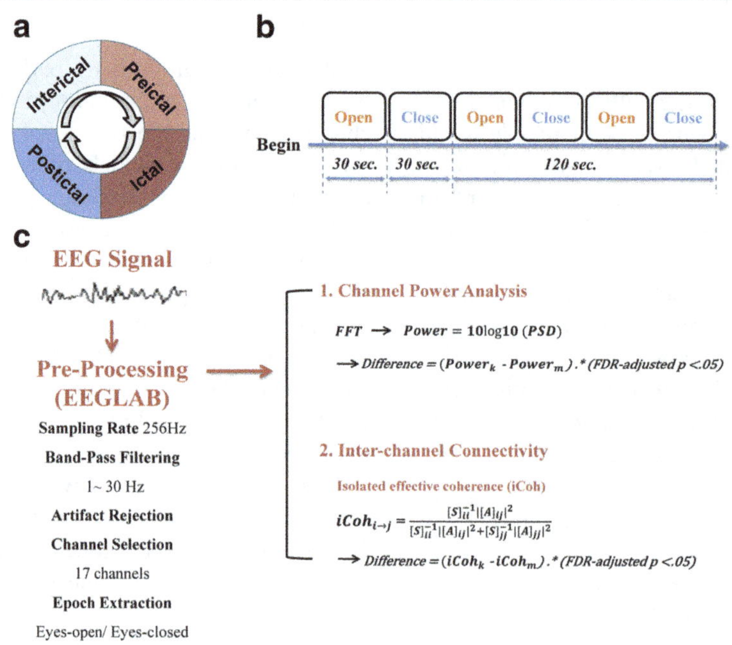

Fig. 1 Analytical procedures. **a**: Migraine cycle; **b**: Resting-state EEG recording; **c**: EEG signal processing

36 h before or after an ictal phase on the day of EEG study, respectively. Inter-ictal phase was coded for patients in a pain-free period between pre-ictal and post-ictal phases.

Subjects were excluded if they had systemic diseases, connective tissue disorders, neurological or psychiatric disorders, as well as other painful conditions according to their self-report. All subjects had normal vision after correction. To prevent the mis-classification of migraine phases or the distracted effect on EEG, patients were requested not to take analgesics within 2 days before EEG recording, nor take any psychotropic drugs within 4 weeks before the EEG study. None of our patients were on any migraine preventive agents.

This study was approved by the Institutional Review Board at Taipei VGH (approved ID: 2011-06-009IC). Informed consent was obtained from all subjects before they joined the study.

Experimental design

Experiments were performed in a quiet, dimly light room in our hospital. During the first 2 min of the experiment, subjects were instructed to take several deep breaths while they adapted to the environment. Next, subjects were instructed to open their eyes for 30 s and close their eyes for 30 s and to repeat this sequence for a total of three times (Fig. 1b). Meanwhile, EEG signals were recorded using Nicolet EEG system (Natus Medical, Incorporated, San Carlos, CA, USA) with Ag/AgCl electrodes. Eighteen EEG electrodes (Fp1, Fp2, F7, F3, Fz, F4, F8, T3, C3, Cz, C4, T4, T5, P3, P4, T6, O1, and O2) were placed according to the conventional 10–20 EEG system [24] and the guideline of American Clinical Neurophysiology Society [25]. Fz was used as the reference channel. The skin under the reference electrodes were abraded and disinfected with a 70 % isopropyl alcohol swab before calibration. The impedance of the electrodes was calibrated under 5 kΩ. The EEG signals were amplified and digitized at a sampling rate of 256 Hz with 16-bit quantization.

EEG data analysis

The EEG data were analyzed with EEGLAB, an open-source MATLAB toolbox for electrophysiological signal processing and analysis [26]. The analytical procedures for EEG signal processing included a band-pass filter, artifact rejection, epoch extraction, time-frequency analysis, and coherence estimation (Fig. 1c). During signal preprocessing, raw EEG signals were subjected to 1-Hz high-pass and 30-Hz low-pass finite impulse response (FIR) filters. For the artifact rejection, firstly, apparent eye contaminations in EEG signals were manually removed by visual inspection. Secondly, Independent Component Analysis (ICA) was applied to the EEG signals and the components responsible for the eye movements and blinks were rejected. Then, the EEG signals without these artifact components was reconstructed using the back-projection method [26]. Finally, the reconstructed EEG signals were inspected again using the "Automatic Channel Rejection (ACR)" function with Kurtosis measurement and Z-score threshold of 5 to remove noisy channels. Eyes-open and eyes-closed resting-state signals of three blocks were extracted and concatenated for further analyses.

EEG power analysis

Processed time-series data were transformed into the frequency domain by a 256-point fast Fourier transform with Welch's method. Specifically, 90-s spans of data were analyzed with a 256-point moving window with a 128-point overlap. Windowed data were extended to 512 points by zero-padding to calculate power spectra, yielding an estimation of the power spectra with 60 frequency bins from 1 to 30 Hz (frequency resolution: 0.5 Hz). Power spectra of these windows were averaged and converted to a logarithmic scale. Mean delta (δ: 1–3.5 Hz), theta (θ: 4–7.5 Hz), alpha (α: 8–12.5 Hz), and beta (β: 13–30 Hz) band powers of 17 channels were visualized on a two-dimensional (2-D) topographic map.

EEG coherence analysis

For all groups (inter-ictal, pre-ictal, ictal, post-ictal, and HCs), we explored the coupling between brain areas within particular frequency bands based on the up-to-date coherence algorithm, named isolated effective coherence (iCoh) [22], which is a multivariate approach to address the effective connectivity. Its advantages not only are insensitive to volume conduction but also can detect direct pathways linking brain regions. Firstly, the Source Information Flow Toolbox (SIFT) [27] in the EEGLAB was used to identify the optimal multivariate autoregressive model. Then, the magnitude of iCoh for channel $j \rightarrow$ channel i at the frequency of w is estimated from the following formula [22].

$$iCoh_{j\rightarrow i}(w) = \frac{[S_\varepsilon]_{ii}^{-1}\left|\left[\hat{A}(w)\right]_{ij}\right|^2}{[S_\varepsilon]_{ii}^{-1}\left|\left[\hat{A}(w)\right]_{ij}\right|^2 + [S_\varepsilon]_{jj}^{-1}\left|\left[\hat{A}(w)\right]_{jj}\right|^2},$$

where $0 \le \boldsymbol{iCoh}_{j\rightarrow i}(w) \le 1$, the autoregressive coefficients $[\mathbf{A}(w)]_{kl} \equiv 0$, for all (k, l) such that $(k, l) \neq (i, j)$ and $k \neq l$ and the spectral density matrix $[\boldsymbol{S}_\varepsilon]_{kl} \equiv 0$, for all (k, l) such that $k \neq l$.

Statistical analysis

Group differences in clinical profiles were analyzed by Student's t-test (migraine patients vs. HCs) or one-way ANOVA (four phases of migraine patients) for continuous variables and chi-square or Fisher's exact tests for categorical variables. Resting-state EEG band power and coherence values were compared across all five groups (HC and 4 migraine phase groups) by the Wilcoxon rank-sum test, followed by calculation of the false discovery rate (FDR) for multiple comparisons. The significance level was set to 0.05. Statistical analysis was performed in the SPSS software package (version 15.0) and MATLAB (2011a) Bioinformatics Toolbox.

Results

Demographic and clinical characteristics

A total of 61 patients with migraine without aura joined the study, of whom, 11 were excluded because of taking analgesic medications within 2 days before the EEG study, yielding a final sample of 50 patients for analysis. These 50 patients were classified into inter-ictal (n = 22), pre-ictal (n = 12), ictal (n = 8), and post-ictal (n = 8) phases. In addition, 20 HCs were also recruited. Demographic and clinical characteristics were similar between the migraine group and HC group and also similar across the four migraine phase groups (Table 1).

Comparisons of resting-state EEG power between migraine patients and HCs

Dynamic changes in EEG power/coherence between migraine patients and HCs or between migraine phases were more robust in the eyes-open (Figs. 2, 3, 4 and 5) than in the eyes-closed condition (Additional file 1: Figures S1, S2, S3 and S4). Therefore, we used EEG data from the eyes-open condition in subsequent analyses.

Significant differences in resting-state EEG power in the eyes-open condition in migraine patients from each phase versus HCs for the delta, theta alpha, and beta domains are shown in Fig. 2. Inter-ictal patients had significantly lower delta, theta, alpha and beta EEG power in the fronto-central (F4, C3, Cz, C4) and parietal (P3, P4) regions, compared to HCs (FDR-adjusted p < .05, Fig. 2a). EEG power values did not differ between pre-ictal patients and HCs in any of the four EEG frequency domains (Fig. 2b). Ictal patients had lower delta, theta, alpha and beta (fronto-central and parietal regions) power than HCs (FDR-adjusted p < .05, Fig. 2c). EEG power variability in post-ictal patients was similar to that in HCs (Fig. 2d).

Comparisons of resting-state EEG power across migraine phases

Significant differences in resting-state EEG power between the four migraine-phase groups are shown in Fig. 3. EEG power intensity of pre-ictal patients in the fronto-central and parietal regions of delta theta, alpha and beta bands were higher than the corresponding values in inter-ictal patients (FDR-adjusted p < .05, Fig. 3a). Compared to pre-ictal patients, ictal patients had lower fronto-central and parieto-occipital delta, theta, alpha, and beta EEG power (FDR-adjusted p < .05, Fig. 3b). Centro-parietal delta, theta, alpha, and beta EEG power intensity were higher in post-ictal patients than in ictal patients (FDR-adjusted p < .05, Fig. 3c). Right centro-parietal delta, theta, alpha, and beta EEG power intensity were lower in inter-ictal patients than in post-ictal patients (FDR-adjusted p < .05, Fig. 3d).

Table 1 Comparisons of demographics, headache profiles, and psychological characteristics between study groups

Characteristic	Migraine patients (*N* = 50)	HCs (*N* = 20)	*P*	Migraine phase groups				*P*
				Inter-ictal (*N* = 22)	Pre-ictal (*N* = 12)	Ictal (*N* = 8)	Post-ictal (*N* = 8)	
Sex, F:M	35:15	11:9	0.24	16:6	6:6	7:1	6:2	0.49
Age, y	36.0 ± 9.9	36.9 ± 6.7	0.63	33.0 ± 9.0	39.0 ± 7.5	40.0 ± 11.5	38.0 ± 12.4	0.27
Migraine headache profile								
Disease duration, y	16.0 ± 9.3	N/A	N/A	15.0 ± 8.1	16.0 ± 7.8	20.0 ± 9.6	16.0 ± 13.8	0.72
Frequency, d/month.	3.8 ± 1.3	N/A	N/A	3.8 ± 1.4	3.8 ± 1.3	3.6 ± 1.3	3.9 ± 1.0	0.81
Pain severity[a]	7.0 ± 1.9	N/A	N/A	8.0 ± 2.1	7.0 ± 1.8	8.0 ± 1.9	6.0 ± 1.7	0.42
MIDAS score[b]	16.3 ± 13.4	N/A	N/A	19.1 ± 16.6	17.8 ± 10.7	11.0 ± 11.8	15.7 ± 13.5	0.59
Psychometric scores								
BDI	8.7 ± 5.7	N/A	N/A	9.4 ± 6.1	7.7 ± 5.6	9.9 ± 5.3	7.9 ± 5.8	0.68
HADS-A	6.7 ± 3.7	N/A	N/A	7.6 ± 3.2	5.5 ± 3.4	6.6 ± 3.0	7.8 ± 5.7	0.41
HADS-D	4.6 ± 3.3	N/A	N/A	4.8 ± 3.4	3.6 ± 2.2	5.0 ± 2.8	4.2 ± 3.3	0.46

Abbreviations: *BDI* Beck Depression Inventory, *F:M* ratio of females to males, *HADS-A* Hospital Anxiety Depression Scale, Anxiety, *HADS-D* Hospital Anxiety Depression Scale, Depression, *HC* healthy controls, *MIDAS* Migraine Disability Assessment Scale. Of note, group differences in clinical profiles were analyzed by Student's *t*-test (migraine patients vs. HCs) or one-way ANOVA (four phases of migraine patients) for continuous variables and chi-square or Fisher's exact tests for categorical variables

[a]0–10 scale. [b]0–270 range

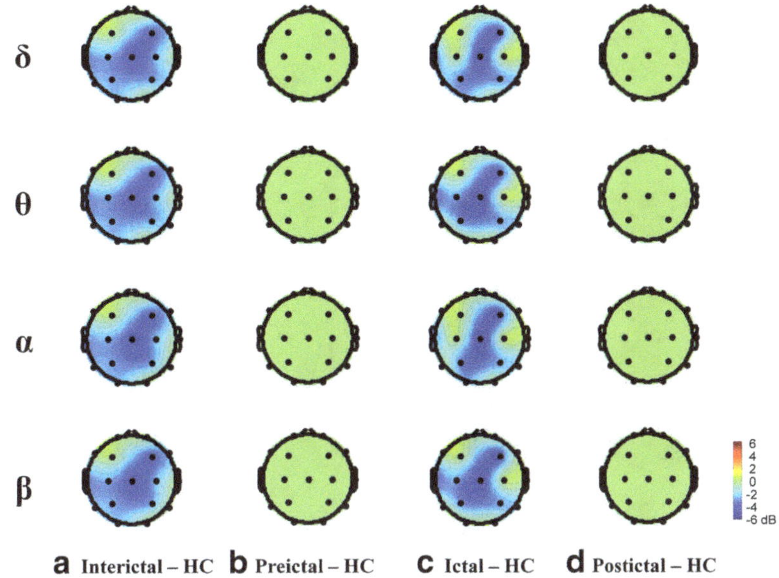

Fig. 2 Topographical comparison of significant EEG power differences ($p < .05$) between migraine patients in different migraine phases and HCs during eyes-open recording. Color intensity indicates the magnitude of the power difference (*red* for increased power, *blue* for decreased power) in each channel

Comparisons of resting-state EEG coherence between migraine patients and HCs

Comparisons of resting-state EEG coherence between migraine patients in each phase of the migraine cycle versus HCs are shown in Fig. 4. Delta, theta, alpha, and beta EEG coherence networks were lower in inter-ictal patients than in HCs (FDR-adjusted $p < .05$; Fig. 4a), with the exception of fronto-occipital network. Specifically, inter-ictal patients had decreased delta EEG coherence in fronto-central network, theta and alpha EEG coherence in fronto-central and posterior networks, and centro-parietal reductions in beta EEG coherence. Of note, the fronto-occipital network showed enhanced EEG coherence in theta, alpha, and beta bands (FDR-adjusted $p < .05$; Fig. 4a). The EEG coherence networks of pre-ictal patients, generally, did not differ from those of HCs, except for a slight increase in

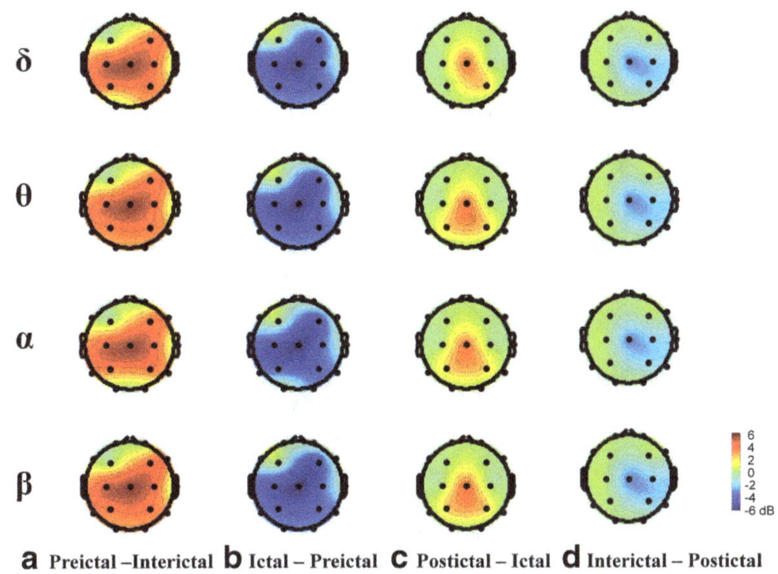

Fig. 3 Topographical comparisons of significant EEG power differences ($p < .05$) between patients in each of the four migraine phases during eyes-open recording. Color intensity indicates the magnitude of the power difference (red for increased power, blue for decreased power) in each channel

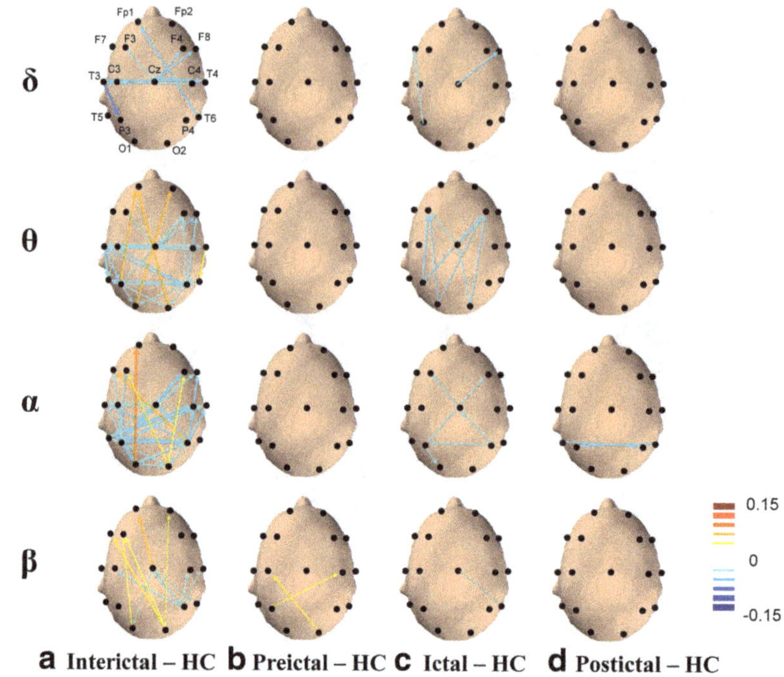

Fig. 4 Topographical comparisons of significant EEG coherence differences ($p < .05$) between patients in different migraine phases and HCs during eyes-open recording. Line sizes and colors reflect the magnitude of the difference in coherence intensity between electrode pairs, with *red* indicating positive differences (more coherent) and *blue* indicating negative differences (more independent). The directions of *arrows* represent the direct paths of inter-channel coupling

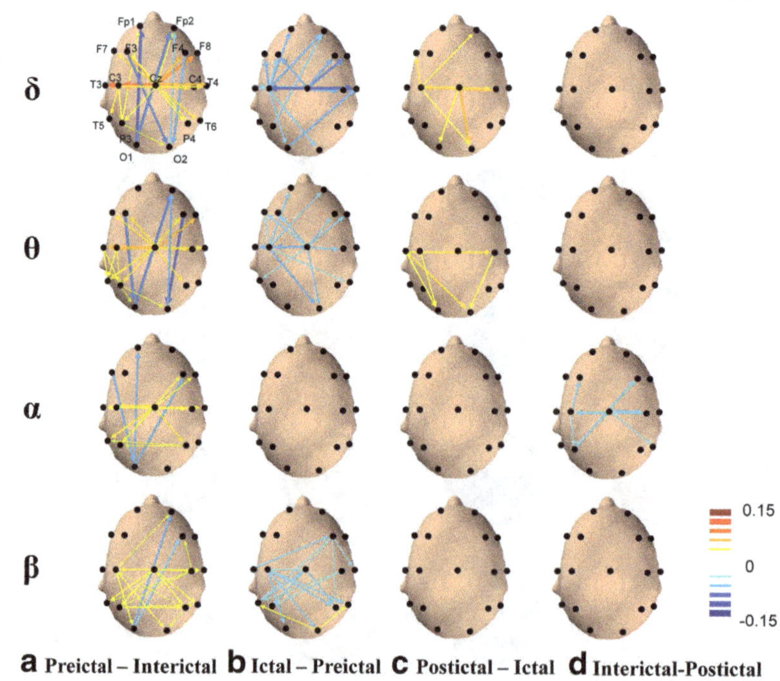

Fig. 5 Topographical comparisons of significant EEG coherence differences ($p < .05$) between migraine patients in each of the four phases of the migraine cycle during eyes-open recording. Line sizes and colors reflect the magnitude of the difference in coherence intensity between electrode pairs, with *red* indicating positive differences (more coherent) and *blue* indicating negative differences (more independent). The directions of *arrows* represent the direct paths of inter-channel coupling

posterior beta EEG coherence (Fig. 4b). The cortical connection intensities of EEG coherence networks for theta and alpha frequency bands in ictal patients were lower than those in HCs (FDR-adjusted $p < .05$; Fig. 4c). Coherence in post-ictal patients was similar to that in HCs, with the exception of a small downtrend in posterior alpha EEG coherence. (Fig. 4d).

Comparisons of resting-state EEG coherence across migraine phases

As demonstrated in Fig. 5, significant differences in resting-state EEG coherence were observed between all pairs of consecutive migraine phases. Large significant differences in EEG coherence networks were observed in the delta, theta, and alpha bands in the frontal, central, temporal, parietal, and occipital regions. Specifically, compared to inter-ictal patients, pre-ictal patients had higher EEG coherence in the delta, theta, alpha, and beta bands (FDR-adjusted $p < .05$; Fig. 5a) except for a reduction of EEG coherence in fronto-occipital network in delta, theta, alpha and beta bands (FDR-adjusted $p < .05$; Fig. 5a). Meanwhile, ictal patients had significantly lower EEG coherence networks in the delta, theta, and beta bands than did pre-ictal patients (FDR-adjusted $p < .05$; Fig. 5b). Moreover, as in Fig. 5c, compared to ictal patients, post-ictal patients had greater EEG coherence, particularly in the delta and theta centro-occipital network (FDR-adjusted $p < .05$). Finally, compared to post-ictal patients, inter-ictal patients had markedly lower EEG coherence networks in the alpha band (FDR-adjusted $p < .05$; Fig. 5d).

Discussion

In the present study, using resting-state EEG, we showed that migraine patients in the inter-ictal and ictal phases, but not in the pre- and post-ictal phases, exhibited lower EEG power and coherence than HCs. Comparing the phase groups in series pairs (inter-ictal, pre-ictal, ictal, post-ictal), we observed increases in EEG power and coherence from the inter-ictal to the pre-ictal phase, decreases from the pre-ictal to the ictal phase, and finally increases from the ictal to the post-ictal phase. The fronto-occipital network in inter-ictal patients showed enhanced EEG coherence as compared to HC or pre-ictal patients. Of note, our results showed higher effect sizes in the eyes-open EEG than eyes-closed EEG. The exact mechanisms are not clear. We do not know whether there is a link to the facts that visual cortical hyperexcitibility is more common in patients with migraine [28] and visual areas in eyes-open condition show greater activation than in eyes-closed condition [29].

Migraine attacks have been hypothesized to start at the cortical level [8, 30, 31]. Previously, the synchronization levels of cortical activity during visual stimulation in migraine patients have been shown to differ from those in HCs [11, 12]. Our findings provide new evidence of cortical abnormalities during a resting state as detected by EEG power spectra and coherence analyses. Furthermore, our findings complement prior resting-state EEG studies demonstrating cortical activity differences between adjacent migraine phases [15, 16].

Extending prior work showing abnormal cortical activity in migraine patients, particularly in the inter-ictal phase [8], we found that the EEG power and coherence, except for the effective connectivity in fronto-occipital network, were lower in the inter-ictal patients than in HCs. That is, migraine patients in the inter-ictal phase exhibited hypo-coupling in the frontal and centro-posterior networks, and hyper-coupling in the fronto-occipital network. Unlike our study results, previous studies showed similar EEG power between inter-ictal patients and HCs [16, 32]. Nevertheless, during the tasks for evoked potentials, inter-ictal patients have been reported to exhibit reduced EEG power [33] and synchronization [11] in relation to HCs. Compared to HCs, migraine patients showed significantly reduced EEG power and coherence during migraine attacks, which normalized after migraine attacks. These power results are in line with the results of two prior studies [34, 35]. Moreover, the decreased EEG coherence in our ictal patients suggests that hypo-coupling may occur during migraine attacks.

Our resting-state EEG results also provide information about the cortical state in the pre-ictal phase. We found significantly higher EEG power and coherence in pre-ictal versus inter-ictal phases. This increased EEG power suggests a relatively excessive cortical power intensity in the pre-ictal phase, which is generally consistent with a higher anterior delta EEG power relative to the inter-ictal phase [15]. Our elevated EEG resting-state coherence in pre-ictal phase points to hyper-coupling of regional brain connectivity, especially in the fronto- and centro-posterior networks. Intriguingly, prior studies have described a pre-ictal "normalization" (towards HCs) of cortical responses to visual and auditory evoked potentials [13, 36, 37]. The exact underlying mechanisms accounting for our findings are not known. In fact, Sakai et al. [38] demonstrated an increase or normalization of cerebral serotonin synthesis from the inter-ictal stage to migraine attacks. Nevertheless, one recent study [39] reported activation of the hypothalamus and brainstem during the prodromal phase (i.e. pre-ictal state) of migraine patients. Because our study did not employ source localization methods, the brain regions responsible for our observations in EEG power and coherence require further investigations.

This study's major strengths were a sizable number of patients in different migraine phases and headache diary recordings for classifications of migraine phases in each patient. However, this study also had limitations. First, it is known that EEG power, concordance and coherence differences were reported in patients with psychiatric disorders, such as unipolar or bipolar disorders, as well as attention deficit hyperactivity disorder [40, 41]. We could not completely exclude the possibility that some of our participants might have such disorders since not all participants had psychiatric consultations. Second, because we recruited low-frequency episodic migraine patients only, one should be cautious about generalizing the findings to other migraine patient groups, such as high-frequency or chronic migraine patients. Third, because we employed a cross-sectional design, it is unknown whether the present results could be repeated in an examination of the same individuals with a longitudinal study design. Fourth, the number of participants and the sex ratio in each group was not fully matched. The imbalance can be explained by the low frequency of migraine attacks in our participants. The sex imbalance in different migraine cycles might be due to the small number in some cycles. Moreover, the vulnerability of coherence measures to volume conduction represents a potential confounder in our study. However, such an influence would be reduced in our study because we calculated differences only between pairs of migraine phases. Last, our study employ EEG, which records signals that are principally of cortical origin. Thus further investigations combining functional MRI with EEG should be pursued to examine the involvement of cortical/subcortical dysfunction in different migraine phases.

Conclusions

The present study revealed dynamic changes in resting-state EEG power and effective connectivity using band power analysis and iCoh, respectively, across different migraine phases in patients with low frequency migraine. EEG effective connectivity in pre-ictal patients showed an augmented coupling in the fronto-central and centro-posterior networks and a reduced coupling in the fronto-occipital network. Such brain network dynamics could have implications for understanding complex neurophysiology of migraine before a headache attack.

Additional file

Additional file 1: Figure S1. Topographical comparison of significant EEG power differences ($p < .05$) between migraine patients in different migraine phases and HCs during eyes-closed recording. Color intensity indicates the magnitude of the power difference (red for increased power, blue for decreased power) in each channel. **Figure S2.** Topographical comparisons of significant EEG power differences ($p < .05$) between patients in each of the four migraine phases during eyes-closed recording. Color intensity indicates the magnitude of the power difference (red for increased power, blue for decreased power) in each channel. **Figure S3.** Topographical comparisons of significant EEG coherence differences ($p < .05$) between patients in different migraine phases and HCs during eyes-closed recording. Line sizes and colors reflect the magnitude of the difference in coherence intensity between electrode pairs, with red indicating positive differences (more coherent) and blue indicating negative differences (more independent). The directions of arrow represent the direct paths of inter-channel coupling. **Figure S4.** Topographical comparisons of significant EEG coherence differences ($p < .05$) between migraine patients in each of the four phases of the migraine cycle during eyes-closed recording. Line sizes and colors reflect the magnitude of the difference in coherence intensity between electrode pairs, with red indicating positive differences (more coherent) and blue indicating negative differences (more independent). The directions of arrow represent the direct paths of inter-channel coupling. (DOCX 2036 kb)

Funding

This study was supported by the Computational Intelligence and Brain Computer Interface (CI&BCI) Centre, University of Technology Sydney, Australian Research Council (ARC) under discovery grant DP150101645, the UST-UCSD International Center of Excellence in Advanced Bioengineering sponsored by the Taiwan National Science Council I-RiCE Program (MOST-103-2911-I-009-101), the Aiming for the Top University Plan of National Chiao-Tung University sponsored by the Ministry of Education of Taiwan (104 W963), the National Science Council of Taiwan (MOST 103-2321-B-010-017), and the Army Research Laboratory (W911NF-10-2-0022). Meanwhile, this study was supported in part by grants from Ministry of Science and Technology of Taiwan (104-2314-B-010-015-MY2, 103-2321-B-010-017), Taipei-Veterans General Hospital (VGHUST104-G7-1-1, V104C-082, V104E9-001), Ministry of Science and Technology support for the Center for Dynamical Biomarkers and Translational Medicine, National Central University, Taiwan (MOST 103-2911-I-008-001), Academia Sinica (IBMS-CRC103-P04), Brain Research Center, National Yang-Ming University, Ministry of Health and Welfare (MOHW104-TDU-B-211-113-003), and a grant from Ministry of Education, Aim for the Top University Plan.

Author' contributions

C-TL and S-JW conceived and designed the experiments. K-LL and S.-JW performed the experiments. ZHC and C-HC analyzed the data. ZHC, C-HC, K-LL and S-JW wrote the paper. A-CY and J-LF revised the manuscript. All authors read and approved the final manuscript.

Competing interests

ZH Cao, C-T Lin, C-H Chuang, K-L Lai and A-C Yang report no conflicts of interest. S-J Wang has served on the advisory boards of Daiichi-Sankyo and Eli Lilly. He has received speaking honoraria from local companies (Taiwan branches) of Pfizer, MSD and GSK. He has received research grants from the Taiwan National Science Council, Taipei-Veterans General Hospital and Taiwan Headache Society. J-L Fuh is a member of a scientific advisory board of Novartis, and has as well received research support from the Taiwan National Science Council and Taipei-Veterans General Hospital.

Author details

[1]Faculty of Engineering and Information Technology, University of Technology Sydney, Sydney, Australia. [2]Department of Electrical and Computer Engineering, Institute of Electrical Control Engineering, National Chiao Tung University, Hsinchu, Taiwan. [3]Brain Research Center, National Chiao Tung University, Hsinchu, Taiwan. [4]Neurological Institute, Taipei Veterans General Hospital, Taipei, Taiwan. [5]Department of Psychiatry, Taipei Veterans General Hospital, Taipei, Taiwan. [6]Faculty of Medicine, National Yang-Ming University School of Medicine, Taipei, Taiwan. [7]Division of Interdisciplinary Medicine and Biotechnology, Beth Israel Deaconess Medical Center/Harvard Medical School, Boston, MA, USA. [8]Brain Research Center, National Yang-Ming University, Taipei, Taiwan.

References

1. Stovner LJ, Hagen K, Jensen R, Katsarava Z, Lipton RB, Scher AI, Steiner TJ, Zwart JA (2007) The global burden of headache: a documentation of headache prevalence and disability worldwide. Cephalalgia 27:193–210
2. Wang SJ, Fuh JL, Young YH, Lu SR, Shia BC (2000) Prevalence of migraine in Taipei, Taiwan: a population-based survey. Cephalalgia 20:566–72

3. Goadsby PJ, Lipton RB, Ferrari MD (2002) Migraine–current understanding and treatment. N Engl J Med 346:257–70
4. Bigal ME, Liberman JN, Lipton RB (2006) Obesity and migraine: a population study. Neurology 66:545–50
5. Queiroz LP, Rapoport AM, Weeks RE, Sheftell FD, Siegel SE, Baskin SM (1997) Characteristics of migraine visual aura. Headache 37:137–41
6. Cady RK, Sheftell F, Lipton RB, O'Quinn S, Jones M, Putnam DG, Crisp A, Metz A, McNeal S (2000) Effect of early intervention with sumatriptan on migraine pain: retrospective analyses of data from three clinical trials. Clin Ther 22:1035–48
7. Aurora S, Wilkinson F (2007) The brain is hyperexcitable in migraine. Cephalalgia 27:1442–53
8. Cosentino G, Fierro B, Brighina F (2014) From different neurophysiological methods to conflicting pathophysiological views in migraine: a critical review of literature. Clin Neurophysiol 125:1721–30
9. Coppola G, Pierelli F, Schoenen J (2007) Is the cerebral cortex hyperexcitable or hyperresponsive in migraine? Cephalalgia 27:1427–39
10. Khedr EM, Ahmed MA, Mohamed KA (2006) Motor and visual cortical excitability in migraineurs patients with or without aura: transcranial magnetic stimulation. Neurophysiol Clin 36:13–8
11. De Tommaso M, Stramaglia S, Marinazzo D, Trotta G, Pellicoro M (2013) Functional and effective connectivity in EEG alpha and beta bands during intermittent flash stimulation in migraine with and without aura. Cephalalgia 33:938–47
12. De Tommaso M, Trotta G, Vecchio E, Ricci K, Van de Steen F, Montemurno A, Lorenzo M, Marinazzo D, Bellotti R, Stramaglia S (2015) Functional connectivity of EEG signals under laser stimulation in migraine. Front Hum Neurosci 9:640
13. Judit A, Sandor PS, Schoenen J (2000) Habituation of visual and intensity dependence of auditory evoked cortical potentials tends to normalize just before and during the migraine attack. Cephalalgia 20:714–9
14. Bruni O, Russo PM, Violani C, Guidetti V (2004) Sleep and migraine: an actigraphic study. Cephalalgia 24:134–9
15. Bjork M, Sand T (2008) Quantitative EEG power and asymmetry increase 36 h before a migraine attack. Cephalalgia 28:960–8
16. Bjork MH, Stovner LJ, Engstrom M, Stjern M, Hagen K, Sand T (2009) Interictal quantitative EEG in migraine: a blinded controlled study. J Headache Pain 10:331–9
17. Van Diessen E, Numan T, Van Dellen E, van der Kooi AW, Boersma M, Hofman D, van Lutterveld R, van Dijk BW, van Straaten EC, Hillebrand A, Stam CJ (2015) Opportunities and methodological challenges in EEG and MEG resting state functional brain network research. Clin Neurophysiol 126:1468–81
18. Schoenen J (2006) Neurophysiological features of the migrainous brain. Neurol Sci 27(Suppl 2):S77–81
19. Sakkalis V (2011) Review of advanced techniques for the estimation of brain connectivity measured with EEG/MEG. Comput Biol Med 41(12):1110–7
20. Russo A, Tessitore A, Giordano A, Corbo D, Marcuccio L, De Stefano M, Salemi F, Conforti R, Esposito F, Tedeschi G (2012) Executive resting-state network connectivity in migraine without aura. Cephalalgia 32:1041–8
21. Schwedt TJ, Larson-Prior L, Coalson RS, Nolan T, Mar S, Ances BM, Benzinger T, Schlaggar BL (2014) Allodynia and descending pain modulation in migraine: a resting state functional connectivity analysis. Pain Med 15:154–65
22. Pascual-Marqui RD, Biscay RJ, Bosch-Bayard J, Lehmann D, Kochi K, Kinoshita T et al (2014) Assessing direct paths of intracortical causal information flow of oscillatory activity with the isolated effective coherence (iCoh). Front Hum Neurosci 8:448
23. The International Classification of Headache Disorders: 2nd edition (2004). Cephalalgia 24 (Suppl 1): 9–160
24. Klem GH, Lüders HO, Jasper H, Elger C (1999) The ten-twenty electrode system of the International Federation. Electroencephalogr Clin Neurophysiol 52:3–6
25. American Clinical Neurophysiology Society (2006) Guideline 6: A proposal for standard montages to be used in clinical EEG. J Clin Neurophysiol 23:111–7
26. Delorme A, Makeig S (2004) EEGLAB: An open source toolbox for analysis of single-trial EEG dynamics including independent component analysis. J Neurosci Methods 134:9–21
27. Delorme A, Mullen T, Kothe C, Akalin Acar Z, Bigdely-Shamlo N, Vankov A et al (2011) EEGLAB, SIFT, NFT, BCILAB, and ERICA: new tools for advanced EEG processing. Comput Intell Neurosci 2011:1–12
28. Aurora SK, Ahmad BK, Welch KM, Bhardhwaj P, Ramadan NM (1998) Transcranial magnetic stimulation confirms hyperexcitability of occipital cortex in migraine. Neurology 50:1111–4
29. Gusnard DA, Raichle ME (2001) Searching for a baseline: functional imaging and the resting human brain. Nat Rev Neurosci 2(10):685–94
30. Sand T, Zhitniy N, White LR, Stovner LJ (2008) Visual evoked potential latency, amplitude and habituation in migraine: a longitudinal study. Clin Neurophysiol 119:1020–7
31. De Tommaso M, Ambrosini A, Brighina F, Coppola G, Perrotta A, Pierelli F, Sandrini G, Valeriani M, Marinazzo D, Stramaglia S, Schoenen J (2014) Altered processing of sensory stimuli in patients with migraine. Nat Rev Neurol 10:144–55
32. Clemens B, Bank J, Piros P, Bessenyei M, Veto S, Toth M, Kondakor I (2008) Three-dimensional localization of abnormal EEG activity in migraine: a low resolution electromagnetic tomography (LORETA) study of migraine patients in the pain-free interval. Brain Topogr 21:36–42
33. Coppola G, Pierelli F, Schoenen J (2009) Habituation and migraine. Neurobiol Learn Mem 92:249–59
34. Sand T (1991) EEG in migraine: a review of the literature. Funct Neurol 6:7–22
35. Siniatchkin M, Gerber WD, Kropp P, Vein A (1999) How the brain anticipates an attack: a study of neurophysiological periodicity in migraine. Funct Neurol 14:69–77
36. Sand T, Vingen JV (2000) Visual, long-latency auditory and brainstem auditory evoked potentials in migraine: relation to pattern size, stimulus intensity, sound and light discomfort thresholds and pre-attack state. Cephalalgia 20:804–20
37. Chen WT, Wang SJ, Fuh JL, Lin CP, Ko YC, Lin YY (2009) Peri-ictal normalization of visual cortex excitability in migraine: an MEG study. Cephalalgia 29:1202–11
38. Sakai Y, Dobson C, Diksic M, Aubé M, Hamel E (2008) Sumatriptan normalizes the migraine attack-related increase in brain serotonin synthesis. Neurology 70:431–9
39. Maniyar FH, Sprenger T, Monteith T, Schankin CJ, Goadsby PJ (2015) The premonitory phase of migraine–what Can We learn from It? Headache 55:609–20
40. Barry R, Clarke A (2012) Resting state brain oscillations and symptom profiles in attention deficit/hyperactivity disorder. Suppl Clin Neurophysiol 62:275–87
41. Tas C, Cebi M, Tan O, Hızlı-Sayar G, Tarhan N, Brown EC (2015) EEG power, cordance and coherence differences between unipolar and bipolar depression. J Affect Disord 172:184–90

9

Altered functional connectivity of amygdala underlying the neuromechanism of migraine pathogenesis

Zhiye Chen[1,2,3], Xiaoyan Chen[2], Mengqi Liu[1,3], Zhao Dong[2], Lin Ma[1*] and Shengyuan Yu[2*]

Abstract

Background: The amygdala is a large grey matter complex in the limbic system, and it may contribute in the neurolimbic pain network in migraine. However, the detailed neuromechanism remained to be elucidated. The objective of this study is to investigate the amygdala structural and functional changes in migraine and to elucidate the mechanism of neurolimbic pain-modulating in the migraine pathogenesis.

Methods: Conventional MRI, 3D structure images and resting state functional MRI were performed in 18 normal controls (NC), 18 patients with episodic migraine (EM), and 16 patients with chronic migraine (CM). The amygdala volume was measured using FreeSurfer software and the functional connectivity (FC) of bilateral amygdala was computed over the whole brain. Analysis of covariance was performed on the individual FC maps among groups.

Results: The increased FC of left amygdala was observed in EM compared with NC, and the decreased of right amygdala was revealed in CM compared with NC. The increased FC of bilateral amygdala was observed in CM compared with EM. The correlation analysis showed a negative correlation between the score of sleep quality (0, normal; 1, mild sleep disturbance; 2, moderate sleep disturbance; 3, serious sleep disturbance) and the increased FC strength of left amygdala in EM compared with NC, and a positive correlation between the score of sleep quality and the increased FC strength of left amygdala in CM compared with EM, and other clinical variables showed no significant correlation with altered FC of amygdala.

Conclusions: The altered functional connectivity of amygdala demonstrated that neurolimbic pain network contribute in the EM pathogenesis and CM chronicization.

Keyword: Migraine, Amygdala, Neurolimbic pain network, Functional connectivity, fMRI

Background

Migraine is a common type of primary headaches with a reported prevalence of about 5.7% in men and 17.0% in women [1], and the prevalence of migraine is 9.3 of general population [2] in China. Migraine is also a major cause of chronic headaches, approximately 2.5% of episodic migraine (EM) is transformed to chronic migraine (CM) [3]. Although the growing studies supported the key roles of cortical spreading depression (CSD) and trigeminovascular system in the migraine pathogenesis, the rigorous neuromechanism of EM and the road to migraine chronicization were not completely understood and became to be worth paying close attention.

Beyond neurovascular model, a dysfunctional neurolimbic pain network model expands the conventional concept about migraine, and it could help understand the migraine attack, the migraine chronicization and refractoriness [4]. Recently, increased connectivity between amygdala and visceroceptive cortex in migraine was observed, and which confirmed the roles of neurolimbic pain network dysfunction in the migraine pain genesis [5]. The central sensitization of migraine was confirmed in the animal model by Malick et al. in 2000 [6], and this model could account for many of the temporal and sysmptomatic features of migraine [7]. Ongoing researches demonstrated

* Correspondence: cjr.malin@vip.163.com; yusy1963@126.com
[1]Department of Radiology, Chinese PLA General Hospital, 28 Fuxing Road, Beijing 100853, China
[2]Department of Neurology, Chinese PLA General Hospital, 28 Fuxing Road, Beijing 100853, China
Full list of author information is available at the end of the article

that central sensitization could reach critical clinical implications for chronic head and neck pain [8]. Therefore, we propose that neurolimbic pain network may bridge the gap between the neurovascular model and central sensitization model.

Based on the current knowledge, the brain regions related with pain processing and modulation mainly included prefrontal cortex, basal ganglia, thalamus, cingulate cortex, insular, cerebellum and periaqueductal gray matter (PAG). Some studies demonstrated that amygdala also involved the migraine pain modulation, such as the modulation of synaptic transmission by CSD [9] and the PAG network [10] and chronic migraine. The amygdala is a large grey matter complex in the limbic system, and it plays a key role in emotion, motivation, learning and memory, and also in migraine [11].

Therefore, the motivation of this study is to investigate the amygdala structural and functional changes in migraine and to elucidate the mechanism of neurolimbic pain-modulating in the migraine pathogenesis. We hypothesized that amygdala was involved in the pain modulation in migraine. To address this hypothesis, we obtained structural and functional MR images for normal controls (NC), episodic migraine (EM) patients, and chronic migraine (CM) patients. Firstly, the amygdala volume was automatically measured based on the structural images using FreeSurfer software, and comparisons of between-group analysis were performed. Secondly, the functional connectivity of bilateral amygdala was computed based on resting-state fMRI, and comparisons of between-group analysis were performed to explore the altered functional connectivity in CM compared with EM.

Methods

Subjects

Fifty-two subjects were enrolled, including 18 patients with EM and 16 patients with CM, and 18 NCs with matched age and gender. Patients were recruited from International Headache Center, Department of Neurology, Chinese PLA General Hospital, and inclusion criteria was based on the International Classification of Headache Disorders, third Edition (beta version) (ICHD -3 beta) [12]. All the subjects underwent a standard categorical four-grade sleep disturbance scale (SDS) (0, normal; 1, mild sleep disturbance; 2, moderate sleep disturbance; 3, serious sleep disturbance), Visual Analogue Scale(VAS), Hamilton Anxiety Scale (HAMA), Hamilton Depression Scale (HAMD) and Montreal Cognitive Assessment (MoCA) evaluation. The exclusion criteria were the following: cranium trauma, illness interfering with central nervous system function, psychotic disorder, and regular use of a psychoactive or hormone medication, and onabotulinumtoxin A medication. All the CM patients did not experience medication overuse. NCs were recruited form hospital staffs and their relatives. All the subjects received general physical examination and neurological examination and were normotensive (≤140/90 mmHg), and free from cardiovascular, metabolic and psychiatric disorders. All the subjects were right-handed and underwent MRI conventional examination to exclude the subjects with cerebral infarction, malacia or occupying lesions. The alcohol, nicotine, caffeine and other substances were avoided at least 12 h before MRI examination. Written informed consent was obtained from all participants according to the approval of the ethics committee of the Chinese PLA General Hospital.

MRI acquisition

MRI scans were taken in the interictal stage at least 3 days after a migraine attack, and no migraine preventive medication was used in the past 3 months. Images were acquired on a GE 3.0T MR system (DISCOVERY MR750, GE Healthcare, Milwaukee, WI, USA) and a conventional eight channel quadrature head coil was used. All the subjects were instructed to lie in a supine position, and form padding was used to limit head movement. Conventional T2-weighted images were obtained first. Then a high resolution three-dimensional T1-weighted fast spoiled gradient recalled echo(3D T1-FSPGR) sequence was performed, which generated 360 contiguous axial slices [TR (repetition time) = 6.3 ms, TE (echo time) = 2.8 ms, flip angle = 15o, FOV (field of view) = 25.6cm × 25.6cm, Matrix = 256 × 256, slice thickness = 1 mm]. Lastly, the resting-state fMRI was performed, where subjects were instructed to relax, keep their eyes closed, stay awake, remain still, and clear their heads of all thoughts. Functional images were obtained by using a gradient echo-planar imaging (EPI) sequence (TR = 2000 ms, TE = 30 ms, flip angle = 90, slice thickness = 4mm, slice gap = 1 mm, FOV = 24cm × 24cm, Matrix = 64 × 64), and 180 continuous EPI functional volumes were acquired axially over 6 min. All the subjects did not complain any discomfort and feel asleep during scanning. No obvious structural damage was observed based on the conventional MR images.

Data processing

MR structural images were processed using Freesurfer software (version 4.3.0) (http://surfer.nmr.mgh.harvard.edu/fswiki/FreeSurfer), which was run using the Linux 2.6.15-2.5 operating system. The amygdala volume could be automatically measured using automated labeling of neuroanatomical structures technique, and the accuracy has been validated comparing with manual labeling [13]. The preprocessing steps have been elucidated in previous studies [13, 14].

Functional images were processed using Statistical Parametric Mapping 8 (SPM8) (http://www.fil.ion.ucl.ac.uk/spm) and resting-state fMRI data analysis toolkit (REST v1.8) [15] running under MATLAB 7.6 (The Mathworks, Natick, MA, USA).

The data preprocessing was carried out as following: (1) The first ten volumes of each functional time course was discarded to allow for T1 equilibrium and the participants to adapt; (2) Slice timing; (3) Head motion correction; (4) Spatial normalization. These steps were performed by SPM8. No subjects had head motion with more than 1.5mm displacement in X, Y, and Z direction or 1.50 of any angular motion throughout the course of the scanning. The linear trend removal and temporal band-pass filtering (0.01–0.08 Hz) was performed by REST [15].

The functional connectivity analysis was performed as following: (1) Spatial smooth (full width at half maximum (FWHM) = 6 mm) using SPM8; (2) Amygdala was defined using AAL template [16] (Fig. 1), then the amygdala was resliced with the brainmask template with 63 × 71 × 63 size to avoid the some voxels outside the brain; (3) Functional connectivity computation of the left and right amygdala were performed using REST(v1.8). The time course of bilateral amygdala were extracted, and Pearson correlation were used to calculated functional connectivity between the extracted time course and the averaged time courses of the whole brain in a voxel-wise manner. The white matter, CSF, and the six head motion parameters were used as covariates. (4) The individual r-maps were normalized to Z-maps using Fisher's Z transformation. (5) The positive clusters based on the statistical parametric mapping were generated binary mask, and the connectivity strength of the positive brain region was extracted based on the Z-maps.

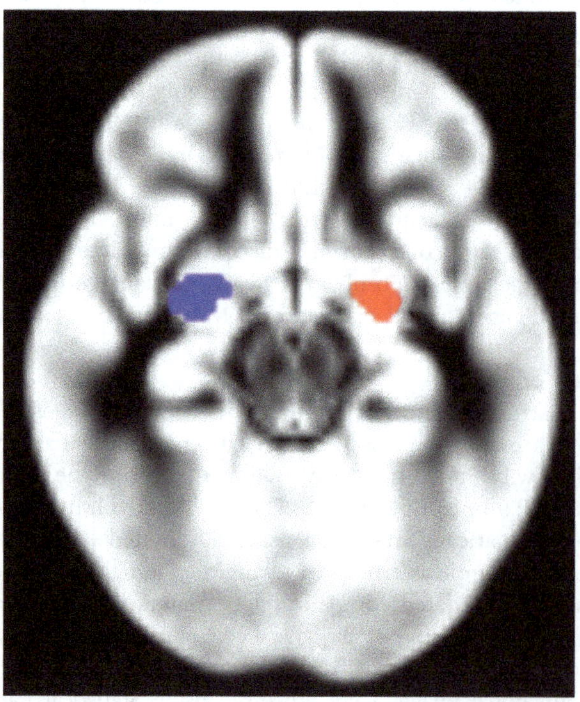

Fig. 1 The bilateral amygdala masks were generated based on the AAL template. *Red*, left amygdala; *Blue*, right amygdala

Statistical analysis

The age, education years, VAS, HAMA, HAMD and MoCA were performed with one-way analysis of variance (ANOVA), disease duration (DD) was performed with two-sample *t* test. Post Hoc multiple comparisons were performed by LSD methods with equal variances and Dunnett's T3 with unequal variances. The amygdala volume was compared using Analysis of covariance (ANCOVA) among each group, covarying for age, gender and education years. The Pearson correlation analysis was performed between disease duration, VAS and amygdala volume. These statistics was processed using IBM SPSS 19.0, and the *P* value of less than 0.05 was considered to indicate a statistically significant difference.

Analysis of covariance (ANCOVA) was performed to identify the regions with significant differences in connectivity to amygdala between groups, covarying for age, gender, education years. Significance was set at a *P* value of < 0.001 without correction. The minimal number of contiguous voxels was set at 10. The statistical maps were masked on SPM8 T1 template.

Bivariate correlation analysis was applied to the connectivity strength of the positive brain region in each compared groups. The Pearson's method was performed for the scaled variable, and the Spearman's method was performed for the ordinal variables. The *P* value of less than 0.05 was considered to indicate a statistically significant difference.

Results

Demography and neuropsychological test

Demography and neuropsychological scores were shown in Table 1. Age, education years, HAMD score and

Table 1 The clinical characteristics of the subjects

	NC	EM	CM
Num(F/M)	18(14/4)	18(14/4)	16(12/4)
Age	39.1 ± 10.0	33.4 ± 11.0	42.4 ± 8.6
DD	NA	12.4 ± 8.1	11.3 ± 9.3
EduYears	13.7 ± 3.2	13.7 ± 3.7	10.8 ± 3.8
SDS	NA	1.27 ± 1.0	2.4 ± 1.1
VAS	NA	8.3 ± 1.5	7.9 ± 1.5
HAMA	9.7 ± 3.2	15.7 ± 9.85	21.6 ± 11.0
HAMD	15.9 ± 2.9	10.9 ± 7.3	16.3 ± 10.5
MoCA	26.9 ± 2.5	29.2 ± 1.5	22.9 ± 5.4

DD disease duration, *EduYears* education years, *SDC* sleep disturbance scale, *VAS* visual analogue scale, *HAMA* Hamilton anxiety scale, *HAMD* Hamilton depression scale, *MoCA* Montreal Cognitive Assessment, *NC* normal control, *EM* episodic migraine, *CM* chronic migraine

MoCA score showed no significant difference among each group ($P > 0.01$). HAMA score in NC (9.7 ± 3.2) was lower than that in CM (21.6 ± 11.0), and other groups showed no significant difference among them.

Comparison of amygdala volume among each group

The amygdala volume showed no significant difference among NC (left, 1.61 ± 0.32 ml; right, 1.64 ± 0.25 ml; mean, 1.62 ± 0.27ml), EM(left, 1.59 ± 0.26ml; right, 1.64 ± 0.21 ml; mean, 1.62 ± 0.23 ml) and CM (left, 1.62 ± 0.23 ml; right, 1.68 ± 0.20 ml; mean, 1.65 ± 0.20 ml), although the amygdala volume in CM showed the increased trend compared with that in NC and EM. The correlation analysis demonstrated that there was no significant correlation between VAS, MMSE, HAMA, HAMD, MoCA score and amygdala volume.

Comparison of functional connectivity of amygdala between NC and EM

It was demonstrated that the brain regions with increased FC of the left amygdala mainly located in the left middle cingulate gyrus ([-18 -45 36], T value 4.18) and left precuneus ([-9 -66 39], T value 4.14) in EM compared with NC (Fig. 2). However, the increased FC of right amygdala could not be revealed in EM compared with NC. The decreased FC of bilateral amygdala was not observed in EM compared with NC.

Comparison of functional connectivity of amygdala between NC and CM

There were no significant changes for FC of left amygdala between NC and CM. The brain regions with decreased FC of the right amygdala mainly located in right inferior occipital lobe ([30 -99 -3], T value 4.26) and right middle occipital lobe ([45 -83 12], T value 4.11) in CM compared with NC (Fig. 2). There was no increased significant change for FC of the right amygdala in CM compared with NC.

Comparison of functional connectivity of amygdala between EM and CM

Table 2 and Fig. 2 showed the increased functional connectivity of bilateral amygdala in CM compared with EM. The common brain regions with increased connectivity located in bilateral inferior temporal gyri.

The difference brain regions with increased connectivity were observed for bilateral amygdala. The remained brain regions with increased connectivity of left amygdala mainly located in the right orbital part of superior frontal gyrus, left fusiform, right postcentral gyrus, left rectus, right amygdala and left precentral gyrus in CM compared with EM. The remained brain regions with increased connectivity of right amygdala mainly located in the left middle cingulate gyrus, left orbital part of medial frontal gyrus, left temporal pole, right orbital part of inferior frontal gyrus, right anterior cingulate gyrus and left orbital part of inferior frontal gyrus. The decreased FC of bilateral amygdala was not observed in CM compared with EM.

Correlation analysis of the connectivity strength of the positive brain regions with the clinical variables

The correlation analysis showed a negative correlation between the score of sleep quality (0, normal; 1, mild

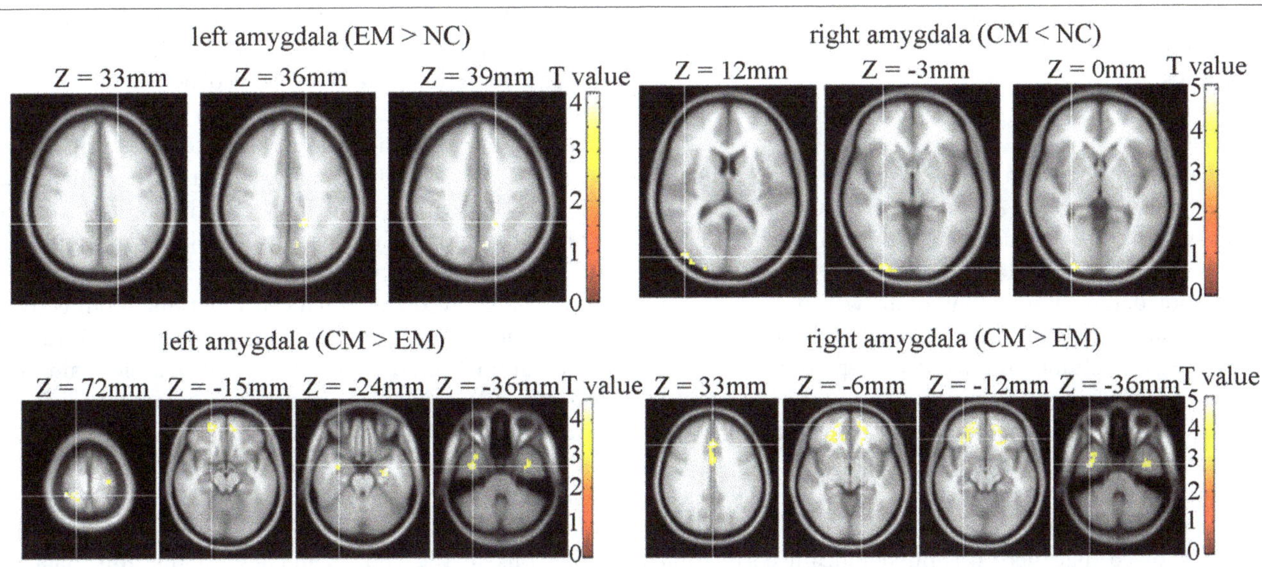

Fig. 2 Comparison of FC of amygdala among NC, EM and CM. Warm color represents altered functional connectivity. EM > NC, increased FC of amygdala in EM compared with NC; CM < NC, decreased FC of amygdala in CM compared with NC; CM > EM, increased FC of amygdala in CM compared with EM

Table 2 The brain regions with increased functional connectivity of bilateral amygdala in CM patients compared with EM in resting state

	Anatomic region	MNI-space			K value	P_{uncorr}value	T value
		X	Y	Z			
L-Amygdala	Temporal_Inf_L	-33	-6	-42	33	0.000	5.90
	Temporal_Inf_R	39	-3	-33	35	0.000	5.72
	Frontal_Sup_Orb_R	21	51	-15	36	0.000	5.08
	Fusiform_L	-33	-9	-24	28	0.000	4.96
	Postcentral_R	18	-38	72	28	0.000	4.58
	Rectus_L	-6	48	-15	19	0.000	4.53
	Amygdala_R	33	0	-24	10	0.000	4.28
	Precentral_L	-24	-18	75	12	0.000	3.85
R-Amygdala	Temporal_Inf_L	-33	-6	-42	47	0.000	6.49
	Cingulum_Mid_L	0	27	33	113	0.000	5.67
	Temporal_Inf_R	42	-3	-36	45	0.000	4.79
	Frontal_Med_Orb_L	-15	54	-6	68	0.000	4.61
	Temporal_Pole_L	-42	15	-33	11	0.000	4.48
	Frontal_Inf_Orb_R	30	33	-12	106	0.000	4.46
	Cingulum_Ant_R	9	36	-6	10	0.000	4.29
	Frontal_Inf_Orb_L	-24	24	-18	45	0.000	4.19

MNI Montreal Neurological Institute, *X, Y, Z* coordinates of the primary maximum of the cluster; ($T > 3.39$, $P < 0.001$) (without correction)

sleep disturbance; 2, moderate sleep disturbance; 3, serious sleep disturbance) and the increased FC of left amygdala in EM compared with NC, and a positive correlation between the score of sleep quality and the increased FC of left amygdala in CM compared with EM (Fig. 3). There was no significant correlation between the score of sleep quality and the altered FC strength of amygdala in CM compared with NC.

VAS, HAMA, HAMD and MoCA showed no significant correlation with altered FC of amygdala in comparison groups.

Discussion

The relationship between pain and limbic system always receives much concern. As an essential element of the limbic system, the amygdala is worth of further study in migraineurs.

Our data demonstrated that there was no significant difference among NC, EM and CM, which demonstrated that amygdala volume could not be regarded as a progressive biomarker in migraine. Although a previous study showed the decreased amygdala volume in CM compared with EM based on voxel-based morphometry [17], the different results may be associated with the heterogeneous migraineurs in the study. The correlation analysis showed that there was no significant correlation between amygdala volume and the neuropsychological scale score, VAS, disease duration, which also suggested that amygdala volume could not be used to monitor the migraine progression. But the increased volume of the amygdala can be seen in the neuropathic pain, either in the study of animal models [18] or human subjects [19]. This hints that additional mechanisms or different influence intensity were involved in the pain of migraine on amygdala.

In our study, the enhanced FC of the left amygdala was observed in EM compared with NC, and the other altered amygdala FC was not revealed, which confirmed that left amygdala may be associated with the genesis of EM, and the enhanced FC may also be relevant to understanding the EM associated with psychopathology. This laterality pattern may be associated with the different functions of bilateral amygdala, and the left amygdala was known to contribute to the brain's reward system. Therefore, the laterality mechanism should be further investigation.

Figure 2 showed the enhanced functional connectivity of bilateral amygdala in CM compared with EM. Just as in the animal modes study of neuropathic pain, the time-dependency of changes in the activity of the amygdala were shown [20]. Our study showed a similar time-dependency tendency and gave a direct evidence of central sensitization. By the ground of this enhanced FC, the animal trial proved that sensitization of neurons in the central nucleus of the amygdala via the decreased GABAergic inhibition contributes to the development of neuropathic pain-related anxiety-like behaviors [21].

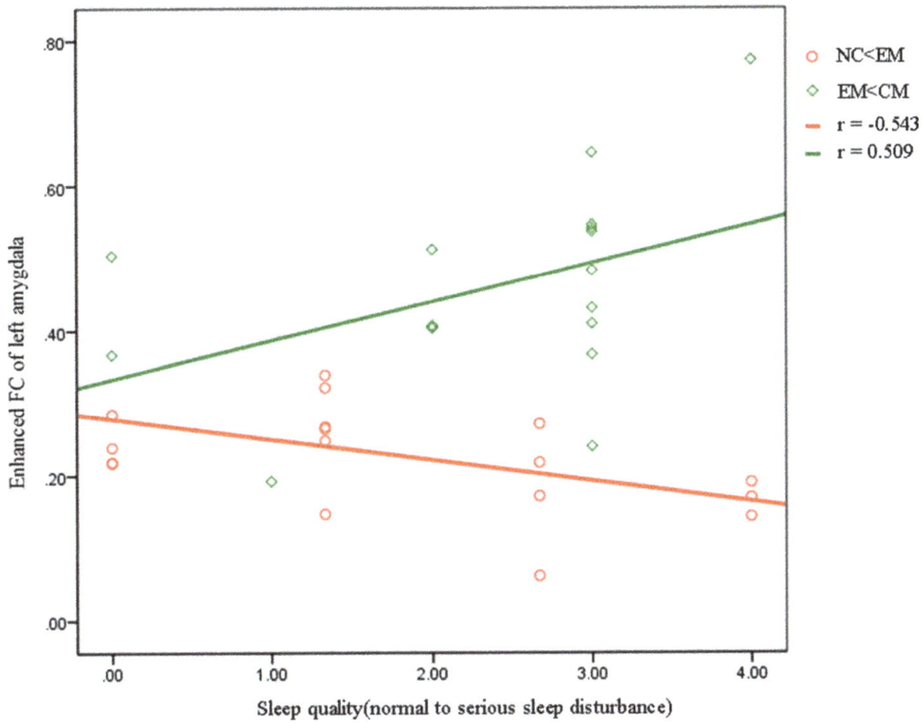

Fig. 3 The correlation of the score of sleep quality with the enhanced FC of left amygdala in EM compared with NC (red circle and line) and in CM compared with EM (green rhombus and line). NC < EM, the increased FC of left amygdala in EM compared with NC; EM < CM, the increased FC of left amygdala in CM compared with EM

This study showed there were no significant changes for FC of the right amygdala in NC vs. EM and EM vs. CM. However, there was a significant decreased FC of right amygdala in CM compared with NC. These altered FC pattern demonstrated that left and right amygdala played different roles in the genesis of EM and CM. The enhanced FC of left amygdala could underlie the genesis of EM, and contribute in the CM chronicization. While the decreased FC of right amygdala also could underlie the genesis of CM, and some brain regions with increased FC of right amygdala may participate in CM chronicization based on the comparison of EM and CM. The altered FC pattern of left and right amygdala may be associated with different functions of bilateral amygdala. The left amygdala mainly induced pleasant or unpleasant emotions, while the right amygdala mainly induced negative emotions such as fear and sadness [22]. Therefore, left and right amygdala played the different roles in the genesis of EM and CM.

Based the Table 2, the brain regions with evident enhanced connectivity were inferior temporal gyrus (ITG) and orbitofrontal gyrus (OFG). ITG is located on the inferior convexity of the temporal lobe in human, and it participated in the analysis of visual form and object recognition, and is considered to be the final stage in the ventral cortical visual system [23]. Voxel-based morphometry demonstrated that gray matter volume decreased in right ITG in CM patients [24], and our study confirmed the enhanced connectivity between ITG and amygdala, which may confirmed that ITG played a crucial role in the neurolimbic pain-modulation network. A study of effects of long-term acupuncture treatment on resting-state brain activity in migraine patients revealed that a decrease in ReHo values was observed after treatment in the left ITG [25], which indicated that the resting activity of ITG could be used for the evaluation of the therapy of migraine, and the enhanced FC between ITG and amygdala may provide a new clue to reveal the neuromechanism of migraine.

Acute and chronic pain may involve multiple brain regions for the pain processing, and they are interconnected to construct the pain network [26]. Regarding migraine, the pain genesis may embrace the acute and chronic process, such as EM and CM. OFG, anatomically called as ventromedial prefrontal cortex, is participated the sensory integration [27] and the expected reward and punishment of an action, and it shares extensive reciprocal connections with the amygdala. Fumal et al. demonstrated that OFG was involved chronic migraine evolving from episodic migraine, and showed persistent orbitofrontal hypofunction after withdrawal of analgesics [28]. The disrupted OFG connectivity or circuitry could affect the decision-making, emotion regulation and reward expectation, however, our study demonstrated the enhanced connectivity was involved between the OFC and amygdala in CM evolving from EM. This connectivity pattern demonstrated that amygdala participated the central sensitization, and the mechanism should be worth further study.

Our data also showed the enhanced connectivity between left amygdala and left middle cingulate cortex (MCC) in EM compared with NC, and between the right amygdala and right anterior cingulate cortex (ACC) and MCC. ACC played a role in pain modulation, analgesia, and attention and anticipation of pain [26, 29]. Although a recent VBM study demonstrated that the decreased ACC grey matter was observed in CM compared with EM [17], our study showed enhanced connectivity of the amygdala with ACC in CM, and this indicated the amygdala played a key role in the pain modulation of ACC. A recent study revealed that MCC also showed pain-induced activation after painful heat stimulus in EM compared with NC [30], and Teutsch et al. demonstrated that increased grey matter was observed after noxious stimuli were applied repetitively to NC [31]. In our study, enhanced connectivity between amygdala and MCC was observed, and this connectivity pattern suggested the amygdala modulation network had a crucial role in the EM and CM genesis.

The relationship between migraine and sleep has been reported, and there was a significant association between severe sleep disturbance and primary headache disorder, especially in CM [32]. The insufficient sleep may induce a migraine attack, and lack of adequate rest might be an attack-precipitating and hyperalgesia-inducing factor [33–35]. A large clinical sample of migraineurs study with 1283 migraineurs revealed the substantial sleep/migraine relationship, and implicate sleep disturbance in specific headache patterns and severity [36]. However, the precise mechanism remained poorly understood up to now.

The amygdala plays a role in REM sleep modulation [37], and functional interactions between the amygdala and the cortex was demonstrated by PET data during REM sleep [38]. An animal study demonstrated that amygdala played a role in sleep regulation and sleep disturbance may be associated with psychopathology [39], and a recent resting-state functional MRI showed that altered amygdala FC was investigated after 36 h of total sleep deprivation [40]. Therefore, sleep disturbance may involve the functions of amygdala. In this study, an increased FC of left amygdala in EM compared with NC and in CM compared with EM. The correlation analysis demonstrated that there was a negative correlation between the degree of sleep disturbance and the increased FC of left amygdala in EM, which suggested that sleep disturbance may play a limited role in the EM attack. However, a positive correlation was investigated between the degree of sleep disturbance and the increased FC of left amygdala in CM compared with EM, which confirmed that sleep disturbance may play a key role in CM genesis evolved from EM. Therefore, these sleep/increased FC of left amygdala relationship could explained the fact that sleep complaints occurred with greater frequency among CM than EM [36]. Although the results were interesting to reveal the role of sleep quality by the enhanced amygdala FC in EM and CM genesis, it should be cautious to explain the relationship between the sleep disturbance and migraine genesis since the left amygdala could induced pleasant or unpleasant emotion [22].

The present study has some limitations. First, the number of EM and CM patients was relatively small, and a large sample study would be need in future study. Second, this study was a cross-sectional study, and the longitudinal observation should be performed to investigate the evolvement of EM to CM. Lastly, the effect of emotion regulation or lability on the change of amygdala FC in migraine would be investigated in the future because of well-known emotional correlates of amygdala [22, 41].

Conclusions

The present study is the first to address the roles of amygdala in the neurolimbic pain-modulating in the migraine pathogenesis. Enhanced FC of the left amygdala in EM and decreased FC of the right amygdala in CM could elucidate the different neuromechanism of migraine. The enhanced FC of bilateral amygdala gave a direct evidence of central sensitization from EM to CM. And the sleep/increased FC of left amygdala relationship further enlightened the neuromechanism of enhanced FC of amygdala in neurolimbic pain network dysfunction. Potential treatment may be supported by the mechanism of this limbic system change.

Abbreviations

CM: Chronic migraine; EM: Episodic migraine; NC: Normal control

Acknowledgements

This work was supported by the National Natural Sciences Foundation of China (81371514), Special Financial Grant from the China Postdoctoral Science Foundation (2014T70960) and the Foundation for Medical and health Sci & Tech innovation Project of Sanya (2016YW37).

Authors' contributions

Category 1: (a) Conception and Design: LM; SYY; (b) Acquisition of Data: ZYC; MQL; XYC, ZD. (c) Analysis and Interpretation of Data: ZYC. Category 2: (a) Drafting the Article: ZYC. (b) Revising it for Intellectual Content: LM; SYY. All authors read and approved the final manuscript.

Competing interests

The authors declare that they have no competing interests.

Author details
[1]Department of Radiology, Chinese PLA General Hospital, 28 Fuxing Road, Beijing 100853, China. [2]Department of Neurology, Chinese PLA General Hospital, 28 Fuxing Road, Beijing 100853, China. [3]Department of Radiology, Hainan Branch of Chinese PLA General Hospital, Beijing 100853, China.

References

1. Scher AI, Gudmundsson LS, Sigurdsson S, Ghambaryan A, Aspelund T, Eiriksdottir G et al (2009) Migraine headache in middle age and late-life brain infarcts. JAMA 301:2563–2570
2. Yu S, Liu R, Zhao G, Yang X, Qiao X, Feng J et al (2012) The prevalence and burden of primary headaches in China: a population-based door-to-door survey. Headache 52:582–591
3. Lipton RB (2009) Tracing transformation: chronic migraine classification, progression, and epidemiology. Neurology 72:S3–S7
4. Maizels M, Aurora S, Heinricher M (2012) Beyond neurovascular: migraine as a dysfunctional neurolimbic pain network. Headache 52:1553–1565
5. Hadjikhani N, Ward N, Boshyan J, Napadow V, Maeda Y, Truini A et al (2013) The missing link: enhanced functional connectivity between amygdala and visceroceptive cortex in migraine. Cephalalgia 33:1264–1268
6. Malick A, Burstein R (2000) Peripheral and central sensitization during migraine. Funct Neurol 15(Suppl 3):28–35
7. Dodick D, Silberstein S (2006) Central sensitization theory of migraine: clinical implications. Headache 46(Suppl 4):S182–S191
8. Curatolo M, Arendt-Nielsen L, Petersen-Felix S (2006) Central hypersensitivity in chronic pain: mechanisms and clinical implications. Phys Med Rehabil Clin N Am 17:287–302
9. Dehbandi S, Speckmann EJ, Pape HC, Gorji A (2008) Cortical spreading depression modulates synaptic transmission of the rat lateral amygdala. Eur J Neurosci 27:2057–2065
10. Mainero C, Boshyan J, Hadjikhani N (2011) Altered functional magnetic resonance imaging resting-state connectivity in periaqueductal gray networks in migraine. Ann Neurol 70:838–845
11. Akcali D, Sayin A, Sara Y, Bolay H (2010) Does single cortical spreading depression elicit pain behaviour in freely moving rats? Cephalalgia 30:1195–1206
12. Headache Classification Committee of the International Headache Society (IHS) (2013) The International Classification of Headache Disorders, 3rd edition (beta version). Cephalalgia 33:629–808.
13. Fischl B, Salat DH, Busa E, Albert M, Dieterich M, Haselgrove C et al (2002) Whole brain segmentation: automated labeling of neuroanatomical structures in the human brain. Neuron 33:341–355
14. Fischl B, Salat DH, van der Kouwe AJ, Makris N, Segonne F, Quinn BT, Dale AM (2004) Sequence-independent segmentation of magnetic resonance images. Neuroimage 23(Suppl 1):S69–S84
15. Song XW, Dong ZY, Long XY, Li SF, Zuo XN, Zhu CZ et al (2011) REST: a toolkit for resting-state functional magnetic resonance imaging data processing. PLoS One 6, e25031
16. Tzourio-Mazoyer N, Landeau B, Papathanassiou D, Crivello F, Etard O, Delcroix N et al (2002) Automated anatomical labeling of activations in SPM using a macroscopic anatomical parcellation of the MNI MRI single-subject brain. Neuroimage 15:273–289
17. Valfre W, Rainero I, Bergui M, Pinessi L (2008) Voxel-based morphometry reveals gray matter abnormalities in migraine. Headache 48:109–117
18. Goncalves L, Silva R, Pinto-Ribeiro F, Pego JM, Bessa JM, Pertovaara A et al (2008) Neuropathic pain is associated with depressive behaviour and induces neuroplasticity in the amygdala of the rat. Exp Neurol 213:48–56
19. Mao C, Wei L, Zhang Q, Liao X, Yang X, Zhang M (2013) Differences in brain structure in patients with distinct sites of chronic pain: A voxel-based morphometric analysis. Neural Regen Res 8:2981–2990
20. Goncalves L, Dickenson AH (2012) Asymmetric time-dependent activation of right central amygdala neurones in rats with peripheral neuropathy and pregabalin modulation. Eur J Neurosci 36:3204–3213
21. Jiang H, Fang D, Kong LY, Jin ZR, Cai J, Kang XJ et al (2014) Sensitization of neurons in the central nucleus of the amygdala via the decreased GABAergic inhibition contributes to the development of neuropathic pain-related anxiety-like behaviors in rats. Mol Brain 7:72
22. Lanteaume L, Khalfa S, Regis J, Marquis P, Chauvel P, Bartolomei F (2007) Emotion induction after direct intracerebral stimulations of human amygdala. Cereb Cortex 17:1307–1313
23. Denys K, Vanduffel W, Fize D, Nelissen K, Peuskens H, Van Essen D, Orban GA (2004) The processing of visual shape in the cerebral cortex of human and nonhuman primates: a functional magnetic resonance imaging study. J Neurosci 24:2551–2565
24. Yu S, Chen X, Chen Z, Dong Z, Ma L (2014) EHMTI-0307. Chronification of migraine: a clinical and voxel-based morphometry study. J Headache Pain 15:1
25. Zhao L, Liu J, Zhang F, Dong X, Peng Y, Qin W et al (2014) Effects of Long-Term Acupuncture Treatment on Resting-State Brain Activity in Migraine Patients: A Randomized Controlled Trial on Active Acupoints and Inactive Acupoints. PLoS One 9, e99538
26. Peyron R, Laurent B, Garcia-Larrea L (2000) Functional imaging of brain responses to pain. A review and meta-analysis (2000). Neurophysiol Clin 30:263–288
27. Kringelbach ML (2005) The human orbitofrontal cortex: linking reward to hedonic experience. Nat Rev Neurosci 6:691–702
28. Fumal A, Laureys S, Di Clemente L, Boly M, Bohotin V, Vandenheede M et al (2006) Orbitofrontal cortex involvement in chronic analgesic-overuse headache evolving from episodic migraine. Brain 129:543–550
29. Tessitore A, Russo A, Esposito F, Giordano A, Taglialatela G, De Micco R et al (2011) Interictal cortical reorganization in episodic migraine without aura: an event-related fMRI study during parametric trigeminal nociceptive stimulation. Neurol Sci 32(Suppl 1):S165–S167
30. Schwedt TJ, Chong CD, Chiang CC, Baxter L, Schlaggar BL, Dodick DW (2014) Enhanced pain-induced activity of pain-processing regions in a case-control study of episodic migraine. Cephalalgia 34:947–958
31. Teutsch S, Herken W, Bingel U, Schoell E, May A (2008) Changes in brain gray matter due to repetitive painful stimulation. Neuroimage 42:845–849
32. Odegard SS, Engstrom M, Sand T, Stovner LJ, Zwart JA, Hagen K (2010) Associations between sleep disturbance and primary headaches: the third Nord-Trondelag Health Study. J Headache Pain 11:197–206
33. Alstadhaug K, Salvesen R, Bekkelund S (2007) Insomnia and circadian variation of attacks in episodic migraine. Headache 47:1184–1188
34. Engstrom M, Hagen K, Bjork MH, Stovner LJ, Gravdahl GB, Stjern M, Sand T (2013) Sleep quality, arousal and pain thresholds in migraineurs: a blinded controlled polysomnographic study. J Headache Pain 14:12
35. Haque B, Rahman KM, Hoque A, Hasan AT, Chowdhury RN, Khan SU et al (2012) Precipitating and relieving factors of migraine versus tension type headache. BMC Neurol 12:82
36. Kelman L, Rains JC (2005) Headache and sleep: examination of sleep patterns and complaints in a large clinical sample of migraineurs. Headache 45:904–910
37. Siegel JM (2006) The stuff dreams are made of: anatomical substrates of REM sleep. Nat Neurosci 9:721–722
38. Maquet P, Franck G (1997) REM sleep and amygdala. Mol Psychiatry 2:195–196
39. Benca RM, Obermeyer WH, Shelton SE, Droster J, Kalin NH (2000) Effects of amygdala lesions on sleep in rhesus monkeys. Brain Res 879:130–138
40. Shao Y, Lei Y, Wang L, Zhai T, Jin X, Ni W et al (2014) Altered resting-state amygdala functional connectivity after 36 h of total sleep deprivation. PLoS One 9, e112222
41. Perlman G, Simmons AN, Wu J, Hahn KS, Tapert SF, Max JE et al (2012) Amygdala response and functional connectivity during emotion regulation: A study of 14 depressed adolescents. J Affect Disord 139:75–84

10

Depression and anxiety behaviour in a rat model of chronic migraine

Mingjie Zhang[1], Yufei Liu[2], Mangsuo Zhao[3], Wenjing Tang[1], Xiaolin Wang[1], Zhao Dong[1] and Shengyuan Yu[1*]

Abstract

Background: Epidemiological and clinical studies have demonstrated comorbidity between migraine and affective disorders. However, it is unclear whether chronic migraine can lead to affective disorders in other animals.

Methods: A classical chronic migraine rat model (repeated dura mater inflammatory soup [IS] infusion) was used to evaluate depression and anxiety behaviour via weight, sucrose preference test, open field test and elevated plus maze test.

Results: We found that sucrose preference, locomotor and rearing behaviours, inner zoon distance percent, open-arm entries percent and serotonin and dopamine levels in the prefrontal cortex decreased significantly in the IS group compared with those in the control group; co-administration of low-dose amitriptyline ameliorated these deficits. However, no differences in weight, inner zone time percent, or open-arm time percent between the IS and control groups. These results were used to create new depression and anxiety scales to comprehensively assess and evaluate the degree of affective disorders in rats. Most of chronic migraine animals showed depression and anxiety like behaviors but a few didn't.

Conclusions: Most of the chronic migraine rats were present depression and anxiety like behaviors. The new scales we created are expected to use in the future studies to find out the potential mechanism of affective disorders' comorbidity.

Keywords: Chronic migraine, Depression, Anxiety, Scale

Background

Epidemiological and clinical studies have demonstrated that primary headache, particularly migraine, has a bidirectional relationship with depression and anxiety [1–5]. Patients with depression have a more than three-fold relative risk of developing migraine compared with non-depressed patients. Similarly, migraineurs have a more than three-fold relative risk of developing depression compared with patients without migraine [6]. More patients with depression and anxiety suffer chronic daily headache than episodic headache, particularly those with a transformed migraine [7]. Comorbidities of depression and anxiety may increase headache frequency in migraineurs [8]. We reported previously that animals with depression (using olfactory bulbectomy or unpredictable chronic mild stress models) elicited severe nociceptive behaviours and had increased plasma levels of substance P [9, 10]. However, it is unknown whether chronic migraine can lead to affective disorders.

Several chronic migraine animal models have been proposed [11, 12]. Repeated inflammatory soup (IS) infusion on the dura mater as meningeal nociception is one of the most widely used models, as it mimics neurogenic inflammation of migraine pathophysiology. Repeated delivery of IS through a pre-implanted cannula daily induces a short-lasting (about 3-6 h) decrease and a long-lasting (>3 weeks) decrease in the facial withdrawal threshold [13]. The animals also exhibit decreased routine physical activity, increased resting behaviour, and specific ipsilateral facial grooming behaviours after IS infusion [11]. In the present study, we used this animal model to study the effects of chronic migraine on affective disorders.

* Correspondence: yusy1963@126.com
[1]Department of Neurology, Chinese PLA General Hospital, 28 Fuxing Road, Beijing 100853, People's Republic of China
Full list of author information is available at the end of the article

The Hamilton Depression Scale, Beck Depression Inventory, and Self-rated Depression Scale are used in the clinic to diagnose and evaluate the degree of depression. Recently, stagnation was used as a scale to assess the psychometric properties in the patients with chronic migraine and medication overused headache [14, 15]. The Hamilton Anxiety Scale and Self-Rating Anxiety Scale are used to evaluate the degree of anxiety. However, it is very difficult to evaluate an affective disorder in animals. Anhedonia is a core symptom of depression and is frequently tested using the sucrose preference test [16]. The open field (OF) test examines exploratory behaviour and tension state in new surroundings, and has been used as a depression and anxiety test [17]. Travel distance is representative of locomotor behaviour, and the number of times the animal stands on its hind legs represents rearing behaviour. This behaviour is similar to psychomotor retardation (decreased motor activity) on the Hamilton Depression Scale. Weight change is also a clinical feature of depression [18]. If a subject loses >2 kg in 3 d, they gain 2 points on the Hamilton Depression Scale; therefore, weight is another index parameter. Researchers use these tests to evaluate the success of establishing depression in an animal model, such as in an unpredictable chronic mild stress model [16]. Depression like behavior was also found in other animal models, but it may be slight and not easily to be discovered. An animal scale is needed to integrate all indices to evaluate the degree of depression and anxiety.

In this study, we used a rat model of chronic migraine to evaluate depression and anxiety behaviours in rats, and created scales for these affective disorders.

Methods

Ethical concerns

The experimental procedures were approved by the Committee on Animal Use for Research and Education of the Laboratory Animals Centre, General Hospital of Chinese People's Liberation Army (Beijing, PR China), and were consistent with the ethical guidelines recommended by the International Association for the Study of Pain in conscious animals [19]. Efforts were made to minimise animal suffering.

Habituation

The experiments were conducted in male Wistar rats (weight, 180–200 g) purchased from the Laboratory Animal Centre, Academy of Military Medical Science of People's Liberation Army. All rats were housed separately at a constant temperature (22–25 °C).

Animal grouping

The IS contained 0.2 mM prostaglandin E_2 and 2 mM each of histamine, serotonin, and bradykinin. The rats were divided into 4 groups: control (CON; $n = 10$); IS ($n = 10$; 1 rat died from intestinal paralysis); IS + amitriptyline (AMI) ($n = 10$); and AMI ($n = 10$). After recovery from the cannula implantation surgery, facial withdraw thresholds were recorded; the sucrose preference, OF, and elevated plus maze (EPM) tests were performed to obtain baseline measurements. We delivered 2 μL IS to the rats in the IS and the IS + AMI groups, and the same volume of saline to the rats in the AMI and CON groups through the cannula using a micro-injector for 21 d. AMI was dissolved in water and given to the rats in the IS + AMI and AMI groups (5 mg/kg, intragastric [i.g.]) [20]. The same volume of water was given to the rats in the IS and CON groups for 21 d. Pain thresholds were tested every day during the 21-d experiment, and weight and sucrose preference was measured and tested every week. The OF and EPM tests were carried out after 21 d.

Surgical procedures

A cannula was implanted as described previously by Su et al. [21]. An absolute diet was given to the rats the day before the surgery to prevent abdominal distention. The rats were anesthetised with 10% chloral hydrate (4 mL/kg, intraperitoneal [i.p.]) and placed in a stereotactic frame. A horizontal incision was made in the head and all connective tissues were removed with 3% hydrogen peroxide to expose the bregma. A drill was used for a 1-mm-diameter craniotomy (+1.5 mm after the bregma, +1.5 mm lateral), so as not to destroy the dura. A plastic cannula, with a stainless steel needle extending 1 mm from the bottom, was inserted into the hole and fixed with the help of 502 glue. A matched cap was used to close the cannula to prevent clogging. We used dental cement for further fixation, and sutured the incision. All rats received prophylactic treatment with an antibiotic (cefdinir 10 mg/kg, i.g.) for 3 d after surgery. Experiments were conducted 4 d after the surgery.

Pain threshold examination

Baseline pressure thresholds were obtained with von Frey filaments using the manufacturer's recommended force values (15, 10, 8, 6, 4, and 2 g), applied perpendicularly to the periorbital region of the rats. A positive response on the von Frey test was documented when the rat stroked its face with the ipsilateral forepaw, and the head recoiled quickly toward the side away from the stimulus, or vocalisation [13]. Facial allodynia was assessed via von Frey testing and calculated as the 50% positive response threshold.

Sucrose preference test

The sucrose preference test was performed before (baseline) and weekly after IS administration. At the start of the experiment, the animals were trained to drink a 1% sucrose solution by exposing them to sucrose instead of water for 48 h. Then, the rats received a series of sucrose preference tests, preceded by 22 h of food and water deprivation. Each animal was presented simultaneously with two weighed bottles: one contained a sucrose solution (1%) and the other contained water. The two bottles were reweighed 1 h later, and the percent preference for sucrose consumption was calculated. Sucrose preference (%) = sucrose solution consumption/(sucrose solution consumption + water consumption) × 100.

OF test

The OF test was designed to analyse locomotor and rearing behaviours of rats. The apparatus comprised a circular black base (90-cm diameter) surrounded by black walls (50 cm), as described previously [22]. The inner space was a 60-cm diameter circle; the outside space was annular and 30-cm wide outside the inner space. Illumination was provided by a 40 W bulb. On the day before (Day 0) and 15 d after the olfactory bulbectomy surgery, all rats were tested in the OF for 5 min. Total distance, inner zone distance and inner zone time were recorded by a computerized video tracking system (Ethovision 2.0; Noldus, Wagenigen, The Netherlands). Rearing behaviour (number) from the video was determined by an experimenter. The OF was wiped with a 5% alcohol solution between each test to remove olfactory cues. The percentage of inner zone time (IT%) was calculated as the time in the inner zone/300 s × 100. The inner zone distance percentage (ID%) was calculated as the inner zone distance/total distance × 100.

EPM test

The EPM test was designed to measure anxiety-like responses and was conducted in a 4-arm maze elevated 70 cm above the floor. The 2 closed arms had 22-cm-high dark walls and the 2 open arms had 0.5-cm-high edges. The angle between the arms was 90°. Illumination was provided by a 40 W bulb. The rats were placed in the centre of the apparatus facing a closed arm for 5 min. The percent of time spent in the open arm, the number of open arm entries, and the total number of arm entries were recorded by a camera mounted 1.3 m above the maze, and analysed using a computerised video tracking system (Ethovision 2.0; Noldus). Time in the open arm, time in the closed arm, open arm entries, and closed arm entries were all recorded by the computerised video tracking system. Open arm time percent (OT%) was calculated as time in the open arm/300 s × 100. Open arm entries percent (OE%) was calculated as entries into the open arm/(entries into the open arm + entries into the closed arm) × 100. These data were analysed by an experimenter blinded to the experimental treatments.

Standard depression and anxiety disorder scales

Loss of interest scores 4 points, slow movement scores 4 points, and weight loss scores 2 points on the Hamilton Depression Rating Scale. We set up a new standard scale using a highest sucrose preference score of 10 points, and a highest OF test score of 10 points (equal for locomotor and rearing behaviours). The highest score for weight change was 5 points. As anxiety indices were based on the same principle (i.e., fear of a new environment), they were given equal scores of 7 points.

The range of normal values was determined by the CON group results, as animals in this group were not exposed to pain, and they were less likely to be affected by mental disorders. The range was >5% or <5%. The CON group indices were normally distributed. High scores indicated normal behaviour and low scores indicated depression or anxiety for indices other than weight. Overweight and underweight are responses to depression; therefore, we used normal weight as the highest score, and overweight and underweight scored fewer points. The specific scale systems are shown below in Results section "Scales of depression and anxiety disorders in rats".

Biochemical analysis of the prefrontal cortex

The rats were sacrificed the day after the depression and anxiety tests. Their skulls were removed, and the prefrontal cortex was dissected and stored at −80 °C for biochemical analyses. Serotonin (5-HT) and dopamine levels were determined in the prefrontal cortex using enzyme linked immunosorbent assay (ELISA) kits (Nanjing Jiancheng Bioengineering Institute, China), according to the manufacturer's instructions (R&D Systems, Minneapolis, MN, USA). Four rats in each group were used for this assay, and each sample was run in duplicate. The prefrontal cortex was weighed and homogenised at 1 g/10 mL in phosphate buffer solution with 1 mM phenylmethylsulfonyl fluoride (PMSF) and 1 mM ethylene glycol-bis(β-aminoethyl ether)-N,N,N',N'-tetraacetic acid (EGTA). The microtiter plates (96-well flat-bottom) were gently shaken for 60 min at 37 °C with 40 μL samples diluted or 50 μL standards at concentrations of 75–1,200 ng/L 5-HT and 62.5–1,000 ng/L dopamine, 10 μL of anti-5-HT or anti-dopamine monoclonal antibody and 50 μL streptavidin-enzyme. The plates were washed 5 times with wash solution, chromogenic reagents A and B were added in turn for 10 min at 37 °C, and the stop solution was added. The hormone levels were determined in a microplate reader at an absorbance of 450 nm. The standard curve demonstrated a direct relationship between optical density and 5-HT or dopamine concentration.

Statistical analysis

SPSS 16.0 was used for data analysis. A one-way analysis of variance (ANOVA) followed by the Student–Newman–Keuls test for multiple comparisons were used to compare differences among groups. Student's t-tests were used when two groups were compared. The relationships between total anxiety and total depression scores were examined with Pearson's correlation coefficient analysis. Data are presented as means ± standard error. $P < 0.05$ was considered significant.

Results

Facial withdrawal threshold

Facial withdrawal threshold was measured the day before administration and everyday just before administration. No significant differences ($P > 0.05$, one-way ANOVA) were detected among the four groups on the first day. After administration, the thresholds decreased significantly in the IS and IS + AMI groups ($P < 0.001$ vs. CON group). Thresholds in the IS group held steady at 2 g after 1 week of administration. However, the thresholds in the IS + AMI group increased gradually and were significantly different on Day 8 ($P < 0.05$, IS vs. IS + AMI). A significant difference was detected between the IS + AMI and the AMI groups during the late half of the first week ($P < 0.001$, IS + AMI vs. AMI) and on Day 21 ($P < 0.05$, IS + AMI vs. AMI) (Fig. 1a).

Depression tests

Body weight, sucrose preference, travel distance, and number of explorations in the OF test were used to evaluate depression. Weight increased as time went on; however, no differences were found among the four groups ($P > 0.05$) (Fig. 1b, d). Sucrose preference, which reflects anhedonia, is a classical method to evaluate depression. Sucrose preference decreased in the IS group during the 21 d. A significant difference was detected between the IS and CON groups after 21 d ($P < 0.05$, IS vs. CON) (Fig. 1c, e). Locomotor and rearing behaviours can also reflect depression. The distance travelled by rats in the IS group was significantly less ($P < 0.001$, IS vs. CON) (Fig. 1f), and they explored less area ($P < 0.05$, IS vs. CON) (Fig. 1g) than rats in the CON group. AMI significantly improved locomotor ($P < 0.01$, IS vs. IS + AMI) and rearing behaviours in the IS group ($P < 0.05$, IS vs. IS + AMI), but not sucrose preference ($P > 0.05$). Administering AMI only did not affect the results ($P > 0.05$).

Anxiety tests

The ID% and IT% value on the OF test and OT% and OE% on the EPM test were used to evaluate anxiety. Anxious rats are afraid to explore and will stand in a safer place, such as the outer perimeter of the OF or the closed arm of the EPM. ID% and OE% were significantly lower in the IS group than those in the CON group ($P < 0.05$, IS vs. CON) (Fig. 1h, k). However, no differences were detected in the IT% or OT% between the CON and IS groups (Fig. 1i, j). AMI significantly improved ID% ($P < 0.01$, IS vs. IS + AMI), IT% ($P < 0.01$, IS vs. IS + AMI), and OE% ($P < 0.05$, IS vs. IS + AMI).

Depression and anxiety scales

Tables 1 and 2 show the depression and anxiety scales for rats, respectively. Fewer points indicate more depression or anxiety. Depression can lead to overweight and underweight [16]. A full score on the new scale was 5 points. Weight of 330–360 g (normal weight for 9–10-week-old rats) = 5. An increase or decrease of 10 g was −1 point for each 10 g increment. A score of 0 was given for weights <300 g or >390 g. On the sucrose preference test, a full score of 10 points was given to >95% sucrose preference; <50% was 0. Each 5% increase was 1 point. On the OF test, locomotor behaviour > 20 m was 5 points, no movement was 0; each 5-m increase was 1 point. A full score for rearing behaviour was also 5 points, >20 times was 5 points, no exploration was 0; every 5× increase was 1 point (Table 1).

A full score for the anxiety scale was 7 points. More than 30% for ID%, IT%, or OT% was scored as 7 points, and <1% was 0. Every 5% increase was 1 point. More than 45% for the OE% was a full score of 7, <1% was 0, and 1–20% was 1 point. Every 5% increase was 1 point (Table 2).

The results were similar to the primary behavioural data (Fig. 2), except IT% (Fig. 2f), which was significantly different, and open-arm entries (Fig. 2h), in which the significant difference disappeared.

Finally, we added all of the scores together. As a result, most of the IS group rats were more depressed and anxious than those in the CON group. However, not all control rats had normal emotions, and not all IS group rats were depressed or anxious. AMI was not only useful for depression, but also anxiety, if used very early in the onset of headache (Fig. 2i, j). We tested the relationship between anxiety and depression, and more depression usually indicated more anxiety. However, a few rats were only anxious or depressed (Fig. 2k).

Concentration of 5-HT and dopamine in the prefrontal cortex

5-HT and dopamine concentrations in the prefrontal cortex decreased consistently in the IS group.

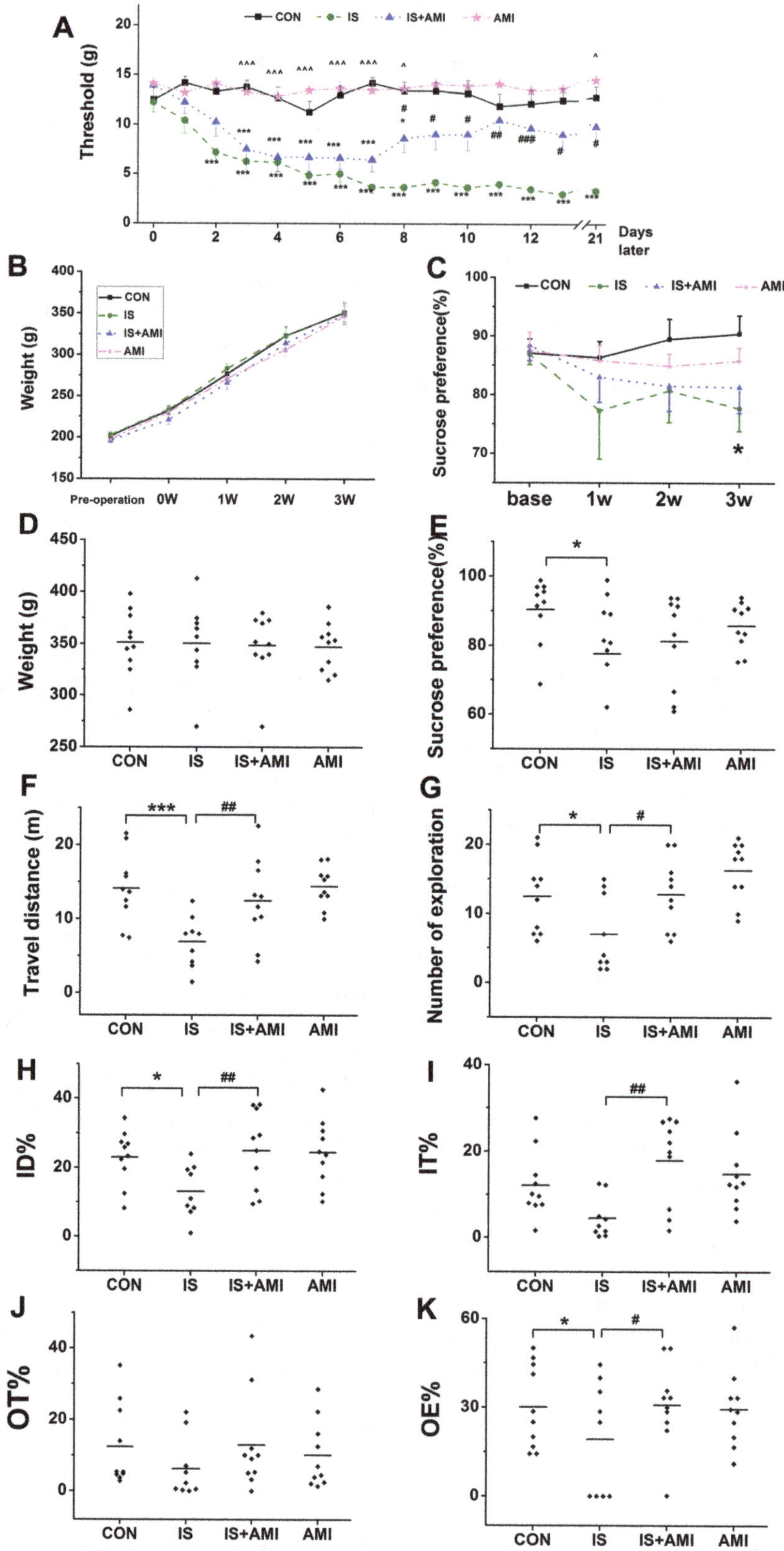

Fig. 1 (See legend on next page.)

(See figure on previous page.)
Fig. 1 Behavioural studies of allodynia, depression, and anxiety. **a**: Facial withdraw threshold. **b**–**e**: Depressive behaviours. **f**–**g**: Anxiety behaviours. **a**–**c**: The horizontal axis shows time, and the vertical axis shows the values. The facial withdraw threshold (**a**) decreased gradually in the inflammatory soup (IS) and IS + amitriptyline (AMI) groups, and was significantly different form the control (CON) group on Day 3 (***$P < 0.001$, IS and IS + AMI group vs. CON group). However, the threshold increased gradually in the IS + AMI group on Day 8 and was significantly different from the IS group (#$P < 0.05$, vs. IS group). No difference in weight was detected among the four groups (**b**, **d**) ($P > 0.05$). Sucrose preference (**c**, **e**) was significantly lower in the IS group than that in the CON group after 21 d of administration (*$P < 0.05$, IS vs. CON); no difference was found between the IS and IS + AMI groups. Travel distances (**f**), number of explorations (**g**), and inner zone distance percent (ID%) (**h**) on the open field (OF) test were all significantly lower in the IS group than those in the CON group but recovered after AMI treatment (*$P < 0.05$ and ***$P < 0.001$, IS vs. CON; #$P < 0.05$ and ##$P < 0.01$, IS vs. IS + AMI). Inner zone time percentage (**i**) tended to be lower in the IS group. Open-arm time percentage (OT%) (**j**) and entry percentage (OE%) (**k**) on the elevated plus maze test were lower in the IS group than those in the CON group; only OE% was significantly different (*$P < 0.05$, IS vs. CON; #$P < 0.05$, IS vs. IS + AMI)

Table 1 Scale of depression in rats

Depression indexes	Interval			Scores
Weight (g)		<300		1
	300 ≤		<310	2
	310 ≤		<320	3
	320 ≤		<330	4
	330 ≤		<340	5
	340 ≤		<350	5
	350 ≤		<360	5
	360 ≤		<370	4
	370 ≤		<380	3
	380 ≤		<390	2
		390≤		1
Sucrose preference (%)	50 ≤		<55	1
	55 ≤		<60	2
	60 ≤		<65	3
	65 ≤		<70	4
	70 ≤		<75	5
	75 ≤		<80	6
	80 ≤		<85	7
	85 ≤		<90	8
	90 ≤		<95	9
		95≤		10
Travel distance (m)		0		0
	0 <		<5	1
	5 ≤		<10	2
	10 ≤		<15	3
	15 ≤		<20	4
		20≤		5
Explpration number		0		0
	0 <		<5	1
	5 ≤		<10	2
	10 ≤		<15	3
	15 ≤		<20	4
		20≤		5

Table 2 Scale of anxiety in rats

Anxiety indexes	Interval			Points
Inner zone distance percent, ID%	0 ≤		<1	0
	1 ≤		<5	1
	5 ≤		<10	2
	10 ≤		<15	3
	15 ≤		<20	4
	20 ≤		<25	5
	25 ≤		<30	6
		30≤		7
Inner zone time percent, IT (%)	0 ≤		<1	0
	1 ≤		<5	1
	5 ≤		<10	2
	10 ≤		<15	3
	15 ≤		<20	4
	20 ≤		<25	5
	25 ≤		<30	6
		30≤		7
Open arm time percent, OT (%)	0 ≤		<1	0
	1 ≤		<5	1
	5 ≤		<10	2
	10 ≤		<15	3
	15 ≤		<20	4
	20 ≤		<25	5
	25 ≤		<30	6
		30≤		7
Open arm entries percent, OE (%)	0 ≤		<1	0
	1 ≤		<20	1
	20 ≤		<25	2
	25 ≤		<30	3
	30 ≤		<35	4
	35 ≤		<40	5
	40 ≤		<45	6
		45≤		7

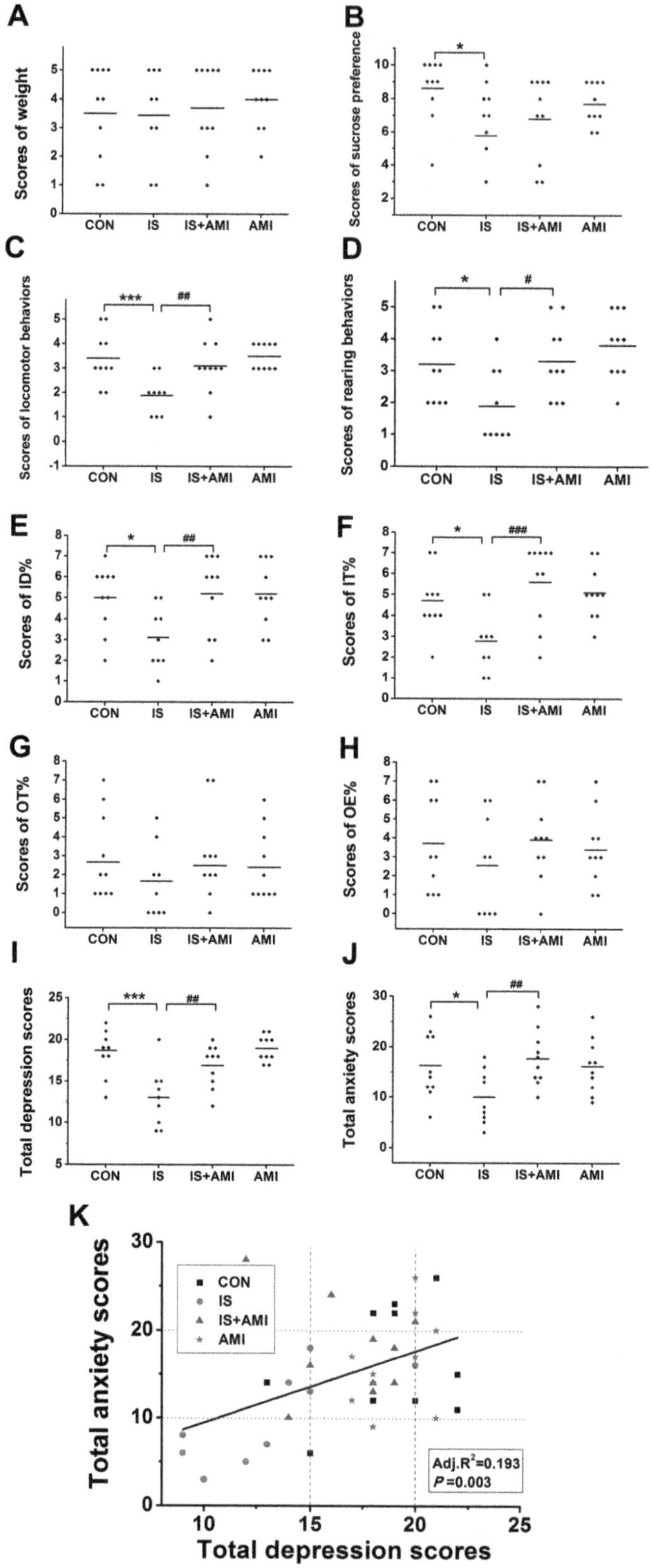

Fig. 2 (See legend on next page.)

(See figure on previous page.)

Fig. 2 Depression and anxiety scale scores. **a**–**d**: Depression-associated scores. **e**–**h**: Anxiety-associated scores. Facial withdraw threshold. **b**–**e**: Depressive behaviours. **i**: All depression scores together. **j**: All anxiety scores together. **k**: Relationship between total anxiety and total depression scores. The results were similar to the primary behavioural data, except for the inner zone time percentage (IT%) (**f**), which was significantly different, and open-arm entries (OE%) (**h**), in which the significant difference disappeared. Total depression (**i**) and anxiety scores (**j**) were significantly lower in the IS group (*$P < 0.05$, ***$P < 0.001$, IS vs. CON) but improved in the IS + AMI group (##$P < 0.01$, IS vs. IS + AMI). More depression paralleled more anxiety in most of the rats (**k**). However, a few rats had only anxiety or only depression

Repeated administration of AMI did not increase 5-HT levels; however, when AMI was used to treat pain, 5-HT and dopamine levels increased significantly (Fig. 3).

Discussion

The present study investigated whether IS leads to depression and anxiety and whether a small dose of AMI can effectively treat depression and anxiety. The results showed that IS group rats had cutaneous allodynia and were depressed and anxious. AMI was able to reverse the allodynia and decreased the occurrence of depression and anxiety.

Affective disorders

Many studies have demonstrated a relationship between migraine and mental disorders. Cohort and epidemiological studies have shown that migraineurs have a higher risk of depression compared with those having no history of headache without exception [23–25] and compared with patients having other severe headache types [26]. This indicates that headache is not the only cause of depression but also the migraine itself [26]. Ratcliffe first reported a large population-based sample investigating physician-diagnosed migraine. The results showed that a past-year migraine was significantly and positively associated with depression, dysthymia, bipolar disorder, panic attacks, panic disorder, agoraphobia, and simple phobia [adjusted odds ratios, 1.74–3.21] [5]. Anxiety differs from depression, but clinical and epidemiological surveys have confirmed that both disorders commonly occur together [27, 28]: 42.3–84.6% of patients with migraine suffer from depression and anxiety, and 66.1–85.7% of patients with anxiety suffer from migraine and depression [3]. All of these studies showed a correlation among migraine, depression, and anxiety in different races and cultural backgrounds using different research methods.

Few animal studies have evaluated the relationship between migraine and mental disorders, possibly because animal models that recapitulate the pathophysiology of migraine are scarce. In this study, we used an accepted chronic migraine IS animal model. IS was administered on the dura matter and caused an instant transient reduction in the pain threshold that lasted approximately 3-6 h. Chronic IS exposure for more than 1 week can lead to a persistently reduced pain threshold [13]. This animal model is reproducible [11]; we used it to demonstrate the relationship between migraine and affective disorders.

Our results showed that rats with chronic migraine were more depressed and showed particularly less locomotor behaviour. Sucrose preference and rearing behaviours were also significantly different compared with those of the control rats. The rats with chronic migraine

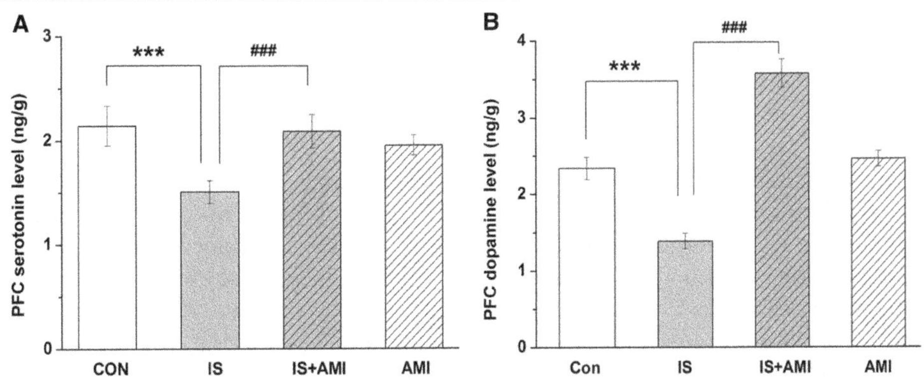

Fig 3 Concentrations of serotonin (**a**) and dopamine (**b**) in the prefrontal cortex measured by ELISA. 5-HT and dopamine concentrations were significantly lower in the IS group than those in the CON and IS + AMI groups in the prefrontal cortex. No differences were found between the CON and AMI groups (***$P < 0.001$, IS vs. CON; ###$P < 0.001$, groups IS vs. IS + AMI.)

were more anxious, as demonstrated by in the IT% and OE% but not the time percentages of the two tests. In addition, concentrations of 5-HT and dopamine in the prefrontal cortex were significantly lower in the IS group than those in the control group. These results are consistent with clinical studies, indicating that this chronic migraine animal model fits the phenotype and can be used to elucidate the molecular mechanism of depression due to chronic migraine. The forced swim test is widely used to assess depression and antidepressant activity. However, we did not use this test because it can lead to depression and may affect the results of other tests.

The scales developed for rats in the present study showed that depression and anxiety were positively correlated. Depression and anxiety are two classes of psychiatric disease. Major depressive disorder is a mood disorder that can be coupled with mania, whereas anxiety is a normal physiological phenomenon; too much anxiety leads to generalised anxiety disorder or panic disorder. Clinical and epidemiological studies have reported that depression and anxiety often co-occur. More than 75% of patients with a depressive disorder also suffer from an anxiety disorder [29]. These comorbidities lead to severe symptoms and increase suicide risk [30]. Most of the rats with chronic headache in the present study suffered from depression and anxiety. A linear relationship was found between the total depression score and the total anxiety score. Rats with a total depression score < 15 points also had <10 points on the total anxiety score, and they were always IS group rats. Rats whose total depression score was >20 points also scored >10 points on the total anxiety score, and they were always from the CON and AMI groups. The comorbidity ratio in these rats was similar to that of patients, which verified the rational and feasibility of our scales.

The risk factors for comorbid depression and anxiety may be related with headache frequency and sex distribution. We plan to change the dosage and frequency of IS and use different sexes of rats to explore the aetiology of this comorbidity.

Effect of low-dosage AMI

AMI is a tricyclic antidepressant that has been widely used for half a century. It has not only been used to treat depression but also to relieve chronic pain, including diabetic peripheral neuropathy, post herpetic neuralgia, fibromyalgia, and migraine. Early research suggested that AMI blocks reuptake of 5-HT and norepinephrine (NE) in the synaptic cleft, which effectively increases their concentrations. The onset time was about 1 month, and the dosage used was 100–300 mg/d. AMI also acts quicker on ion channels by blocking both tetrodotoxin-sensitive (TTX-s) and TTX-resistant (TTX-R) Na + currents in the dorsal root ganglion [31]. It also blocks TTX-s Nav1.4 current in gene-transfected HEK293T [32] and TTX-R Na + channels in trigeminal ganglion neurons (TG) [33]. Our team reported previously that AMI blocks the TTX-R Nav1.8 and TTX-R Nav1.9 current in TG [34, 35].

In the present study, 5-HT concentration in the cortex did not increase after 21 d of AMI administration alone, perhaps because the effect of blocking reuptake didn't occur within 3 weeks. However, 5-HT and DA concentrations did increase when AMI and IS were co-administered compared with IS alone. This result may be due to an indirect effect of relieving pain first, and then reducing depression and increasing 5-HT and DA concentrations. Next, we wanted to demonstrate and observe nociceptive behaviour immediately after AMI administration. However, the rats were sleepy and were less active after being given the AMI; therefore, it was very difficult to distinguish whether the decrease in nociceptive behaviour was caused by being pain-free or sleepy.

Depression and anxiety disorder scales

Many indices have been used to evaluate affective disorders in animals; however, some studies have shown that some of these indices are significantly different, whereas others are not. All kinds of scales are used to evaluate disorders clinically and can also be used to evaluate animals. The most interesting finding of the present study was that not all IS rats developed depression or anxiety. All data mean something, even outliers. Therefore, a future study is necessary to find out the reason.

Limitations

The present study has some limitations. First, female animals didn't contain in this study, but it may relate to migraine and affective disorders, so female rats would be added in future studies. Second, the scales was not wide application and needed to be confirmed. Lastly, the present study only found out the behaviors and the mechanism need to be study in the future.

Conclusions

The present study evaluated the depression and anxiety behaviors on a chronic migraine animal model and the therapeutic effects of low-dose amitriptyline. Most of the chronic migraine rats were present depression and anxiety like behaviors, but not all. We used new scales of depression and anxiety to comprehensively assess and wanted to find out the differences between depression and non-depression rats in the chronic migraine in the future study.

Abbreviations
5-HT: serotonin; AMI: amitriptyline; CON: control; EPM: elevated plus maze; ID%: inner zone distance percent; IS: inflammatory soup; IT%: inner zone time percent; OE%: open arm entries percent; OF: open field; OT%: open arm time percent

Acknowledgements
This work was supported by the National Natural Science Foundation of China (grants 81600952, 81471147, 81671077, 81471146, 81500966 and 81500943), Beijing Science and Technology Project (grant Z161100002616013), the Capital Development Scientific Research (grant 2014-4-5013) and Beijing Natural Science Foundation (grants 7162178 and 7164268). We are grateful to Professor Zhuo Yang and other people in the Laboratory of Neurophysiology, School of Medicine, Nankai University for direction of behavior tests.

Authors' contributions
Category 1: (a) Conception and Design: SYY, MJZ; (b) Acquisition of Data: MJZ, YFL, MSZ. (c) Analysis and Interpretation of Data: WJT, XLW, ZD. Category 2: (a) Drafting the Article: MJZ. (b) Revising it for Intellectual Content: SYY, WJT. All authors read and approved the final manuscript.

Competing interests
The authors declare that they have no competing interests.

Author details
[1]Department of Neurology, Chinese PLA General Hospital, 28 Fuxing Road, Beijing 100853, People's Republic of China. [2]Department of Neurology, Tianjin Third Center Hospital, Tianjin 300170, People's Republic of China. [3]Department of Neurology, Yuquan Hospital, Medical Center, Tsinghua University, Beijing 100049, People's Republic of China.

References
1. Beghi E, Bussone G, D'Amico D, Cortelli P, Cevoli S, Manzoni GC, Torelli P, Tonini MC, Allais G, De Simone R, D'Onofrio F, Genco S, Moschiano F, Beghi M, Salvi S (2010) Headache, anxiety and depressive disorders: the HADAS study. J Headache Pain 11(2):141–50
2. Breslau N, Schultz LR, Stewart WF, Lipton RB, Lucia VC, Welch KM (2000) Headache and major depression: is the association specific to migraine? Neurology 54(2):308–13
3. Jette N, Patten S, Williams J, Becker W, Wiebe S (2008) Comorbidity of migraine and psychiatric disorders–a national population-based study. Headache 48(4):501–16
4. Lanteri-Minet M, Radat F, Chautard MH, Lucas C (2005) Anxiety and depression associated with migraine: influence on migraine subjects' disability and quality of life, and acute migraine management. Pain 118(3):319–26
5. Ratcliffe GE, Enns MW, Jacobi F, Belik SL, Sareen J (2009) The relationship between migraine and mental disorders in a population-based sample. Gen Hosp Psychiatry 31(1):14–9
6. Torelli P, D'Amico D (2004) An updated review of migraine and co-morbid psychiatric disorders. Neurol Sci 25(Suppl 3):S234–5
7. Juang KD, Wang SJ, Fuh JL, Lu SR, Su TP (2000) Comorbidity of depressive and anxiety disorders in chronic daily headache and its subtypes. Headache 40(10):818–23
8. Oh K, Cho SJ, Chung YK, Kim JM, Chu MK (2014) Combination of anxiety and depression is associated with an increased headache frequency in migraineurs: a population-based study. BMC Neurol 14:238
9. Zhang M, Dai W, Liang J, Chen X, Hu Y, Chu B, Pan M, Dong Z, Yu S (2013) Effects of UCMS-induced depression on nociceptive behaviors induced by electrical stimulation of the dura mater. Neurosci Lett 551:1–6
10. Liang J, Yu S, Dong Z, Wang X, Liu R, Chen X, Li Z (2011) The effects of OB-induced depression on nociceptive behaviors induced by electrical stimulation of the dura mater surrounding the superior sagittal sinus. Brain Res 1424:9–19
11. Melo-Carrillo A, Lopez-Avila A (2013) A chronic animal model of migraine, induced by repeated meningeal nociception, characterized by a behavioral and pharmacological approach. Cephalalgia 33(13):1096–105
12. Pradhan AA, Smith ML, McGuire B, Tarash I, Evans CJ, Charles A (2014) Characterization of a novel model of chronic migraine. Pain 155(2):269–74
13. Oshinsky ML, Gomonchareonsiri S (2007) Episodic dural stimulation in awake rats: a model for recurrent headache. Headache 47(7):1026–36
14. Innamorati M, Pompili M, Erbuto D, Ricci F, Migliorati M, Lamis DA, Amore M, Girardi P, Martelletti P (2015) Psychometric properties of the stagnation scale in medication overuse headache patients. J Headache Pain 16:1052
15. Innamorati M, Pompili M, Fiorillo M, Lala N, Negro A, Del Bono SD, Lester D, Girardi P, Martelletti P (2013) Overattachment and perceived disability in chronic migraineurs. Clin Neurol Neurosurg 115(7):954–8
16. Willner P (2005) Chronic mild stress (CMS) revisited: consistency and behavioural-neurobiological concordance in the effects of CMS. Neuropsychobiology 52(2):90–110
17. Mattioli L, Funari C, Perfumi M (2009) Effects of Rhodiola rosea L. extract on behavioural and physiological alterations induced by chronic mild stress in female rats. J Psychopharmacol 23(2):130–42
18. Gibson-Smith D, Bot M, Milaneschi Y, Twisk JW, Visser M, Brouwer IA, Penninx BW (2016) Major depressive disorder, antidepressant use, and subsequent 2-year weight change patterns in the Netherlands Study of Depression and Anxiety. J Clin Psychiatry 77(2):e144–51
19. Zimmermann M (1983) Ethical guidelines for investigations of experimental pain in conscious animals. Pain 16(2):109–10
20. Pringsheim T, Diksic M, Dobson C, Nguyen K, Hamel E (2003) Selective decrease in serotonin synthesis rate in rat brainstem raphe nuclei following chronic administration of low doses of amitriptyline: an effect compatible with an anti-migraine effect. Cephalalgia 23(5):367–75
21. Su M, Ran Y, Han X, Liu Y, Zhang X, Tan Q, Li R, Yu S (2016) Rizatriptan overuse promotes hyperalgesia induced by dural inflammatory stimulation in rats by modulation of the serotonin system. Eur J Neurosci 44(4):2129–38
22. Wang W, Qi WJ, Xu Y, Wang JY, Luo F (2010) The differential effects of depression on evoked and spontaneous pain behaviors in olfactory bulbectomized rats. Neurosci Lett 472(2):143–7
23. Radat F, Swendsen J (2005) Psychiatric comorbidity in migraine: a review. Cephalalgia 25(3):165–78
24. Antonaci F, Nappi G, Galli F, Manzoni GC, Calabresi P, Costa A (2011) Migraine and psychiatric comorbidity: a review of clinical findings. J Headache Pain 12(2):115–25
25. Lipton RB, Hamelsky SW, Kolodner KB, Steiner TJ, Stewart WF (2000) Migraine, quality of life, and depression: a population-based case-control study. Neurology 55(5):629–35
26. Breslau N, Lipton RB, Stewart WF, Schultz LR, Welch KM (2003) Comorbidity of migraine and depression: investigating potential etiology and prognosis. Neurology 60(8):1308–12
27. McWilliams LA, Goodwin RD, Cox BJ (2004) Depression and anxiety associated with three pain conditions: results from a nationally representative sample. Pain 111(1-2):77–83
28. Schoevers RA, Beekman AT, Deeg DJ, Jonker C, van Tilburg W (2003) Comorbidity and risk-patterns of depression, generalised anxiety disorder and mixed anxiety-depression in later life: results from the AMSTEL study. Int J Geriatr Psychiatry 18(11):994–1001
29. Hirschfeld RM (2001) The Comorbidity of Major Depression and Anxiety Disorders: Recognition and Management in Primary Care. Prim Care Companion J Clin Psychiatry 3(6):244–254
30. Cyranowski JM, Schott LL, Kravitz HM, Brown C, Thurston RC, Joffe H, Matthews KA, Bromberger JT (2012) Psychosocial features associated with lifetime comorbidity of major depression and anxiety disorders among a community sample of mid-life women: the SWAN mental health study. Depress Anxiety 29(12):1050–7
31. Song JH, Ham SS, Shin YK, Lee CS (2000) Amitriptyline modulation of Na(+) channels in rat dorsal root ganglion neurons. Eur J Pharmacol 401(3):297–305
32. Wang GK, Russell C, Wang SY (2004) State-dependent block of voltage-gated Na + channels by amitriptyline via the local anesthetic receptor and its implication for neuropathic pain. Pain 110(1-2):166–74
33. Hur YK, Choi IS, Cho JH, Park EJ, Choi JK, Choi BJ, Jang IS (2008) Effects of carbamazepine and amitriptyline on tetrodotoxinresistant Na + channels in immature rat trigeminal ganglion neurons. Arch Pharm Res 31(2):178–82
34. Liang J, Liu X, Pan M, Dai W, Dong Z, Wang X, Liu R, Zheng J, Yu S (2014) Blockade of Nav1.8 currents in nociceptive trigeminal neurons contributes to anti-trigeminovascular nociceptive effect of amitriptyline. Neuromolecular Med 16(2):308–21
35. Liang J, Liu X, Zheng J, Yu S (2013) Effect of amitriptyline on tetrodotoxin-resistant Nav1.9 currents in nociceptive trigeminal neurons. Mol Pain 9:31

11

Disrupted functional connectivity of periaqueductal gray subregions in episodic migraine

Zhiye Chen[1,2,3], Xiaoyan Chen[2], Mengqi Liu[1,3], Shuangfeng Liu[1], Lin Ma[1*] and Shengyuan Yu[2*]

Abstract

Background: The periaqueductal gray (PAG) dysfunction was recognized in migraine, and the altered dysfunction of PAG subregions were not totally detected up to now. The aim of this study is to investigate the altered functional connectivity of PAG subregions in EM patients.

Methods: The brain structural images and resting state functional MR imaging (rs-fMRI) data were obtained from 18 normal controls (NC) and 18 EM patients on 3.0 T MR system. Seven subregions of PAG were classified as bilateral ventrolateral PAG (vlPAG), lateral PAG (lPAG), dorsolateral PAG (dlPAG) and dorsomedial PAG (dmPAG). The functional connectivity maps of each PAG subregion were calculated, and Two sample *t*-test was applied with age and sex as covariables.

Results: Bilateral vlPAG and left dlPAG presented decreased functional connectivity, and the other subregions (bilateral lPAGs, right dlPAG and dmPAG) showed no significant altered functional connectivity in EM compared with NC. The brain regions with decreased functional connectivity mainly located in bilateral prefrontal cortex(PFC), middle temporal gyrus, primary motor area (PMA) and supplementary motor area (SMA) and right ventrolateral PFC (vlPFC) in EM patients in this study. Disease duration was positively related to the functional connectivity of bilateral vlPAG on the bilateral thalamus and putamen, left pallidum and right medial orbitofrontal gyrus in EM patients.

Conclusion: The present study suggested that the dysfunction of bilateral vlPAG and left dlPAG presented in EM, and functional evaluation of PAG subregions may be help for the diagnosis and understanding of EM pathogenesis.

Keywords: Episodic migraine, Functional connectivity, Magnetic resonance imaging, Periaqueductal gray, Resting-state functional MRI

Background

Periaqueductal gray (PAG) was a center with powerful descending antinociceptive neuronal network [1, 2], and the dysfunction in migraine [3] may be considered as a possible "generator" of migraine attacks [1, 4, 5]. Current studies [6, 7] supported that PAG network participated in the migraine, which may impair the descending pain modulatory. In episodic migraine (EM) paitents, it had been detected for the nonspecific PAG lesions on T2WI [8], impaired iron homeostasis of PAG [1], and increased mean kurtosis and mean diffusivity on diffusion kurtosis imaging [9].

PAG is a small mesencephalic brain structure, and the different subregions may present different specific function. Existing concepts recognized that the anatomical organization of PAG mainly included seven parts: bilateral ventrolateral PAG (vlPAG), bilateral lateral PAG (lPAG), bilateral dorsolateral PAG (dlPAG) and dorsomedial PAG (dmPAG), and PAG connections could also be identified by diffusion tractography and functional connectivity in mammals [10].

The previous document [11] demonstrated that the vlPAG was functionally connected to brain regions associated with descending pain modulation (anterior cingulate cortex (ACC), upper pons/medulla), lPAG and dlPAG

* Correspondence: cjr.malin@vip.163.com; yusy1963@126.com
[1]Department of Radiology, Chinese PLA General Hospital, 28 Fuxing Road, Beijing 100853, China
[2]Department of Neurology, Chinese PLA General Hospital, 28 Fuxing Road, Beijing 100853, China
Full list of author information is available at the end of the article

were connected to brain regions with executive functions (prefrontal cortex, striatum, hippocampus). However, the precise neuromechanism of PAG subregions in the descending pain modulatory system [7] in migraine is not clear.

To investigate the descending pain modulatory circuitry of PAG subregions in migraine, we hypothesize that PAG subregions present different functional connectivity patterns in migraine. To address this hypothesis, we prospectively obtained high resolution structural images and resting state functional MR imaging (rs-fMRI) from 18 EM patients and 18 age- and sex-matched normal controls at first. Secondly, the seed points of PAG subregions were defined, and the functional connectivity was computed. Last, analysis of covariance was performed with age and sex as covariates, and voxel-based correlation was also applied between the functional connectivity of PAG subregions and the clinical variables.

Methods

Subjects

Written informed consent was obtained from all participants according to the approval of the ethics committee of the local institutional review board. Eighteen EM patients (15 EM patients without aura and 3 EM patients with aura) were recruited from the International Headache Center, Department of Neurology, Chinese PLA General Hospital from 2014 to 2015. All the following inclusion criteria should be fulfilled: 1) EM is defined as migraine attack days being less than 15 days per month. The definition of migraine refers to 1.1 Migraine without aura and 1.2 Migraine with aura in (ICHD-III beta) [12]; 2) no migraine preventive medication used in the past 3 months; 3) absence of any chronic disorders, including hypertension, hypercholesterolemia, diabetes mellitus, cardiovascular diseases, cerebrovascular disorders, neoplastic diseases, infectious diseases, connective tissue diseases, other subtypes of headache, chronic pain other than headache, severe anxiety or depression preceding the onset of headache, psychiatric diseases, etc.; 4) absence of alcohol, nicotine, or other substance abuse. Eighteen NCs were recruited from the hospital's staff and their relatives. Inclusion criteria were similar to those of patients, except for the first two items. NCs should never have had any primary headache disorders or other types of headache in the past year. The exclusion criteria were the following: cranium trauma, illness interfering with central nervous system function, psychotic disorder, and regular use of a psychoactive or hormone medication. The anxiety, depression, and cognitive function of all the participants were evaluated with the Hamilton Anxiety Scale (HAMA) [13], the Hamilton Depression Scale (HAMD) [14], and the Montreal Cognitive Assessment (MoCA) Beijing Version (http://www.mocatest.org). All the patients were given with the Visual Analogue Scale (VAS) and the Migraine Disability Assessment Scale (MIDAS). MRI scans were taken in the interictal stage at least 3 days after a migraine attack for EM patients. All the subjects were right-handed and underwent conventional MRI examination to exclude the subjects with cerebral infarction, malacia, or occupying lesions. Alcohol, nicotine, caffeine, and other substances were avoided for at least 12 h before MRI examination.

MRI acquisition

Images were acquired on a GE 3.0 T MR system (DISCOVERY MR750, GE Healthcare, Milwaukee, WI, USA) and a conventional eight-channel quadrature head coil was used. All subjects were instructed to lie in a supine position, and formed padding was used to limit head movement. Conventional T2weighted image (TR = 5000 ms, TE = 113.4 ms, FOV = 24 cm × 24 cm, Matrix = 384 × 384) and T1-FLAIR (TR = 2040 ms, TE = 6.9 ms, FOV = 24 cm × 24 cm, Matrix = 384 × 256) were obtained first. Then, the rs-fMRI was performed, during which subjects were instructed to relax, keep their eyes closed, stay awake, remain still, and clear their heads of all thoughts. Functional images were obtained using a gradient echo-planar imaging (EPI) sequence (TR = 2000 ms, TE = 30 ms, flip angle = 90, slice thickness = 3 mm, slice gap = 1 mm, FOV = 24 cm × 24 cm, Matrix = 64 × 64), and 180 continuous EPI functional volumes were acquired axially over 6 min. Finally, a high resolution three-dimensional T1-weighted fast spoiled gradient recalled echo (3D T1-FSPGR) sequence was performed, which generated 360 contiguous axial slices [TR (repetition time) = 6.3 ms, TE (echo time) = 2.8 ms, flip angle = 15°, FOV (field of view) = 25.6 cm × 25.6 cm, Matrix = 256 × 256, slice thickness = 1 mm]. None of the subjects complained of any discomfort or fell asleep during scanning. No obvious structural damage was observed based on the conventional MR images.

MR image processing

All MR structural and functional images were processed using Statistical Parametric Mapping 12 (SPM12) (http://www.fil.ion.ucl.ac.uk/spm) and the rs-fMRI data analysis toolkit (REST v1.8) [15] running under MATLAB 7.6 (The Mathworks, Natick, MA, USA). The data preprocessing was carried out as follows: (1) The first ten volumes of each functional time course was discarded to allow for T1 equilibrium and the participants to adapt; (2) Slice timing; (3) Head motion correction; (4) Spatial normalization. These steps were performed by SPM12. No subjects had head motion with more than 1.5 mm displacement in X, Y, and Z direction or 1.50 of any angular motion throughout the course of the scanning. The linear trend removal and temporal band-pass filtering (0.01–0.08 Hz) was performed by REST [15].

The functional connectivity analysis was performed as follows: (1) Spatial smooth (full width at half maximum (FWHM) = 6 mm) using SPM8; (2) The subregions of PAG were classified as seven seeds based on the previous studies [6, 10, 16–19]: 1) left ventrolateral PAG (l_vlPAG)(MNI coordinates: l_vlPAG = –4; –26; –14 with 2 mm radius); 2) right ventrolateral PAG(r_vlPAG) (MNI coordinates: r_vlPAG = 4; –26; –14 with 2 mm radius); 3) left lateral PAG(l_lPAG) (MNI coordinates: l_lPAG = –3; –28; –10 with 2 mm radius); 4) right lateral PAG (r_lPAG) (MNI coordinates: r_lPAG = 3; –28; –10 with 2 mm radius); 5) left dorsolateral PAG(l_dlPAG) (MNI coordinates: l_dlPAG = –3; –30; –6 with 2 mm radius); 6) right dorsolateral PAG (r_dlPAG) (MNI coordinates: l_dlPAG = 3; –30; –6 with 2 mm radius); 7) dorsomeidal PAG (dmPAG) (MNI coordinates: dmPAG = 0; –30; –6 with 2 mm radius) (Fig. 1); (3) Functional connectivity computation of the seven subregions of PAG were performed using REST (v1.8). The time courses of subregions of PAG were extracted, and Pearson's correlations were used to calculate the functional connectivity between the extracted time courses and the averaged time courses of the whole brain in a voxel-wise manner. The white matter, cerebrospinal fluid (CSF), and the six head motion parameters were used as covariates. (4) The individual r-maps were normalized to Zmaps using Fisher's Z-transformation.

Statistical analysis

An independent sample *t*-test was applied to the comparison of the age, HAMA, HAMD and MoCA score between NC and EM group. Significant difference was set at a *P* value of < 0.05. The statistical analysis was performed using SPSS 19.0. Two-sample t-tes was performed to identify the regions with significant differences in connectivity to subregions of PAG, covarying for age and sex, and significance was set at a *P* value of <0.001 without correction. Voxel-based correlation analysis was performed using multiple regression model, and significance was set a *P* value of < 0.05 with FDR correction. The minimal number of contiguous voxels was set based on the expected voxels per cluster. The statistical analysis was performed by SPM 12 software.

Results

Demography and neuropsychological test

Eighteen EM patients (F/M = 14/4) and 18 NCs (F/M = 14/4) were enrolled. There was no significant difference for age between EM (33.39 ± 10.69 years old) and CM (39.11 ± 9.99 years old). There was a significant difference for HAMA between NC(9.67 ± 3.16) and EM (15.67 ± 9.85), HAMD between NC(10.89 ± 7.26) and EM(15.89 ± 2.89) and MoCA between NC (27.00 ± 2.46) and EM (29.17 ± 1.47) ($P < 0.05$)(Table 1).

Comparison of the functional connectivity of the subregions of PAG between NC and EM

Table 2 demonstrated that only right vlPAG, left vlPAG and left dlPAG presented decreased functional connectivity in EM compared with NC, and the other subregions (bilateral lPAGs, right dlPAG and dmPAG) showed no significant altered functional connectivity in EM compared with NC.

The decreased functional connectivity of right vlPAG located in left precentral gyrus (Fig. 2), and the decreased functional connectivity of left vlPAG located in left precentral gyrus, left middle frontal gyrus, left inferior parietal gyrus, bilateral middle temporal gyrus, right superior frontal gyrus and right supplementary motor area (Fig. 3). Figure 4 revealed that the decreased

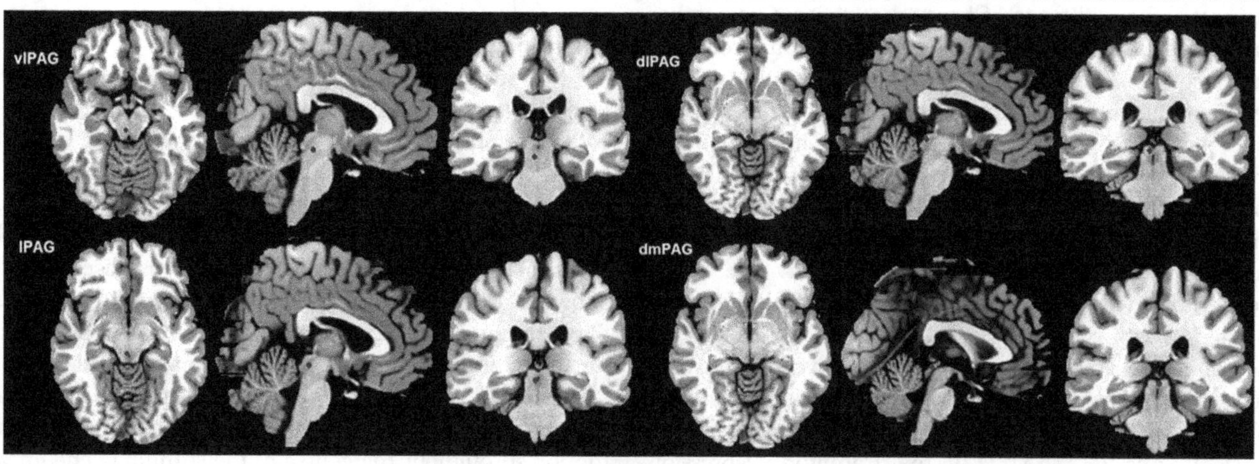

Fig. 1 The seed points of the subregions of PAG. right vlPAG, MNI coordinate:[4–26 -14] with 2 mm radius; right lPAG, MNI coordinate: [3–28 -10] with 2 mm radius; right dlPAG, MNI coordinate: [3–30 -6] with 2 mm radius; dmPAG, MNI coordinate: [0–30 -6] with 2 mm radius

Table 1 The clinical characteristics of normal controls and EM patients

	EM	NC
Num(F/M)	18(14/4)	18(14/4)
Age	33.39 ± 10.69	39.11 ± 9.99
HAMA	15.67 ± 9.85	9.67 ± 3.16
HAMD	15.89 ± 2.89	10.89 ± 7.26
MoCA	29.17 ± 1.47	27.00 ± 2.46
DD(yrs)	12.44 ± 8.07	NA
VAS	8.33 ± 1.50	NA
MIDAS	16 ± 17.94	NA

EM episodic migraine, *NC* normal control, *HAMA* hamilton anxiety scale, *HAMD* hamilton depression scale, *MoCA* montreal cognitive assessment, *DD* disease duration, *VAS* visual analogue scale, *MIDAS* migraine disability assessment questionnaire, *NA* not available

functional connectivity of left dlPAG located in the right parts triangularis of inferior frontal gyrus and medial superior frontal gyrus.

Correlation analysis between the functional connectivity of the bilateral vlPAG and left dlPAG and the clinical variables

Only disease duration was positively related with the functional connectivity of bilateral vlPAG, and the other clinical variables showed no significant correlation with the functional connectivity of vlPAG (Table 3). Figure 5 demonstrated that the brain regions with positive correlation located in bilateral thalamus and left pallidum between the functional connectivity of left vlPAG and disease duration in EM patients. The brain regions with positive correlation with disease duration located in bilateral thalamus, putamen, and right medial orbitofrontal gyrus for the functional connectivity of right vlPAG

Table 2 The brain regions with altered functional connectivity of PAG over the whole brain between EM and NC

Group	BA	Anatomic region	MNI-space			Cluster size	P_{uncorr}	Peak T value
			X	Y	Z			
Right_vlPAG								
NC > EM	BA6	Precentral_L	−21	−15	60	14	0.000	4.53
NC < EM		NA	NA	NA	NA	NA		NA
Left_vlPAG								
NC > EM	BA21	Temporal_Mid_R	48	−42	3	13	0.000	4.86
	BA6	Precentral_L	−36	−9	39	20	0.000	4.26
	BA6	Frontal_Sup_R	21	−9	66	24	0.000	3.9
	BA6	Supp_Motor_Area_R	3	12	63	12	0.000	4.16
	BA21	Temporal_Mid_L	−54	−51	9	12	0.000	4.16
	BA46	Frontal_Sup_R	27	48	12	15	0.000	4.14
	BA40	Parietal_Inf_L	−36	−39	42	17	0.000	4.09
	BA46	Frontal_Mid_L	−30	45	21	20	0.000	3.97
NC < EM		NA	NA	NA	NA	NA		NA
Right_lPAG								
NC > EM		NA	NA	NA	NA	NA		NA
NC < EM		NA	NA	NA	NA	NA		NA
Left_lPAG								
NC > EM		NA	NA	NA	NA	NA		NA
NC < EM		NA	NA	NA	NA	NA		NA
Right_dlPAG								
NC > EM		NA	NA	NA	NA	NA		NA
NC < EM		NA	NA	NA	NA	NA		NA
Left_dlPAG								
NC > EM	BA45	Frontal_Inf_Tri_R	48	27	9	12		5.14
	BA8	Frontal_Sup_Medial_R	6	27	57	14		5.13
NC < EM		NA	NA	NA	NA	NA		NA
dmPAG								
NC > EM		NA	NA	NA	NA	NA		NA
NC < EM		NA	NA	NA	NA	NA		NA

NC normal control, *EM* episodic migraine, *vlPAG* ventrolateral PAG, *lPAG* lateral PAG, *dlPAG* dorsolateral PAG, *dmPAG* dorsomedial PAG

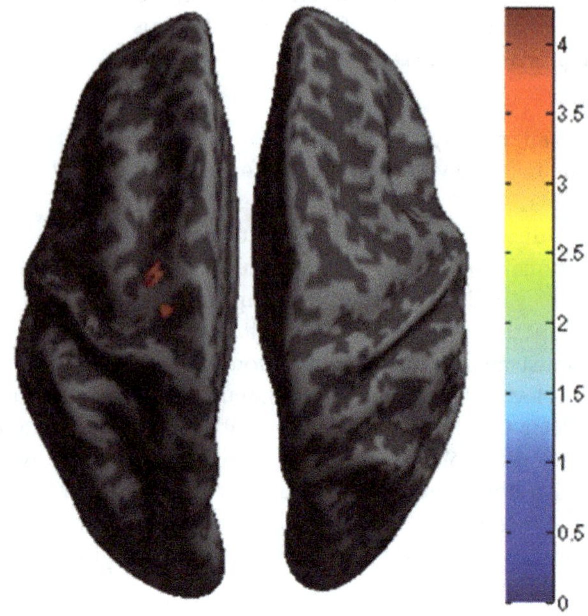

Fig. 2 The decreased functional connectivity of right ventrolateral PAG in EM compared with NC

(Fig. 6). There was no significant correlation between the functional connectivity of left dlPAG and the clinical variables.

Discussion

This study demonstrated that bilateral vlPAG and left dlPAG may play a role in the descending pain modulatory circuit in EM patients, and the other PAG subregions did not show significant altered functional connectivity in EM. This altered functional connectivity pattern established a concept that PAG subregion analysis may be adapted to the investigation of the pain modulatory in EM while not a whole PAG region analysis. Based on the anatomical organization of PAG, different PAG subregions had different cytoarchitecture and neural connections, therefore, different PAG subregions presented different physiological function [20, 21], which may be used to explain the altered functional connectivity of some selected PAG subregions.

In this study, bilateral vlPAG dysfunction were involved with the disrupted functional connectivity in EM patients, especially presented the left predominance. It was known that PAG contains neural circuits that participate in descending antinociception [22], and vlPAG release the antinociceptive peptides Met-enkephalin and neurotensin, which were released when nociception occurred and would result in greater sensitivity of PAG enkephalinergic neurons and greater excitability of the descending PAG output neurons that are responsible for antinociception [23]. The output of vlPAG neurons could also be influenced by GABA recptors, and would disrupt the descending pain control system to spinal dorsal horn in a rat experiments [24]. Furthermore, PAG regions receive the projection from spinothalamic tract via the spinomesencephalic tract to transmit the ascending pain and temperature information [25]. Therefore, vlPAG dysfunction may be considered as an important targeted impaired PAG subregion in EM patients.

In this study, right vlPAG only presented the decreased functional connectivity with left precentral gyrus (BA6, premotor cortex), and left vlPAG showed the decreased functional connectivity with left precentral gyrus, right superior frontal gyrus (BA6, premotor cortex, PMC) and right supplementary motor area (SMA). The decreased functional connectivity between motor cortex and PAG was also demonstrated in fibromyalgia patients [26], which

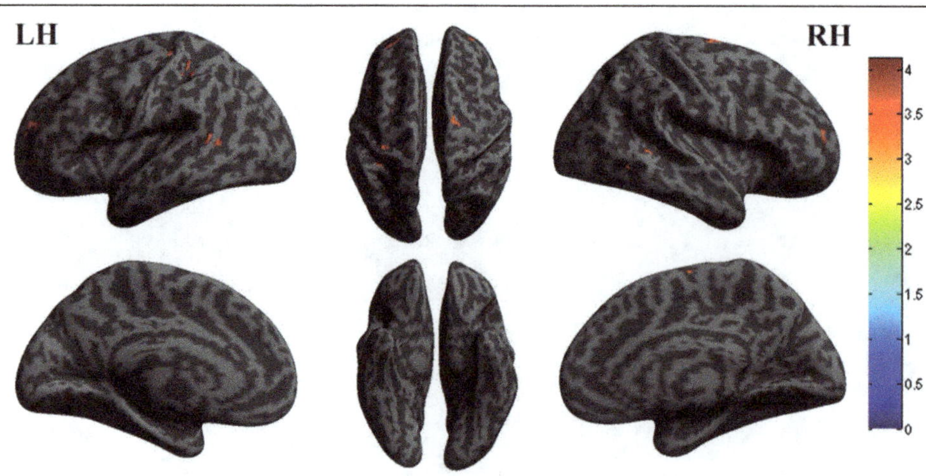

Fig. 3 The decreased functional connectivity of left ventrolateral PAG in EM compared with NC

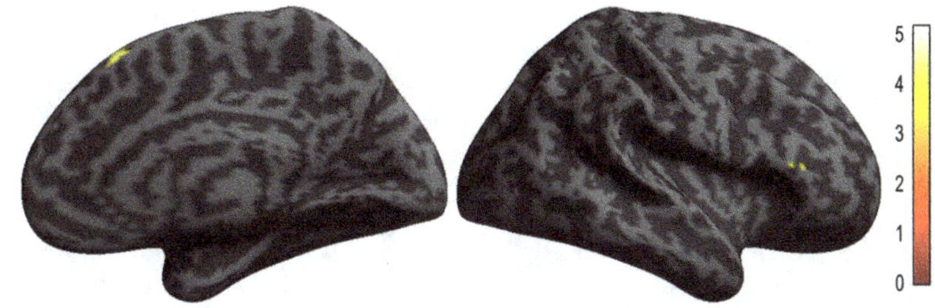

Fig. 4 The decreased functional connectivity of left dorsolateral PAG in EM compared with NC

was also demonstrated in this study and it suggested that vlPAG dysfunction manifested as decreased contralateral functional output from premotor and SMA, and the neuromechanism should further be elucidated.

Left vlPAG presented the decreased functional connectivity with bilateral mid-dorsolateral prefrontal cortex (dlPFC) (BA46) and left dlPAG presented the decreased functional connectivity with right posterior dlPFC (BA8) based on the functional parcellation of PFC. dlPFC mainly lies in the middle frontal gyrus, and it is connected to multiple brain regions, thalamus, basal ganglia and hippocampus, and its function included working memory [27], cognitive flexibility [28], planning [29] and emotion [30]. Although previous document confirmed that PFC dysfunction may be impaired in migraine [7, 31], the precise PFC functional location was not involved in these studies,

Table 3 The voxel-based correlation analysis between the functional connectivity of left ventrolateral PAG(vlPAG) and right vlPAG and the clinical variables

Group	Anatomic region	Cluster size	MNI-space			P_{uncorr}	Peak T value
			X	Y	Z		
Left_vlPAG							
DD							
Positive							
	Thalamus_R	23	9	−3	3	0.000	7.39
			6	−15	6	0.000	5.38
	Pallidum_L	15	−12	3	0	0.000	5.8
	Thalamus_L		−12	−12	0	0.000	5.68
Right_vlPAG							
DD							
Positive							
	Putamen_L	104	−21	9	−9	0.000	8.75
	Frontal_Med_Orb_R	12	12	57	0	0.000	6.31
	Thalamus_L	14	−6	−12	3	0.000	6.06
	Putamen_R	14	24	21	−3	0.000	5.49
	Thalamus_R	15	6	−15	6	0.000	5.12

vlPAG ventrolateral PAG, *DD* disease duration, *Positive* positive correlation

and a recent study demonstrated that migraine without aura showed decreased functional connectivity between PAG and medial PFC (mPFC). In this study, mid-dlPFC and posterior dlPFC presented decreased functional connectivity with left vlPAG and left dlPAG in EM patients, which might be associated with higher HAMA and HAMD scores in EM patients since the dlPFC participated the emotion-nmodulated performance and activity [30]. Therefore, this study suggested that dlPFC might be the targeted impaired brain region in the disrupted vlPAG dysfunction network.

Also, the left dlPAG showed the decreased functional connectivity with right ventrolateral prefrontal cortex (vlPFC) (BA45) in EM patients (Fig. 4). vlPFC was located in the inferior frontal gyrus, and including anterior (BA47), middle (BA45) and posterior (BA44) PFC, which presented different function [32–34]. It was known that right and left vlPFC showed the different specific functions [35], and right vlPFC was thought be play a key role in the motor control [36], and its involvement was not still reported in migraine, and it may be associated with the study methods. In a previous study [37], right anterior vlPFC (BA47) was involved in the integration of emotional processing using a parametric mediation analysis of fMRI. However, right middle (BA45) vlPFC presented decreased functional connectivity with left dlPAG region in the current study. Although it was not consistent with the previous document, it might speculate that middle vlPFC participate in the emotional processing in EM patients since the HAMA and HAMD scores were higher in migraineurs.

Based on two-streams hypothesis [38, 39], dlPFC was the endpoint of the dorsal stream, and vlPFC was the endpoint of the ventral stream. Herein, it could recognize that the endpoints of dorsal and ventral stream were disrupted for the functional connectivity with vlPAG and dlPAG in EM patients, and which may be associated with the visual processing in migraine. In this study, bilateral middle temporal gyrus (BA21) presented decreased functional connectivity with left vlPAG, and BA21 region mainly take part in the processing of visual information, which indicated that disrupted visual information processing may

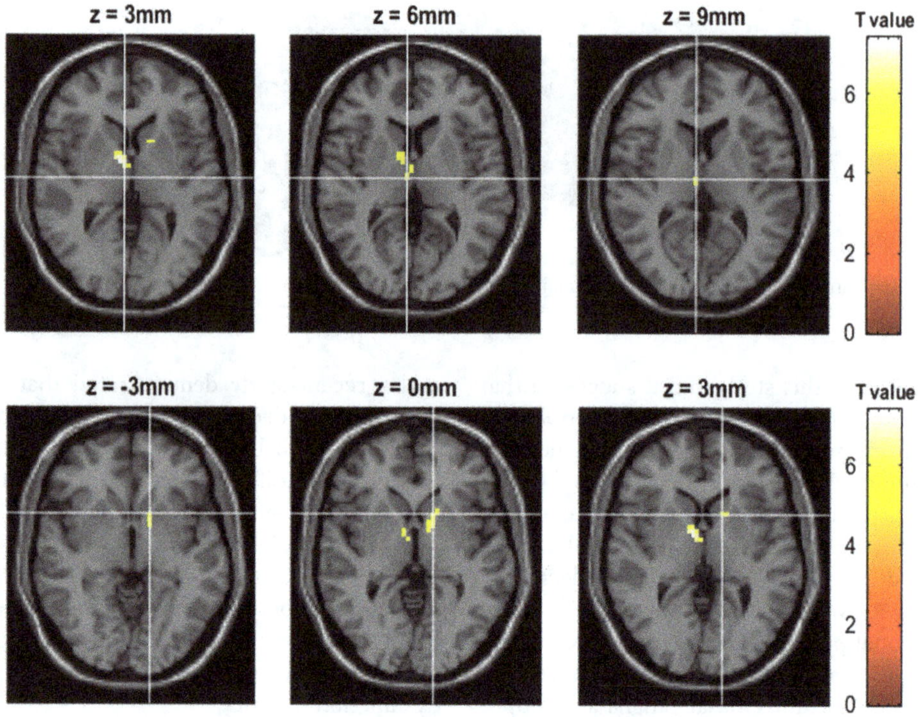

Fig. 5 The brain regions with positive correlation between the functional connectivity of left ventrolateral PAG and disease duration in EM patients

occur in EM patients, and may be associated ventral and dorsal stream.

Voxel-based correlation analysis demonstrated the positive correlation of the diseased duration with the altered functional connectivity of vlPAG, while clinical variables such as VAS, onset frequence, and neuropsychological scale scores were not related with the PAG functional connectivity. These findings indicated that vlPAG dysfunction may be associated with the disease duration, and disease duration may indirectly be used to predict the severity of vlPAG dysfunction in EM patients. A previous study demonstrated that basal ganglia played a significant role in the pathophysiology of the episodic migraine [40], and it also revealed that the disrupted connection with the subcortical gray matter structures (bilateral thalamus and putamen) may be the primary impaired neuromechanism for the descending pain modulation for vlPAG in EM patient.

Conclusions

In conclusion, disrupted functional connectivity of bilateral vlPAG and left dlPAG presented in bilateral dlPFC, right vlPFC, blilateral PMC and right SMA, bilateral middle temporal gyri in EM patients, and the

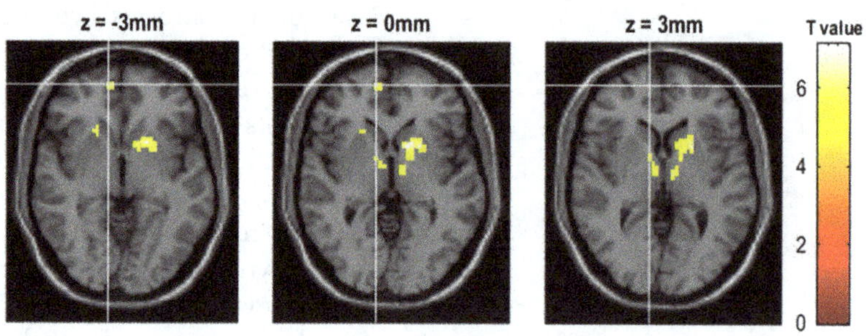

Fig. 6 The brain regions with positive correlation between the functional connectivity of right ventrolateral PAG and disease duration in EM patients

disease duration was positively related to the functional connectivity of bilateral vlPAG on the bilateral thalamus and putamen, left pallidum and right medial orbitofrontal gyrus in EM patients. These findings suggested that functional evaluation of PAG subregion may be contributed to the diagnosis and understanding of EM pathogenesis.

Abbreviations

dlPAG: Dorsolateral PAG; dmPAG: Dorsomedial PAG; EM: Episodic migraine; lPAG: Lateral PAG; NC: Normal controls; PAG: Periaqueductal gray; PFC: Prefrontal cortex; PMA: Primary motor area; SMA: Supplementary motor area; vlPAG: Ventrolateral PAG

Acknowledgments

This work was supported by the National Natural Sciences Foundation of China (81371514), the Special Financial Grant from the China Postdoctoral Science Foundation (2014 T70960) and the Foundation for Medical and health Sci & Tech innovation Project of Sanya (2016YW37).

Authors' contributions

Category 1: (a) Conception and Design: LM; SYY. (b) Acquisition of Data: ZYC; MQL; SFL; XYC. (c) Analysis and Interpretation of Data: ZYC. Category 2: (a) Drafting the Article: ZYC. (b) Revising It for Intellectual Content: LM; SYY. All authors read and approved the final manuscript.

Competing interests

The authors declare that they have no competing interests.

Author details

[1]Department of Radiology, Chinese PLA General Hospital, 28 Fuxing Road, Beijing 100853, China. [2]Department of Neurology, Chinese PLA General Hospital, 28 Fuxing Road, Beijing 100853, China. [3]Department of Radiology, Hainan Branch of Chinese PLA General Hospital, Sanya 572013, China.

References

1. Welch KM, Nagesh V, Aurora SK, Gelman N (2001) Periaqueductal gray matter dysfunction in migraine: cause or the burden of illness? Headache 41:629–37
2. Smith GST, Savery D, Marden C, Costa JJL, Averill S, Priestley JV, Rattray M (1994) Distribution of messenger RNAs encoding enkephalin, substance P, somatostatin, galanin, vasoactive intestinal polypeptide, neuropeptide Y, and calcitonin gene-related peptide in the midbrain periaqueductal grey in the rat. J Comp Neurol 350:23–40
3. Raskin NH, Yoshio H, Sharon L (1987) Headache may arise from perturbation of brain. Headache 27:416–20
4. Kruit MC, Launer LJ, Overbosch J, van Buchem MA, Ferrari MD (2009) Iron accumulation in deep brain nuclei in migraine: a population-based magnetic resonance imaging study. Cephalalgia 29:351–9
5. Tepper SJ, Lowe MJ, Beall E, Phillips MD, Liu K, Stillman MJ et al (2012) Iron deposition in pain-regulatory nuclei in episodic migraine and chronic daily headache by MRI. Headache 52:236–43
6. Mainero C, Boshyan J, Hadjikhani N (2011) Altered functional MRI resting-state connectivity in periaqueductal gray networks in migraine. Ann Neurol 70:838–45
7. Li Z, Liu M, Lan L, Zeng F, Makris N, Liang Y et al (2016) Altered periaqueductal gray resting state functional connectivity in migraine and the modulation effect of treatment. Sci Rep 6:20298
8. Chen Z, Chen X, Liu M, Liu S, Ma L, Yu S (2016) Nonspecific periaqueductal gray lesions on T2WI in episodic migraine. J Headache Pain 17:101
9. Ito K, Kudo M, Sasaki M, Saito A, Yamashita F, Harada T et al (2016) Detection of changes in the periaqueductal gray matter of patients with episodic migraine using quantitative diffusion kurtosis imaging: preliminary findings. Neuroradiology 58:115–20
10. Menant O, Andersson F, Zelena D, Chaillou E (2016) The benefits of magnetic resonance imaging methods to extend the knowledge of the anatomical organisation of the periaqueductal gray in mammals. J Chem Neuroanat 77:110–20
11. Coulombe MA, Erpelding N, Kucyi A, Davis KD (2016) Intrinsic functional connectivity of periaqueductal gray subregions in humans. Hum Brain Mapp 37:1514–30
12. Headache Classification Committee of the International Headache Society (IHS) (2013) The International Classification of Headache Disorders, 3rd edition (beta version). Cephalalgia 33:629–808
13. Maier W, Buller R, Philipp M, Heuser I (1988) The Hamilton anxiety scale: reliability, validity and sensitivity to change in anxiety and depressive disorders. J Affect Disord 14:61–8
14. Hamilton M (1967) Development of a rating scale for primary depressive illness. Br J Soc Clin Psychol 6:278–96
15. Song XW, Dong ZY, Long XY, Li SF, Zuo XN, Zhu CZ et al (2011) REST: a toolkit for resting-state functional magnetic resonance imaging data processing. PLoS One 6:e25031
16. Yu R, Gollub RL, Spaeth R, Napadow V, Wasan A, Kong J (2014) Disrupted functional connectivity of the periaqueductal gray in chronic low back pain. Clin Neuropathol 6:100–8
17. Zyloney CE, Jensen K, Polich G, Loiotile RE, Cheetham A, Laviolette PS et al (2010) Imaging the functional connectivity of the Periaqueductal Gray during genuine and sham electroacupuncture treatment. Mol Pain 6:1–11
18. Menke RA, Jbabdi S, Miller KL, Matthews PM, Zarei M (2010) Connectivity-based segmentation of the substantia nigra in human and its implications in Parkinson's disease. Neuroimage 52:1175–80
19. Kong J, Tu PC, Zyloney C, Su TP (2010) Intrinsic functional connectivity of the periaqueductal gray, a resting fMRI study. Behav Brain Res 211:215–9
20. Hamilton BL (1973) Cytoarchitectural subdivisions of the periaqueductal gray matter in the cat. J Comp Neurol 149:1–27
21. Hamilton BL (1973) Projections of the nuclei of the periaqueductal gray matter in the cat. J Comp Neurol 152:45–57
22. Depaulis A, Keay KA, Bandler R (1994) Quiescence and hyporeactivity evoked by activation of cell bodies in the ventrolateral midbrain periaqueductal gray of the rat. Exp Brain Res 99:75–83
23. Williams FG, Mullet MA, Beitz AJ (1995) Basal release of Met-enkephalin and neurotensin in the ventrolateral periaqueductal gray matter of the rat: a microdialysis study of antinociceptive circuits. Brain Res 690:207–16
24. Yang K, Furue H, Kumamoto E, Dong YX, Yoshimura M (2003) Pre- and postsynaptic inhibition mediated by GABA(B) receptors in rat ventrolateral periaqueductal gray neurons. Biochem Biophys Res Commun 302:233–7
25. Reddi D, Curran N, Stephens R (2013) An introduction to pain pathways and mechanisms. Br J Hosp Med (Lond) 74(Suppl 12):C188–91
26. Cummiford CM, Nascimento TD, Foerster BR, Clauw DJ, Zubieta JK, Harris RE, Dasilva AF (2016) Changes in resting state functional connectivity after repetitive transcranial direct current stimulation applied to motor cortex in fibromyalgia patients. Arthritis Res Ther 18:1–12
27. Barbey AK, Koenigs M, Grafman J (2013) Dorsolateral prefrontal contributions to human working memory. Cortex 49:1195–205
28. Goldman-Rakic PS (1995) Architecture of the prefrontal cortex and the central executive. Ann N Y Acad Sci 769:71–83
29. Chan RC, Shum D, Toulopoulou T, Chen EY (2008) Assessment of executive functions: review of instruments and identification of critical issues. Arch Clin Neuropsychol 23:201–16
30. Herrington JD, Mohanty A, Koven NS, Fisher JE, Stewart JL, Banich MT et al (2005) Emotion-modulated performance and activity in left dorsolateral prefrontal cortex. Emotion 5:200–7
31. Maniyar FH, Sprenger T, Monteith T, Schankin CJ, Goadsby PJ (2015) The premonitory phase of migraine–what can we learn from it? Headache 55:609–20
32. Gold BT, Balota DA, Jones SJ, Powell DK, Smith CD, Andersen AH (2006) Dissociation of automatic and strategic lexical-semantics: functional magnetic resonance imaging evidence for differing roles of multiple frontotemporal regions. J Neurosci 26:6523–32
33. Badre D, Wagner AD (2007) Left ventrolateral prefrontal cortex and the cognitive control of memory. Neuropsychologia 45:2883–901
34. Danker JF, Gunn P, Anderson JR (2008) A rational account of memory predicts left prefrontal activation during controlled retrieval. Cereb Cortex 18:2674–85

35. Levy BJ, Wagner AD (2011) Cognitive control and right ventrolateral prefrontal cortex: reflexive reorienting, motor inhibition, and action updating. Ann N Y Acad Sci 1224:40–62
36. Aron AR, Robbins TW, Poldrack RA (2004) Inhibition and the right inferior frontal cortex. Trends Cogn Sci 8:170–7
37. Kida I, Hoshi Y (2016) Right ventrolateral prefrontal cortex involvement in the integration of emotional processing: Parametric mediation analysis of fMRI. Neurosci Lett 615:92–7
38. Mishkin M, Ungerleider LG (1982) Contribution of striate inputs to the visuospatial functions of parieto-preoccipital cortex in monkeys. Behav Brain Res 6:57–77
39. Schenk T, Mcintosh RD (2010) Do we have independent visual streams for perception and action? Cogn Neurosci 1:52–62
40. Maleki N, Becerra L, Nutile L, Pendse G, Brawn J, Bigal M et al (2011) Migraine attacks the basal ganglia. Mol Pain 7:71

Duration and frequency of migraines affect cognitive function: evidence from neuropsychological tests and event-related potentials

Lifang Huang†, Hong juan Dong†, Xi Wang, Yan Wang and Zheman Xiao*

Abstract

Background: The aim of this study was to evaluate the changes in the cognitive performance of migraine patients using a comprehensive series of cognitive/behavioral and electrophysiological tests.

Method: A randomized, cross-sectional, within subject approach was used to compare neuropsychological and electrophysiological evaluations from migrane-affected and healthy subjects.

Results: Thirty-four patients with migraine (6 males, 28 females, average 36 years old) were included. Migraineurs performed worse in the majority of the Montreal Cognitive Assessment (MoCA) ($p = 0.007$) compared to the healthy subjects, significantly in language ($p = 0.005$), memory ($p = 0.006$), executive functions ($p = 0.042$), calculation ($p = 0.018$) and orientation ($p = 0.012$). Migraineurs had a lower score on the memory trial of the Rey–Osterrieth complex figure test (ROCF) ($p = 0.012$). The P3 latency in Fz, Cz, Pz was prolonged in migraineurs compared with the normal control group ($P < 0.001$). In addition, we analyzed significant correlations between MoCA score and the duration of migraine. We also observed that a decrease in the MoCA-executive functions and calculation score and in the ROCF-recall score were both correlated to the frequency of migraine. Migraineurs were more anxious than healthy subjects ($p = 0.001$), which is independent of cognitive testing. Differences were unrelated to age, gender and literacy.

Conclusions: Cognitive performance decreases during migraine, and cognitive dysfunction can be related to the duration and frequency of a migraine attack.

Keywords: Migraine, Duration, Frequency, Cognitive deficits, Event-related potentials

Background

Migraine is the second most prevalent type of primary headache disorder, which affects approximately 14.7% of both males and females [1]. Migraine is characterized by moderate to severe throbbing pain with sensitivity or intolerance to light and sound during the headache and is often accompanied by nausea and vomiting. Migraine, especially chronic migraine, is often comorbid with psychiatric disorders that exhibit affective temperament dysregulation and suicidal behaviors [2, 3]. Migraine has been associated with an increased risk of vascular events, specifically cardiovascular disease [4]. Vascular pathology is a strong risk factor for cognitive dysfunction [5, 6].

In addition, migraine has been linked to an increased prevalence of clinically silent brain lesions and subtle gray matter damage which affect the cognitive processes [7, 8]. These associations suggest that individuals with migraines have impaired cognitive function due to these structural lesions. However, previous studies of migraine and cognition have been contradictory. Some studies suggest that migraineurs have subtle interictal cognitive abnormalities aligning with attentional deficits [9–11]. Some studies have reported improved performance [12]. Some longitudinal studies have suggested fewer dysfunctions in the Mini Mental State Examination (MMSE) and executive functions in migraineurs. In addition,

* Correspondence: zmxiao@whu.edu.cn
†Equal contributors
Department of Neurology, Renmin Hospital of Wuhan University, Wuhan 430060, Hubei Province, People's Republic of China

some studies have not found any significant differences in cognitive performance between migraine patients and controls [13]. These inconsistencies could be due to methodological issues including different migraine assessment methods and the program of cognitive assessment.

Given the high prevalence of migraine in the general population, it is clear that the relationship between cognitive dysfunction and migraines present a significant public health interest.

Event-related potentials (ERPs) are one of the most useful tools in investigating neural substrates and cerebral regions involved in specific cognitive function because of the objectivity and noninvasiveness of the method. Undoubtedly, the P3 is the most studied cerebral wave used for evaluating cerebral information processing during the course of various neurological diseases because of its easy recording and reliability.

This study aimed to characterize cognitive testing and P3 in migraineurs. We hypothesized that migraine patients have cognitive dysfunction and P3 abnormalities, such as reduced P3 amplitude and/or a prolonged latency, suggesting alterations in the cognitive-evaluative component.

Methods

Participants

We recruited 34 migraine patients (6 males, 28 females; mean age 36 years; range between 20 to 55 years) from the Renmin Hospital of Wuhan University, 10 with aura and 24 without aura. Patients were not receiving prophylactic therapy, were medicine-free for at least 24 h and were in the interictal period when recruited. We also recruited 24 healthy age-matched participants (6 males, 18 females; mean age 36 years; range between 22 to 58 years) with no history of headache or drug/alcohol abuse. Patients and controls had normal or corrected-to-normal vision. We excluded participants who were illiterate or suffering from depression, stroke, or brain injuries. All participants provided written and informed consent prior to commencement of the experiment.

Assessment of migraines

Participants were diagnosed based on diagnostic criteria of the International Classification of Headache Disorders (ICHD-3 beta).

Evaluation of cognitive functions

The Montreal Cognitive Assessment (MoCA) was included as a screening test of general cognitive abilities. Several separate domains of cognitive function were covered including visuospatial functions, attention, language, memory, executive functioning, calculation and orientation. It took approximately 10 min to administer the MoCA. The maximum possible score was 30 points, and a score of 26 or above was considered normal. The Rey–Osterrieth Complex Figure Test (ROCF) was used to assess visual perception, constructional praxis, and visuo-spatial memory, and was adapted from Osterrieth [14]. First, subjects were given the ROCF stimulus card, and they were asked to draw the same figure. Then, after a delay of 20 min, they were required to draw what they remembered. Study variables were as follows: (a) copy accuracy: quality of the copy as a reflection of visuo-constructive ability; (b) delayed recall: accuracy of the figure after the 20 min delay. According to the scoring system, the figure contained 18 elements, each of which received a score of 0.5, 1 or 2, depending on the accuracy, deformation, and location of each element. The full score was 36 for each of the 2 tasks. Basic information processing speed was measured with the Digit Symbol Substitution Test (DSST). In this test, the time needed to copy symbols in boxes that were indexed by digits, according to a key of digit/symbol combinations at the top of a sheet of paper. Under each digit, the corresponding symbol should be written as fast as possible. The time for completion of all symbols was measured. A history of depression and anxiety was determined based on the responses of the participants to a series of questions used to diagnose these mental disorders, called the Self-Rating Anxiety Scale and Self-Rating Depression Scale.

Electrophysiological study

Procedure

The experiment was performed in a sound-attenuated room with a dim light. Participants were seated in a comfortable armchair and were presented with a white fixation cross at the center of a 19 in computer monitor placed 50 cm in front of them. Two hundred stimuli were presented in a random fashion. Stimuli were comprised of target stimuli (the number "2", 20% probability of presentation) and standard stimuli (the number "8", 80% probability of presentation). The duration of each stimulus was 50 ms, and the inter-stimulus interval was randomly varied between 800 ms and 1200 ms. All the stimuli were generated using the E-prime software. Participants were instructed to press the button as quickly and accurately as possible when they viewed the target stimuli. Accuracy was defined as the rate of pressing the button when viewed the target stimuli. Reaction time was defined as the length between viewing the target stimuli and pressing the button accurately. The accuracy and reaction time recordings were accomplished using E-prime software 2.0.

ERP recording and measurement

The electroencephalogram (EEG) was continuously recorded at Fz, Cz and Pz electrode sites according to the 10–20 International System with 36 Ag/AgCl active electrodes via NuAmps EEG/ERPs 36 Channel Amplifier of NEURO SCAN LABS. The electrode site on the scalp was prepared with alcohol and scraped with scrub cream to remove cutin resulting in an electrode impedance of less than 10 kΩ. Electrode impedance was kept below 10 kΩ throughout the experiment. All scalp electrodes were referenced to the average of the left and right mastoid signals. To ensure proper eye fixation and to allow for the removal of events associated with eye movement artifacts, vertical and horizontal eye movements were recorded with two pairs of electrodes, one placed above and below the left eye, and the other 10 mm from the lateral canthus of both eyes. High-pass and low-pass filters were set at 1.0 Hz and 30.0 Hz, respectively. The sampling rate was 1000 Hz.

For each participant, the EEG was segmented into the epoch from 200 ms pre-stimulus to 800 ms post-stimulus via Curry7.0 software. These single-subject waveforms were then used to generate the group-averaged waveforms for display and analysis. A -200 to 0 ms pre-stimulus baseline was used for all ERP waveform measurement and displays. Trials with signal exceeding ±200 mV amplitude in any recording channel were excluded from averaging. The EEG segments were averaged separately for target and standard stimuli. Only correctly detected responses were averaged. The number of averaged trials left after removal of the artifacts was 40 (target) and 160 (standard).

The difference waveform was obtained by subtracting ERPs in response to standard stimuli from those in response to target stimuli. The positive peak between 300 and 500 ms were used to define the P3 component. The peak amplitudes and latencies for the P3 component were measured relative to the pre-stimulus baseline period.

Statistical analysis

We first used the Shapiro-Wilk test to assess the distribution of the variables. Quantitative data were presented as the mean ± standard deviation or median. Student's *t*-test for independent samples (two-tailed) was used to compare the two groups in the scores of cognitive test, p3 amplitude and latency. Correlations between clinical (illness duration and frequency of attacks), cognitive test (MoCA, ROCF, DSST) and electrophysiological (ERP components amplitude and latency) data were computed. Pearson product-moment correlation coefficients (r) were reported. Statistical calculations were carried out using SPSS20.0. All the results were considered to be significant at $p < 0.05$.

Results

Sample characteristics

Table 1 shows demographic and clinical characteristics of migraine. There was no statistically significant difference between migraineurs and healthy subjects in age and education level.

In our study, migraineurs suffered 3.532 (SD 3.956) headaches a month, with the average headache lasting 23.4 h (SD 24.197). On average, migraine participants had been having migraines for 11 years.

Emotional characteristics of both groups were compared: the migraine group was significantly more anxious than the healthy groups.

Comparisons of cognitive testing

Mean scores on the MoCA, digit symbol substitution test and Rey–Osterrieth complex figure test are shown in Table 2. Significant differences were observed in the MoCA ($p = 0.007$), especially in language, memory, executive functions, calculation and orientation. Migraineurs had a lower score on the memory trial of Rey–Osterrieth complex figure test compared to healthy controls ($p = 0.012$). Performance on the digit symbol substitution test and copy trial of Rey–Osterrieth complex figure test was not significantly different.

ERP data

There was no significant group difference in accuracy (migraineurs, 97.41%; healthy subjects, 98.38%; $P = 0.187$), or in the appropriate reaction time between migraineurs (449.1 ms) and healthy subjects (445.1 ms; $P = 0.272$).

Table 3 shows the results of P3 amplitude and latency between the migraine group and healthy group. The latency was longer in the migraine group compared to the healthy subjects ($P < 0.001$). In the migraine group, the P3 amplitude varied between sites, was maximal in the parietal lobe (Pz: 9.906 μV) and minimal in the frontal lobe (Fz: 8.243 μV), with intermediate values at Cz (8.735 μV), but the difference did not reach statistical significance ($P = 0.319$). There was no significant difference between the location of recording: left (Pz3) vs. right (Pz4) vs. midline (Pz).

Correlations between cognitive scores and headache characteristics

We observed that the MoCA score showed a significant, negative and moderate correlation with the duration of migraine, especially in the aspects of language, executive functions, calculation and memory. In addition, the time for the digit symbol substitution test showed a positive correlation with duration of headache. We also observed a significant relationship between MoCA-executive functions, calculation score, ROCF-recall score and the frequency of migraine, whereas the remaining cognitive measures and the results of ERP did not correlate with headache characteristics (Table 4).

Discussion

The present study revealed that migraine patients had significantly lower scores than controls on cognitive tests

Table 1 Sample Characteristics

	Migraineurs Mean ± SD	Healthy subjects Mean ± SD	*P*
N	34	24	
Age, years	36.065 ± 10.046	36.052 ± 12.968	0.997
Education, years	13.032 ± 4.231	13.790 ± 5.298	0.580
Headache score,	6.383 ± 1.670	–	–
Headache frequency, per month	3.532 ± 3.956	– –	– –
Duration of headache, hours	23.4 ± 24.197	–	–
Headache history, years	11.25 ± 9.290	–	–
SCL anxiety score	33.667 ± 8.671	26.737 ± 3.769	0.001*
SCL depression score	33.000 ± 9.390	28.368 ± 5.479	0.064

SCL symptom checklist, **P* < .05

and increased P3 latencies. Our findings suggest that migraineurs are associated with cognitive dysfunctions. Previously, Freitas and colleagues found that 49% of MoCA score variability was attributed to age and education [15]. To exclude the influence of age and education on cognitive function, we had to balance age and education level between migraineurs and healthy subjects when we collected subjects. All participant ages were below 55 years old, and all had at least five years of primary education. For the psychological profile, migraineurs reported higher scores on the symptom checklist for anxiety. Some studies have shown that even subclinical levels of anxiety may negatively impact cognitive ability [16, 17]. To eliminate the effect of psychology, Spearman's correlations were calculated between cognitive tests and psychology tests, and we did not find any correlation between cognitive tests and severity of psychological impairment. The poorer cognitive performance exhibited by migraineurs was not determined by the emotional variables.

The present study revealed that migraineurs had significantly lower scores than healthy subjects on the delayed recall of ROCF test, the total MoCA and in five out of seven cognitive subdomains (i.e., language, executive functions, calculation, memory and orientation domains). The MoCA was included as a screening test for general cognitive abilities and out of a maximum score of 30 points, the cut-off value was 26 points [18]. Eight migraineurs achieved scores below the available cut-off values in the MoCA test, but all of the scores were within two standard deviations of the mean. Four of them had low education, and two were elder than 50 years old. Most of the participants' scores were not lower than the cut-off value reported in normative studies. Thus, we deemed that the reduced efficiency in selected cognitive domains did not correspond to a clinically relevant cognitive deterioration.

The longer durations and the increased frequency of migraine attacks were correlated with decreased cognitive performance. This indicates that the reduced scores on cognitive tests observed in migraineurs compared with controls is directly related to the length of time and the frequency of patient's suffering from migraine.

Gil-Gouveia R aimed to document changes in cognitive performance of migraineurs under two conditions-during a naturally occurring untreated migraine attack and during a headache-free period. It was found that cognitive performance decreased during migraine attacks, especially in reading and processing speed, verbal memory and learning, supporting patients' subjective complaints. Differences were found unrelated to pain intensity or

Table 2 The Cognitive Outcome measures between migraine group and control group

	Migraineurs Mean ± SD	Healthy subjects Mean ± SD	F	*P*
MoCA	25.677 ± 4.291	28.048 ± 1.829	7.664	0.007*
Visuospatial function	3.618 ± 0.604	3.550 ± 0.999	2.252	0.817
Attention	2.706 ± 0.676	2.850 ± 0.366	5.218	0.248
Language	4.971 ± 1.243	5.714 ± 0.643	5.687	0.005*
Executive functions	6.824 ± 1.714	7.600 ± 0.940	6.717	0.042*
Calculation	2.735 ± 0.618	3.000 ± 0.000	19.349	0.018*
Memory	4.029 ± 1.507	5.096 ± 0.995	3.677	0.006**
Orientation	5.824 ± 0.387	6.000 ± 0.00	25.357	0.012*
DSST's	122.917 ± 46.404	106.684 ± 36.002	0.090	0.217
ROCF-copy	35.792 ± 0.833	35.684 ± 0.946	0.684	0.694
ROCF-recall	20.688 ± 6.129	25.316 ± 5.218	0.308	0.012*

Visuospatial function refers to the copy cube and draw a clock test; Attention refers to the vigilance test and digit span test; Language function refers to naming, sentence repetition and verbal fluency test; Executive functions refers to the alternating trail making, abstraction, verbal fluency, copy cube and draw a clock test; Calculation refers to serial 7 s test; Memory contains delayed recall and verbal fluency test; **P* < .05, ***P* < 0.001

Table 3 Results of P3 amplitude and latency between migraine group and control group

ERP		Migraineurs	Healthy subjects	F	P
P3		Mean ± SD	Mean ± SD		
Amplitude (μV)	Fz	8.243 ± 3.964	9.318 ± 3.106	2.474	0.285
	Cz	8.735 ± 4.262	8.973 ± 3.055	1.515	0.820
	Pz	9.906 ± 4586	10.859 ± 3.191	3.337	0.394
Latency (ms)	Fz	406.517 ± 37.552	368.417 ± 12.552	16.253	0.000**
	Cz	406.207 ± 38.097	366.833 ± 17.189	10.775	0.000**
	Pz	408.724 ± 36.748	367.792 ± 17.290	7.814	0.000**

*P < .05, **P < 0.001

duration of the attack [19]. Riva D assessed the effect of migraine on the interictal functioning of children and adolescents and observed that both patient groups had cognitive performance within a normal range, except for a significant delay in the reaction time task. These researchers considered that slower reaction time to simple visual stimuli may be an early sign of a subclinical neuropsychological dysfunction, significantly correlated with the frequency of headache attacks [20]. These data, together with our findings, would favor the view of some neuropsychological abnormalities in migraineurs as a consequence of the disease, or a perpetuating factor.

P3 is a generic name for a variety of relatively late, positive components with a centro-parietal midline distribution. Two principal electrophysiological markers have been considered as an objective index of cognitive processing: latency and amplitude. It is widely accepted that P3 latency reflects the length of stimulus evaluation processes [21], when two choice reaction time (RT) is required and its amplitude is largely determined by stimulus relevance, the amount of attention allocated to the stimulus, working memory and the task's complexity [22, 23].

In our study, the latency for ERP components was significantly increased in migraine subjects. According to the previously mentioned facts, it could be suggested that migraineurs have a prolonged latency of P3, which represents a prolonged cognitive processing time. Some studies have shown that the amplitudes of P3 were significantly decreased in migraine patients compared with the healthy subjects, but the latencies of P3 did not show any significant effects [24, 25]. Other results show significant elongation of latencies and a dysfunction in P3 amplitudes in the migrant group during headache attacks [26]. However, several results have shown that migraine sufferers had longer P3 latencies, which is consistent with our findings.

The divergence among other studies and ours might be due to the different patient selection procedures. In our study, migraine patients were identified by expert neurologists according to established diagnostic criteria of the International Classification of Headache Disorders (ICHD-3 beta), while in previous studies, migraine patients were selected from a cohort of subjects on the basis of self-report measures. This procedure might have led to a misclassification of the non-migraine subjects.

Table 4 Correlation between cognitive scores and headache characteristics in migraine patients

	Migraine score	Migraine frequency	Duration of migraine	Migraine history	SDS	SAS
Cognitive domains	r (p value)	r (p value)	r (p value)	r (p value)	r (p value)	r (p value)
MoCA	−0.194(0.270)	−0.311(0.073)	−0.478(0.004)**	−0.093(0.601)	−0.154(0.454)	−0.193(0.345)
Visuospatial functions	−0.030(0.865)	−0.290(0.096)	−0.257(0.142)	−0.201(0.255)	−0.296(0.142)	−0.315(0.117)
Attention	−0.054(0.762)	−0.143(0.420)	−0.186(0.293)	−0.162(0.361)	−0.283(0.161)	−0.208(0.308)
Language	−0.257(0.142)	−0.221(0.209)	−0.430(0.011)*	−0.149(0.401)	−0.195(0.339)	−0.232(0.255)
Executive functions	−0.165(0.351)	−0.458(0.006)**	−0.405(0.018)*	−0.037(0.835)	−0.228(0.262)	−0.225(0.268)
Calculation	−0.148(0.405)	−0.350(0.042)*	−0.446(0.008)**	−0.221(0.209)	−0.319(0.112)	−0.304(0.132)
Memory	−0.073(0.683)	0.042(0.815)	−0.374(0.030)*	0.058(0.746)	0.1490.468)	0.007(0.974)
Orientation	0.259(0.139)	−0.081(0.649)	−0.115(0.516)	0.059(0.741)	0.178(0.383)	0.238(0.243)
DSST	0.300(0.107)	0.132(0.486)	0.446(0.014)*	−0.175(0.355)	0.207(0.343)	0.270(0.212)
ROCF-recall	−0.318(0.087)	−0.415(0.023)*	−0.078(0.683)	0.075(0.692)	−0.207(0.344)	−0.336(0.117)
ERP Amplitude	−0.173(0.371)	0.136(0.371)	−0.029(0.881)	0.000(0.998)	−0.382(0.072)	−0457(0.028)*
ERP Latency	0.017(0.931)	−0.070(0.718)	−0.100(0.606)	0.093(0.630)	0.316(0.141)	0.312(0.147)

*P < .05, **P < 0.001

Furthermore, some articles have studied the cognition of children and adolescents. Cognition in children is immature, and we cannot compare it with adult cognitive function. Another potentially important factor is the procedure used for ERP. Differences in the tasks may probe different cognitive domains, and may lead to different conclusions.

In our study, ERP latency did not correlate with headache characteristics. This finding is not consistent with our expectations. ERP latency is a sensitive index, which is affected by many factors. The prolongation of latency may be affected by the migraine itself, but not by any characteristic of the headache.

In summary, the electrophysiological and behavioral data suggest that migraine is associated with cognitive dysfunctions, particularly, that cognitive dysfunctions can be related to the duration and the frequency of headache. Previously, people paid more attention to the pain of migraines and usually ignored the impairments of cognitive function in migraineurs. Although this functional phenomenon is present in the absence of clinically relevant deficits, it may reflect a vulnerability to executive high-demanding conditions of daily living activities in patients with migraine.

The strengths of this study include its standardized assessment of migraine status, information on migraine characteristics, and the availability of validated cognitive function measures. We discussed the correlations between neuropsychology, electrophysiology and migraine characteristics. We ruled out the effect of emotion on cognition. Our study had several limitations when interpreting our results. The study sample limited the ability to examine the effects of gender, age and education. Additionally, a previous study has shown that migraineurs with aura tend to exhibit even less decline over time than migraineurs overall [27]. We did not find differences in mean cognitive scores between migraineurs with and without aura. However, this was likely to due to the sample sizes and resulting low statistical power. De Tommaso and colleges found that the changes in brain responsivity are associated with various stages of the migraine cycle, since migraine patients seem to have a response augmentation and poor habituation that normalizes just before/during attacks [28]. In our study, patients were observed outside migraine attacks, but they could be at different points of a migraine cycle. We did not record the last time that they had a migraine attack. Furthermore, we did not observe the cognition of migraine patients at multiple time points, which limited us from examining the change in cognitive function over time.

Conclusions

Cognitive performance decreases during migraine, especially in language, memory, executive functions, calculation and orientation, and cognitive dysfunctions can be related to the duration and the frequency of headache. These findings suggest the existence of brain dysfunction during attacks of migraine, which can relate specifically to migraine. We believe that it is necessary to shorten the duration and reduce the frequency of migraine attack. Careful clinical evaluation should be performed in migraine patients in order to diagnose early cognitive dysfunction and, if available, have them treated properly.

Acknowledgments

We wish to thank the control subjects and the patients who participated in this experiment. This study was supported by the National Natural Science Foundation of China (81471133, 30900459) and the Natural Science Foundation of Hubei Province (2014CFB734).

Authors' contributions

LF carried out the studies and drafted the manuscript. HD participated in the study design and recorded patients. YW performed the statistical analysis. XW helped LF with the recordings of patients. ZX participated in the design of the study, patient recruitment, the results discussion, manuscript drafting and revision. All authors read and approved the final manuscript.

Competing interests

The authors declare that they have no competing interests.

References

1. Bigal ME, Lipton RB (2009) The epidemiology, burden, and comorbidities of migraine. Neurol Clin 27:321–34
2. Serafini G, Pompili M, Innamorati M, Gentile G, Borro M, Lamis DA, Lala N, Negro A, Simmaco M, Girardi P, Martelletti P (2012) Gene variants with suicidal risk in a sample of subjects with chronic migraine and affective temperamental dysregulation. Eur Rev Med Pharmacol Sci 16:1389–98
3. Pompili M, Di Cosimo D, Innamorati M, Lester D, Tatarelli R, Martelletti P (2009) Psychiatric comorbidity in patients with chronic daily headache and migraine: a selective overview including personality traits and suicide risk. J Headache Pain 10:283–90
4. Vetvik KG, MacGregor EA (2017) Sex differences in the epidemiology, clinical features, and pathophysiology of migraine. Lancet Neurol 16:76–87
5. Vermeer SE, Prins ND, den Heijer T, Hofman A, Koudstaal PJ, Breteler MM (2003) Silent brain infarcts and the risk of dementia and cognitive decline. N Engl J Med 348:1215–22
6. Leys D, Henon H, Mackowiak-Cordoliani MA, Pasquier F (2005) Poststroke dementia. Lancet Neurol 4:752–9
7. Schwedt TJ, Dodick DW (2009) Advanced neuroimaging of migraine. Lancet Neurol 8:560–8
8. de Groot JC, de Leeuw FE, Oudkerk M, van Gijn J, Hofman A, Jolles J, Breteler MM (2000) Cerebral white matter lesions and cognitive function: the Rotterdam scan study. Ann Neurol 47:145–51
9. Demarquay G, Caclin A, Brudon F, Fischer C, Morlet D (2011) Exacerbated attention orienting to auditory stimulation in migraine patients. Clin Neurophysiol 122:1755–63
10. Mickleborough MJ, Truong G, Handy TC (2011) Top-down control of visual cortex in migraine populations. Neuropsychologia 49:1006–15
11. Mickleborough MJ, Hayward J, Chapman C, Chung J, Handy TC (2011) Reflexive attentional orienting in migraineurs: the behavioral implications of hyperexcitable visual cortex. Cephalalgia 31:1642–51
12. Wen K, Nguyen NT, Hofman A, Ikram MA, Franco OH (2016) Migraine is associated with better cognition in the middle-aged and elderly: the Rotterdam study. Eur J Neurol 23:1510–6

13. Martins IP, Gil-Gouveia R, Silva C, Maruta C, Oliveira AG (2012) Migraine, headaches, and cognition. Headache 52:1471–82
14. Shin MS, Park SY, Park SR, Seol SH, Kwon JS (2006) Clinical and empirical applications of the Rey-Osterrieth complex figure test. Nat Protoc 1:892–9
15. Freitas S, Simoes MR, Alves L, Santana I (2012) Montreal cognitive assessment: influence of sociodemographic and health variables. Arch Clin Neuropsychol 27:165–75
16. Stillman AN, Rowe KC, Arndt S, Moser DJ (2012) Anxious symptoms and cognitive function in non-demented older adults: an inverse relationship. Int J Geriatr Psychiatry 27:792–8
17. Wetherell JL, Reynolds CA, Gatz M, Pedersen NL (2002) Anxiety, cognitive performance, and cognitive decline in normal aging. J Gerontol B Psychol Sci Soc Sci 57:P246–55
18. Nasreddine ZS, Phillips NA, Bedirian V, Charbonneau S, Whitehead V, Collin I, Cummings JL, Chertkow H (2005) The montreal cognitive assessment, MoCA: a brief screening tool for mild cognitive impairment. J Am Geriatr Soc 53:695–9
19. Gil-Gouveia R, Oliveira AG, Martins IP (2015) Cognitive dysfunction during migraine attacks: a study on migraine without aura. Cephalalgia 35:662–74
20. Riva D, Aggio F, Vago C, Nichelli F, Andreucci E, Paruta N, D'Arrigo S, Pantaleoni C, Bulgheroni S (2006) Cognitive and behavioural effects of migraine in childhood and adolescence. Cephalalgia 26:596–603
21. McCarthy G, Donchin E (1981) A metric for thought: a comparison of P300 latency and reaction time. Science 211:77–80
22. Wang R, Dong Z, Chen X, Liu R, Zhang M, Wu J, Yu S (2014) Cognitive processing of cluster headache patients: evidence from event-related potentials. J Headache Pain 15:66
23. Kok A (2001) On the utility of P3 amplitude as a measure of processing capacity. Psychophysiology 38:557–77
24. Chen W, Shen X, Liu X, Luo B, Liu Y, Yu R, Sun G, Shen M, Wang W (2007) Passive paradigm single-tone elicited ERPs in tension-type headaches and migraine. Cephalalgia 27:139–44
25. Wang R, Dong Z, Chen X, Zhang M, Yang F, Zhang X, Jia W, Yu S (2014) Gender differences of cognitive function in migraine patients: Evidence from event-related potentials using the oddball paradigm. J Headache Pain 15:6
26. Titlic M, Mise NI, Pintaric I, Rogosic V, Vanjaka-Rogosic L, Mihalj M, Jurinovic P, Katic AC, Andjelinovic M (2015) The event-related potential p300 in patients with migraine. Acta Inform Med 23:339–42
27. Kalaydjian A, Zandi PP, Swartz KL, Eaton WW, Lyketsos C (2007) How migraines impact cognitive function: findings from the Baltimore ECA. Neurology 68:1417–24
28. de Tommaso M, Ambrosini A, Brighina F, Coppola G, Perrotta A, Pierelli F, Sandrini G, Valeriani M, Marinazzo D, Stramaglia S, Schoenen J (2014) Altered processing of sensory stimuli in patients with migraine. Nat Rev Neurol 10:144–55

13

The role of attachment insecurity in the emergence of anxiety symptoms in children and adolescents with migraine

Riccardo Williams[1], Luigi Leone[2], Noemi Faedda[3], Giulia Natalucci[4], Benedetta Bellini[4], Elisa Salvi[4], Paola Verdecchia[4], Rita Cerutti[1], Marco Arruda[5] and Vincenzo Guidetti[4*]

Abstract

Background: It is widely recognised that there are associations between headache, psychiatric comorbidity and attachment insecurity in both adults and children. The aims of this study were: 1) to compare perceived attachment security and anxiety in children and adolescents with migraine without aura and a healthy control group; 2) to test whether the child's perceived security of attachment to the mother and the father mediated the association between migraine and anxiety.

Methods: One hundred children and adolescents with Migraine without Aura were compared with a control group of 100 children without headache. The Security Scale (measures perceived security of attachments) and the Self-Administered Psychiatric Scales for Children and Adolescents, a measure of anxiety symptoms, were administered to all participants.

Results: The clinical group had lower attachment security than the control group and higher scores on all anxiety scales. Anxiety was negatively correlated with attachment. Children's attachment to their mother mediated the increase in global anxiety in the clinical group. Insecure paternal attachment was associated with greater insecurity in maternal attachment, suggesting that there is a complex pathway from migraine to anxiety symptoms mediated by perceived insecurity of paternal attachment and hence also by perceived insecurity of maternal attachment.

Conclusion: These results suggest that insecure parental attachment may exacerbate anxiety in children and adolescents with migraine and point to the importance of multimodal interventions, perhaps taking account of family relationships, for children and adolescents with migraine.

Keywords: Migraine, Anxiety, Attachment, Developmental age, Perception of security

Background

The prevalence of migraine in children and adolescents is about 7.7–9.1% [1]. It is widely recognised that headache, in particular migraine, is associated with psychiatric comorbidity in both adults and children [2–4]. The most frequently described psychiatric comorbidities are: anxiety disorders and scholastic anxiety [2], mood disorders [5], sleep disorders [6] and eating disorders [7]. However, some recent studies [8, 9] have called into question the relationship between migraine and psychiatric disorders, especially in children and adolescents with migraine. Given this controversy and its possible implications for treatment and prognosis, it is important to establish the extent of psychiatric problems in patients with migraine, and to understand their origin.

Attachment is defined as a behavioural and cognitive system that regulates an individual's sense of internal security. In infancy, attachment security has been defined as a child's confidence that his or her caregiver will be available and responsive in times of distress [10]. A secure

* Correspondence: vincenzo.guidetti@uniroma1.it
[4]Department of Paediatrics and Child and Adolescent Neuropsychiatry, Sapienza University of Rome, Via dei Sabelli 108, 00185 Rome, Italy
Full list of author information is available at the end of the article

pattern of attachment in childhood with an adult caregiver is a central element in the healthy development, to build self- efficacy and a good level of self-esteem, to protect the individual against stressful events and develop the foundations for mature relationships [11]. On the contrary, insecure models of attachment have to be considered as an important factor of vulnerability for psychopathology when other important stressful events and risk factors occur. In particular, attachment theorists argue that the formation of attachments is the key developmental process with regard to regulation of anxiety. Empirical research has shown that attachment insecurity in childhood and adolescence is an important correlate of anxiety disorder diagnoses, regardless of parental anxiety and psychopathological diagnoses [12]. Moreover, recent research has shown that insecure attachment may exacerbate the frequency and intensity of headache attacks, as well as contributing to associated psychopathology [13].

Given that early attachment is relevant to psychopathology and anxiety regulation during development, this pattern of findings appears consistent with the notion that children's perceived attachment security mediates the emergence of higher anxiety levels in children and adolescents with MoA. Mediation appears a fruitful conceptual and empirical tool to investigate the hypothesized mechanism that transmits an association between an independent variable and a dependent variable (X → Y), introducing a third variable (M) - the mediator [14]. The mediation pattern would thus be represented by: X → M → Y. In our case, the mediation we anticipated would take the form: MoA → attachment security → anxiety. The empirical tenability of such an hypothesis would help further efforts to understand the mechanisms underpinning the association of migraine with anxiety.

Some findings appear consistent with such a mediation. Previous research [13] suggests that migraine has a negative effect on children's perception of the security of their attachment relationships, and that – in turn – perceived attachment insecurity is related to anxiety. This pattern of associations suggests that attachment insecurity partially mediates the association between migraine and anxiety. To the best of our knowledge, no previous study has specifically investigated the role of children's attachment insecurity as a potential mediator of the relationship between anxiety and migraine in children and adolescents. Our aim was to determine whether there was empirical evidence for such a mediation pattern.

We were also interested in investigating whether there were differences in how the perceived security of maternal and paternal attachments affected the migraine-anxiety association. Some evidence from longitudinal research suggests that there are distinct models of attachment for the mother and the father, respectively, and that such distinct models do not coalesce into a single model of attachment until late adolescence [15]. This implies that in an investigation of how attachment security influences anxiety in a paediatric population of migraine sufferers it is important to distinguish between maternal and paternal attachment.

To summarise, the aims of this study were: 1) to compare perceived attachment security and anxiety in a group of children and adolescents with MoA and a group of healthy controls; 2) to test whether children's perceptions of the security of their maternal and paternal attachments mediated the migraine → anxiety association.

Method

Sample and procedure

We investigated these two questions via a case-control study. The clinical group was recruited consecutively from admissions to the Paediatric Headache Centre of Department of Paediatrics and Child and Adolescent Neuropsychiatry, "Sapienza" University of Rome, Policlinico Umberto I. All subjects were recruited in the period between January and December 2011 and met the following inclusion criteria: (a) Diagnosis of MoA (1.1) according to the ICHD–III criteria [16]; (b) aged between 8 and 18 years old; (c) had experienced headaches for at least 6 months; and (d) a minimum of 2 attacks per month over the last 3 months. This latter criterion was adopted in order to avoid having a heterogeneous clinical group containing patients with both sporadic and very frequent migraine episodes.

The exclusion criteria were: (a) diagnosis of secondary headache; (b) diagnosis of other types of primary headache; (b) presence of medical or psychiatric comorbidities (e.g., coeliac disease, epilepsy, diabetes, attention deficit hyperactivity disorder, depression), as these conditions could affect attachment and anxiety. The control group was instead recruited from primary and secondary schools in the province of Rome. All subjects came from the same urban area, were of Caucasian origin and from families with middle class socio-economic status (Class 2: household income = €28,000–55,000 p.a.; Class 3: household income = €55,000–75.000 p.a.; current Italian economic parameters). Both the subjects and their parents were required to give active, informed consent to participation. The study was conducted according to the criteria set out in the Declaration of Helsinki [17].

The size of the groups was sufficient to detect group differences in means of medium magnitude (Cohen's $d \geq .5$) with a power of .80. This level of power appeared adequate given the magnitude of anxiety scores differences between clinical and control groups generally reported in the literature on migraine [9]. As for the association between migraine and attachment security, the sample size guaranteed a power of .80 for correlations as small as 0.2, which also appeared a reasonable minimum, given the variables involved [13, 18–20].

Measures

Anxiety was measured using the Self-Administered Psychiatric Scales for Children and Adolescents (SAFA) battery [21–24].

Perceived attachment security was evaluated using the Italian translation (Calvo V. (1998) Italian translation of the Security Scale by Kerns, Klepac e Cole, Unpublished Manuscript; Calvo V. (2008a) Description and evaluation form of the Security Scale], Unpublished Manuscript; Calvo V. (2008b) Aspects of validation of the Security Scale in Italy: internal consistency and scores distribution. Unpublished Manuscript) of the Security Scale [25]. The *SAFA* [22] is a self-report scale for children and adolescents that assesses six types of psychopathology (anxiety, depression, somatisation, obsessive-compulsive symptoms, psychogenic eating disorders and specific phobias). The psychometric properties of the battery are satisfactory: it has good internal consistency (α = .80), acceptable test-retest stability and satisfactory convergent and discriminant validity [24]. For the purposes of this study we only used the anxiety disorders scale (SAFA-A) which assesses symptoms of generalised anxiety disorder (GAD), social anxiety disorder (SAD), separation (from parents) and loss anxiety (SLA), and scholastic anxiety (SA). The total scale score provides global measure of anxiety.

The *Security Scale* is a 15-item self-report scale used to measure children and adolescents' perceptions of the security within th relationships with their father and mother. The notion of perceived attachment security refers to the degree in which the children or adolescents feel and believe their parents are able to detect and effectively regulate their states of distress [26]. The Security scale is thus composed of two separate scales that measure the level of perceived attachment security with each parent (maternal and paternal security scales), as evaluated by the child and adolescent. A third scale is then reckoned (total scale of perceived security) by cumulating the scores of maternal and paternal scales. The reliability and validity of the Security Scale have been assessed in both child and adolescent samples [26] and it has shown satisfactory stability and internal consistency (maternal attachment: α = .64–.90; paternal attachment: α = .81–.88). The Security Scale has shown convergence with other middle-childhood measures of attachment as well as with observations of children's interactions with their parents [25].

Statistical analyses

We used independent-samples *t*-tests to assess differences between the clinical and control groups. Effect sizes were computed in terms of Cohen's *d* [27], which scales mean differences relative to the pooled standard deviation of the two groups. We also anticipated a mediation pattern. Mediation represents a chain of relations where an antecedent variable relates to a mediating variable, which in turn is associated with an outcome variable [28]. The models in Fig. 1 depict the basic mediation pattern we tested. The mediation hypotheses showed in Fig. 1 were tested using the SPSS PROCESS macro (Hayes, 2013), a procedure implemented under the SPSS statistical package to compute and test mediation effects. Results of the mediation analysis allow to partition the total association of Migraine with Anxiety into an indirect association channeled by attachment (the mediator), and a direct association of migraine with anxiety that is not channeled by attachment.

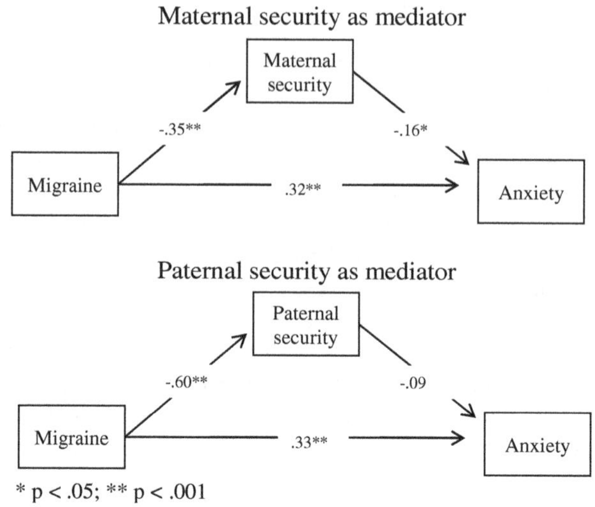

Fig. 1 Maternal security as mediator (*upper panel*), Paternal security as mediator (*lower panel*)

Results

Table 1 reports correlations and descriptive statistics for the pooled groups.

The clinical migraine group was composed of 100 children and adolescents (48 boys; 52 girls) with a mean age of 10.64 (*SD* = 2.85 years), instead the control group was composed of 100 children and adolescents (49 girls; 51 boys), with a mean age of 10.16 years (*SD* = 2.01).

The two groups had similar age ($t < 1$, *ns*) and gender distributions ($\chi^2_{(1)} = 0.18, p = .67$).

Mean differences across groups

Table 2 presents group means for anxiety and attachment and the *t*-statistic for each comparison. Because we tested six comparisons, we set the maximum acceptable type I error rate for each *t*-test at .008 (.05/8) in order to bring the acceptable overall type I error rate close to the nominal .05 level. As Table 2 shows, all group differences were significant using this conservative criterion.

An inspection of the figures in Table 2 reveals that there were remarkable group differences on all SAFA-A

Table 1 Correlations, means and standard deviations for the variables in the study ($N = 200$)

	Group	Gender	Age	TA	GAD	SAD	SLA	SA	PSM	PSF
Group	1	-	-	-	-	-	-	-	-	-
Sex	–.030	1	-	-	-	-	-	-	-	-
Gender	.000	0	1	-	-	-	-	-	-	-
TA	.371**	.016	.131	1	-	-	-	-	-	-
GAD	.337**	–.004	.12	.811**	1	-	-	-	-	-
SAD	.372**	.023	.031	.756**	.521**	1	-	-	-	-
SLA	.240**	.083	–.003	.677**	.443**	.411**	1	-	-	-
SA	.309**	.004	.104	.762**	.560**	.490**	.380**	1	-	-
PSM	–.330**	–.135	–.009	–.259**	–.226**	–.218**	–.099	–.284**	1	-
-PSF	–.600**	–.102	.042	–.281**	–.265**	–.362**	–.116	–.248**	.372**	1
M(SD)	-	-	10.97(2.17)	44.42 (9.62)	44.69 (9.50)	46.15 (8.87)	43.05 (9.31)	48.12 (9.46)	47.41 (9.22)	47.66 (10.26)

Legend: Group: Control Group(0); Clinical Group (1); Gender: Female(0); Male (1); Total anxiety (TA), Generalized Anxiety Disorder (GAD), Social Anxiety Disorder (SAD), Separation and Loss Anxiety; (SLA), Scholastic Anxiety (SA); Security Perception toward the Mather (PSM); Security Perception toward the Father (PSF)
** $p < 0.01$ (two-tailed)

subscales. For all scales the clinical group showed higher anxiety scores compared with the control group, and the differences were all highly significant (all *ps* < .001). To better gauge the size of the reported mean-differences we relied on Cohen's *d* [27]. By this metric, values about .5 indicate medium effects, and values above .8 suggest large effects [27]. Medium-to-large effects were found for GAD ($d = .71$), SA ($d = .80$), SLA ($d = .49$) and SAD ($d = .65$) scores. Therefore one might conclude that the differences in anxiety across groups were considerable. As for the attachment scores, the clinical group showed lower levels of security for both Mother and Father attachment security scores, compared with the control group. The effect sizes were medium-to-large ($d = .70$) for maternal attachment, and very large ($d = 1.50$) for paternal attachment. Such differences suggest a strong discrimination across the clinical and control groups on attachment-related dimensions.

These findings are consistent with the results of earlier studies and provide support for the hypothesis that migraine would be positively associated with anxiety, and negatively associated with attachment security. The magnitude of the differences detected was remarkable, with the majority of effect sizes above the threshold for a medium effect ($d = .5$), and some above the threshold for a large effect ($d = .8$) [27].

Table 2 Mean differences between clinical and control groups on anxiety and attachment security measures

Variable	Clinical Group Mean (SD)	Control Group Mean (SD)	t(df)	p (2-tailed)
GAD	47.92 (9.65)	41.53 (8.26)	5.00 *(196)*	<.0001
SA	49.48 (10.32)	42.89 (5.53)	5.61 *(196)*	<.0001
SLA	45.31 (8.32)	40.85 (9.76)	3.46 *(196)*	<.001
SAD	51.07 (9.93)	45.24 (8.04)	4.54 *(196)*	<.0001
PSM	44.31 (7.18)	50.39 (9.98)	*4.87 (194)*	<.0001
PSF	41.36 (7.77)	53.66 (8.64)	10.43 (193)	<.0001

Legend: Generalized Anxiety Disorder (GAD), Social Anxiety Disorder (SAD), Separation and Loss Anxiety (SLA), Scholastic Anxiety (SA); Security Perception toward the Mather (PSM); Security Perception toward the Father (PSF)

Mediation

Turning to our second aim, we tested a model in which the association between migraine (X) and anxiety (Y) was mediated by attachment (the mediator, M). Fig. 1 depicts a simplified representation of the model Fig. 1. We relied on the SPSS PROCESS macro (Hayes, 2013 – Model #4) to estimate the direct and indirect associations. We controlled for gender and age effects in estimating the model, but such effects are not represented in Fig. 1 for the sake of simplicity.[1]

First we analysed the role of maternal attachment. As for the covariates, anxiety levels were not affected by gender ($t < 1$, $p > .80$), nor by age ($\beta = .12$, $p > .05$). Security of maternal attachment was related to gender ($\beta = -.31$, $p < .05$), with girls expressing more insecurity about this attachment relationship than boys.

Turning to mediation, the results showed (Fig. 1, upper panel) that migraine was negatively associated with maternal attachment security ($\beta = -.35$, $p < .0001$), and in turn maternal attachment security was negatively related to anxiety ($\beta = -.16$, $p < .03$). Such pattern yield an estimate of the indirect effect of migraine through maternal attachment of .057, a significant indirect association because the its 95% confidence interval did not include zero (95% CI: .009, .129). Along with the indirect effect through attachment, a direct association of migraine with anxiety was found ($\beta = .32$, $p < .0001$).

Descriptively, it was possible to compute how much of the total association between migraine and anxiety followed a direct route, and the proportion of the association that was instead mediated by attachment insecurity.

The total effect can be computed by the sum of the direct (.32) and indirect association (.057), and therefore the total effect in this case equaled about .38. Hence, 84% of the total association between migraine and anxiety was attributable to a direct association, and the remaining 16% of the total association was attributable to an indirect path via maternal attachment.

We turned next to the role of paternal attachment (Fig. 1, lower panel)..The mediation model included also the age and gender as covariates (omitted in Fig. 1). Gender did not affect anxiety levels ($t < 1$, $p > .80$), but age was positively associated with anxiety ($\beta = .14$, $p < .04$). As found for maternal attachment security, girls expressed more insecurity about the paternal attachment relationship than boys ($\beta = -.13$, $p < .03$).

Turning to mediation, migraine was strongly negatively associated with paternal attachment security ($\beta = -.60$, $p < .0001$), but paternal attachment security was not associated with anxiety ($\beta = -.09$, $t = 1.08$ $p > .25$). As a consequence, the indirect effect of migraine through paternal attachment was not significant (indirect effect = .054, 95% CI: −.041, .164), and only the direct association of migraine with anxiety could be detected in this model ($\beta = .33$, $p < .0001$).

An exploratory model

The two mediation models suggest different conclusions for the role of maternal and paternal attachment. Maternal attachment security was a stronger correlate of anxiety than perceived paternal attachment security, whereas perceived paternal attachment security was more closely associated with migraine. Combining the results of the two models might suggest a more complex pattern of associations, where the association of migraine with anxiety is channeled through two mediators, first paternal attachment and secondly maternal attachment. We investigated thus in a frankly explorative fashion the possibility that migraine would relate with paternal attachment, paternal attachment would then relate to maternal attachment, which in turn would be connected with anxiety (Fig. 2).

We found that migraine was related with paternal attachment ($\beta = -.60$, $p < .001$), paternal attachment was connected with maternal attachment ($\beta = .37$, $p < .001$), and in turn maternal attachment was associated with anxiety ($\beta = -.25$, $p < .01$). This esplorative model might offer a more nuanced interpretation of the processes that may be at play, suggesting avenues for futire research. Insecure maternal attachment appeared to play a pivotal role channeling the association of paternal attachment, and migraine and eventually relating to anxiety.

Discussion

This study had two objectives. The first was to compare anxiety and perceived attachment security in a group of children and adolescents suffering from MoA and a healthy control group. The second was to test whether the observed group differences in anxiety were mediated by perceived attachment security.

Between-group differences in anxiety levels and perceived attachment security

With respect to the first objective, our results were in line with most previous studies, confirming that children and adolescents with MoA show higher anxiety levels than their healthy peers [2, 9, 29]. More specifically, our findings replicated previous reports of associations between headache and GAD [30], SAD [31], SA [32–34] and SLA [21, 23] in children and adolescents. Analysis revealed differences between the clinical and control groups with respect to security of attachment to both parental figures. It is well documented that attachment insecurity is associated with several organic conditions of infancy and adolescence, in particular conditions in which emotional triggers have a role, such as headache and abdominal pain [19, 35]. Previous studies [36, 37] have suggested that dysfunctional family relationships are associated with greater pain and disability, in particular migraine [13, 18].

The association between headache and attachment insecurity can be seen as originating from the role of early insecure models for the development and maintenance of migraine symptoms, but also materializing because the enduring stressful condition shapes the child's perception of availability of attachment figures. We contend that the mediation results we present are consistent with the latter process, which assumes that chronic stress eventually affects attachment beliefs, as discussed below.

The mediating role of attachment insecurity

As to the second objective of the study, investigating the mediating effect of attachment insecurity on the anxiety symptoms associated with migraine, there were strong negative associations between the paternal and maternal

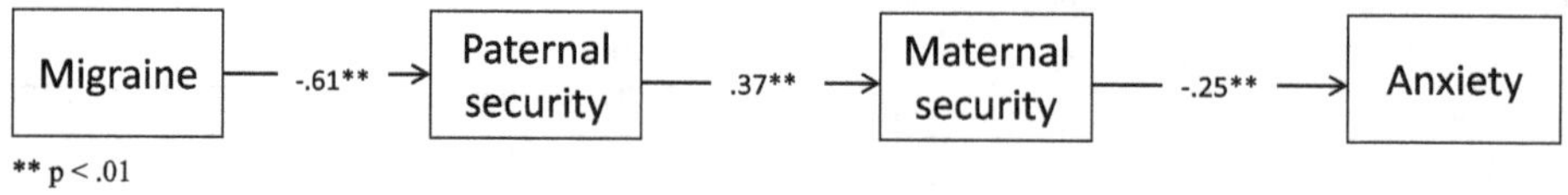

Fig. 2 Chain of associations

dimensions of attachment security evaluated by the Security Scale and all four forms of anxiety. Our results also indicate that the attachment security dimensions seem to mediate some of the group differences in anxiety. These results provide some support for our mediation hypothesis, which was that the migraine-anxiety association would be at least partially mediated by attachment security. Empirical research has suggested various mechanisms for such a mediation pattern [13]. The role of attachment in increasing anxiety in migraine patients could be attributed to two cumulating sources. On the one hand, insecure attachment developed as a result of the pattern of early interactions might make more severe the child's anxiety responses to stressful events. Previous studies have evaluated the relationship between attachment styles and pain, showing that perceptions of pain and the related anxious distress might be influenced by attachment models [18, 19]. A recent study found that the anxious-ambivalent attachment style was positively associated with symptoms of anxiety, depression and somatization in children and adolescents diagnosed with migraine [13]. On the other hand, developmental research has demonstrated that stressful events, in turn, can modify extant attachment models. In other words, it seems that, like other organic diseases, headache episodes might represent stressors and thus trigger anxiety responses, which in turn over-activate the attachment system. The tendency to activate the attachment system in order to regulate distress engendered by physical pain is thought to be particularly strong during development. The level of distress young patients experience due to headache episodes is modulated by their perception of the security of their attachment relationships [20, 21]. It should also be noted that children's lack of trust in parental availability and effectiveness can have a negative impact on the extent to which parental actions modulate their anxiety and distress. The peculiar conditions of headache-related distress may thus activate the attachment system, and the difficulties in meeting the child's proximity request may bring about an insecure anxious attachment style. A recent study by Barone et al. [38] showed that that migraine attacks weaken children's attachment security toward their parents, thus undermining the parental confidence in exerting an effective regulatory function on their children's distress.

The second mediation model evidenced in our results focused on both paternal and maternal attachment and showed that the somatic condition of migraine acted as a stressor, reducing children's perception of the security of their parental attachments. This result confirms that a state of chronic helplessness and pain constitute a major challenge for the attachment system and family interactions. Interestingly enough, our mediation analysis highlighted differences between the networks of associations involving maternal and paternal attachment. Our clinical group perceived their fathers as much less available and much less emotionally reliable than did the control group, yet such lower paternal attachment security did not have a direct effect on anxiety symptoms. However, paternal attachment insecurity did relate with children's trust in their mothers, the ultimate buffer of children's distress, and maternal attachment security in turn was related with anxiety levels. It could be that a child's loss of trust in his or her father results in a heavy burden being placed on the mother; such burden may become apparent the mother could be thus perceived by the child as being less available and less able to regulate his or her fears and distress, all of which leads to an increase in anxiety symptoms. Recent research [38] highlights how that insecure attachment may hinder parental attempts to reduce children's distress in the presence of headache attacks.

Overall our results are in keeping with the reported relationship between attachment insecurity and anxiety symptoms, but to the best of our knowledge this is the first study to provide empirical evidence that attachment mediates the association between pediatric headache disorders and anxiety. Our mediation model also suggested that there are differences between the roles played by perceived maternal and paternal attachment security.

Limitations

We deem the results of this study as potentially fruitful. Of course, further research is needed to allow more detailed conclusions to be drawn. Furthermore, some limitations should be acknowledged. Our sample was relatively modest in size and limited to a specific clinical population, namely children and adolescents with MoA, under observation in a third-level centre, which may increase referral bias. Furthermore, the healthy control group was a convenience sample, and thus subject to the problems inherent in the use of such samples (e.g. relatively high sampling error, selection bias, and other biases). However, the sample size was large enough to guarantee 80% power for the detection of effects in the range suggested by the extant literature.

A second obvious limitation is that our research design cannot be used as the basis for causal inferences. We wish to clarify that the associations and mediation patterns we specified should be considered simply as a summary of a network of associations, and by no means indicative of causal mechanism. The observed network of associations can, nevertheless, be used as the basis for hypotheses about causal relationships that can then be tested using the appropriate experimental designs.

It should also be acknowledged that the measures we used are indicative rather than exhaustive in their respective domains. The Security Scale measures the perceived security of attachment relationships but not attachment style and the SAFA test is a screening instrument rather than a diagnostic instrument. In the future we plan to compare groups of children diagnosed with tension headache, migraine with aura and other chronic conditions. Measures of migraine severity and objective assessments of the psychological traits of clinical subjects and their parents, as well as measures of depression, somatisation and specific phobias would also be useful for characterising parent-child relationships in clinical settings.

Conclusions

Overall this study provides further confirmation of the established association between MoA diagnosis and anxiety symptoms in childhood and adolescence. Secondly, attachment insecurity can be regarded as one of the factors mediating this association. These conclusions may buttress the importance of individual psychotherapy as a treatment for anxiety in children and adolescents with migraine, as well as highlighting the relevance of psychosocial interventions including family interventions [39].

Abbreviations

GAD: Generalised anxiety disorder; MoA: Migraine without aura; SA: Scholastic anxiety; SAD: Social anxiety disorder; SAFA: Self Administered Psychiatric Scales for Children and Adolescents; SLA: Separation and loss anxiety

Funding

This research received no specific grant from any funding agency in the public, commercial, or not-for-profit sectors.

Authors' contributions

RW and VG conceived and designed the study. ES, RC and MA were responsible for critical revision of this manuscript. NF, GN, BB, and PV were responsible for data acquisition. LL was responsible for the statistical analysis. All authors approved the final version of this manuscript.

Competing interests

The authors declare that they have no competing interests.

Author details

[1]Department of Dynamic and Clinical Psychology, Sapienza University of Rome, Rome, Italy. [2]Department of Social and Developmental Psychology, Sapienza University of Rome, Rome, Italy. [3]Phd program in Behavioural Neuroscience, Department of Paediatrics and Child and Adolescent Neuropsychiatry, Sapienza University of Rome, Rome, Italy. [4]Department of Paediatrics and Child and Adolescent Neuropsychiatry, Sapienza University of Rome, Via dei Sabelli 108, 00185 Rome, Italy. [5]Glia Institute, Ribeirão Preto, São Paulo, Brazil.

References

1. Wöber-Bingöl C (2013) Epidemiology of migraine and headache in children and adolescents. Curr Pain Headache Rep 17(6):341
2. Bellini B, Arruda M, Cescut A et al (2013) Headache and comorbidity in children and adolescents. J Headache Pain 14:79
3. Egger HL, Angold A, Costello EJ (1998) Headaches and psychopathology in children and adolescents. J Am Acad Child Adolesc Psychiatry 37(9):951–958
4. Egger HL, Costello EJ, Erkanli A, Angold A (1999) Somatic complaints and psychopathology in children and adolescents: stomach aches, musculoskeletal pains, and headaches. J Am Acad Child Adolesc Psychiatry 38(7):852–860
5. Mazzone L, Vitello B, Incorpora G, Mazzone D (2005) Behavioral and temperamental characteristics of children and adolescents suffering from primary headache. Cephalalgia 26:194–201
6. Bruni O, Russo PM, Ferri R et al (2008) Relationship between headache and sleep in a non-clinical population of children and adolescents. Sleep Med 9: 542–548
7. Bigal ME, Lipton RB, Holland RP et al (2007) Obesity, migraine and chronic migraine: possible mechanisms of interaction. Neurology 68:1851–1861
8. Bruijn J, Locher H, Passchier J, Dijkstra N, Arts WF (2010) Psychopathology in children and adolescents with migraine in clinical studies: a systematic review. Pediatrics 126(2):323–332
9. Antonaci F, Nappi G, Galli F, Manzoni GC, Calabresi P, Costa A (2011) Migraine and psychiatric comorbidity: a review of clinical findings. J Headache Pain 12(2):115–125
10. Bowlby J (1988) A secure base: clinical applications of attachment theory. Routledge, London
11. Sroufe A, Egeland B, Carlson E, Collins A (2005) The development of the person: the Minnesota study of risk and adaptation from birth to adulthood. Guilford Press, New York
12. DeKlyen M, Greenberg MT (2008) Attachment and psychopathology in childhood. In: Cassidy J, Shaver PR (eds) Handbook of attachment: theory, research and clinical applications, 2nd edn. Guilford Press, New York, pp 637–665
13. Tarantino S, De Ranieri C, Dionisi C, Gagliardi V, Paniccia MF, Capuano A, Frusciante R, Balestri M, Vigevano F, Gentile S, Valeriani M (2017) Role of the attachment style in determining the association between headache features and psychological symptoms in migraine children and adolescents. An analytical observational case-control study Headache, doi:10.1111/head.13007.
14. Hafeman DM, Schwartz S (2009) Opening the black box: a motivation for the assessment of mediation. Int J Epidemiol 38:838–845
15. Bretherton I, Munholland K (2008) Internal working models in attachment relationships. In: Cassidy J, Shaver P (eds) Handbook of attachment: theory, research and clinical application, 2nd edn. Guilford Press, New York, pp 102–130
16. Headache Classification Committee of the International Headache Society (IHS) (2013) The international classification of headache disorders, 3rd edition (beta version). Cephalalgia 33(9):629–808
17. World Medical Association (WMA): WMA Declaration of Helsinki – Ethical Principles for Medical Research Involving Human Subjects. Ferney-Voltaire: World Medical Association (2008). Available from: http://ethics.iit.edu/ecodes/node/4618 Accessed 20 Oct 2016
18. Esposito M, Parisi L, Gallai B et al (2013) Attachment styles in children affected by migraine without Aura. Neuropsychiatr Dis Treat 9:1513–1519
19. Savi L, Buccheri R, Tambornini A et al (2005) Attachment styles and headache. J Headache Pain 6:254–257
20. Berry JK, Drummond PD (2014) Does attachment anxiety increase vulnerability to headache? J Psychosom Res 76(2):113–120
21. Tarantino S, De Ranieri C, Dionisi C et al (2015) Migraine equivalents and related symptoms, psychological profile and headache features: which relationship? J Headache Pain 16:536
22. Cianchetti C, Sannio-Fancello G (2001) Scale Psichiatriche di Autosomministrazione per Fanciulli e Adolescenti. O. S. Organizzazioni Speciali, Firenze
23. Tarantino S, De Ranieri C, Dionisi C et al (2013) Clinical features, anger management and anxiety: a possible correlation in migraine children. J Headache Pain 14:39
24. Franzoni E, Monti M, Pellicciari A et al (2009) SAFA: a new measure to evaluate psychiatric symptoms detected in a sample of children and adolescents affected by eating disorders. Correlations with risk factors. Neuropsychiatr Dis Treat 5:207–214

25. Kerns KA, Klepac L, Cole A (1996) Peer relationships and preadolescents' perceptions of security in the child-mother relationship. Dev Psychol 32: 457–466
26. Van Ryzin MJ, Leve LD (2012) Validity evidence for the security scale as a measure of perceived attachment security in adolescence. J Adolesc 35(2):425–431
27. Cohen J (1992) A power primer. Psychol Bull 112(1):155–159
28. MacKinnon DP, Fairchild AJ, Fritz MS (2007) Mediation analysis. Annu Rev Psychol 58:593–614
29. Powers SW, Gilman DK, Hershey AD (2006) Headache and psychological functioning in children and adolescents. Headache 46(9):1404–1415
30. Lee SM (2015) Screening for depression and anxiety disorder in children with headache. Korean J Pediatr 58(2):64–68
31. Jette N, Patten S, Williams J, Becker W, Wiebe S (2008) Comorbidity of migraine and psychiatric disorders: a national population-based study. Headache 48:501–516
32. Masruha MR, Lin J, Minett TS et al (2012) Social anxiety score is high in adolescents with chronic migraine. Pediatr Int 54(3):393–396
33. Assa A, Ish-Tov A, Rinawi F et al (2015) School attendance in children with functional abdominal pain and inflammatory bowel diseases. J Pediatr Gastroenterol Nutr 61(5):553–557
34. Rousseau-Salvador C, Amouroux R, Annequin D et al (2014) Anxiety, depression and school absenteeism in youth with chronic or episodic headache. Pain Res Manag 19(5):235–240
35. Tremblay I, Sullivan MJL (2010) Attachment and pain outcomes in adolescents: the mediating role of pain catastrophizing and anxiety. J Pain 11:160–171
36. Palermo TM, Putnam J, Armstrong G et al (2007) Adolescent autonomy and family functioning are associated with headache-related disability. Clin J Pain 23(5):458–465
37. Logan DE, Scharff L (2005) Relationships between family and parent characteristics and functional abilities in children with recurrent pain syndromes: an investigation of moderating effects on the pathway from pain to disability. J Pediatr Psychol 30(8):698–670
38. Barone L, Lionetti F, Dellagiulia A et al (2015) Behavioural problems in children with headache and maternal stress: is Children's attachment security a protective factor? Inf Child Dev. doi:10.1002/icd.1950
39. Ng QX, Venkatanarayanan N, Kumar L (2017) A systematic review and meta-analysis of the efficacy of cognitive behavioral therapy for the management of pediatric migraine. Headache 57(3):349–362

14

De novo exonic duplication of ATP1A2 in Italian patient with hemiplegic migraine

Stella Gagliardi[1*†], Gaetano Salvatore Grieco[1†], Francesca Gualandi[2], Luisa Maria Caniatti[3], Elisabetta Groppo[3], Marialuisa Valente[1], Giuseppe Nappi[4], Marcella Neri[2] and Cristina Cereda[1]

Abstract

Background: Sporadic Hemiplegic Migraine is a rare form of migraine headache. Mutations in three different genes, two ion-channel genes and one encoding an ATP exchanger, *CACNA1A*, *ATP1A2* and *SCN1A* are all responsible for the FHM phenotype, thus indicating a genetic heterogeneity for this disorder. Here, we described a de novo exonic duplication of *ATP1A2* in an Italian patient with Hemiplegic Migraine.

Case presentation: We describe the case of a young woman (33 year old) who suffered from the age of 8 years of episodic weakness of the limbs, associated to other subjective and objective features. From aged 25, she developed neurological symptoms, like dizziness, blurred vision and an MRI scan revealed aspecific peritrigonal white matter hyperintensities. Aged 32 she suffered of right hemisomatic sudden-onset paresthesias, hypoesthesia and hyposthenia and the patient was genetically investigated for sporadic hemiplegic migraine.

Conclusions: Here we report, for the first time, an exonic duplication in the *ATP1A2* associated with hemiplegic migraine. The variation identified involves exon 21 of the *ATP1A2* and is expected to alter the function of the alpha(2) subunit of the Na(+)/K(+) pump; the de novo nature of the duplication further supports its pathogenic role. To date, no other CNVs have been described in the *ATP1A2* but only point mutations are reported. The novel mutation may result impaired M9 transmembrane domain, in a loss-of-function of the alpha(2) Na(+)/K(+)-ATPase with glutamate accumulation, alteration of synaptic function and neurotransmission.

Keywords: ATP1A2, Duplication, Hemiplegic migraine, De novo

Background

Hemiplegic migraine (HM) is a rare form of migraine headache. There are two types of hemiplegic migraine–familial hemiplegic migraine (FHM) and sporadic hemiplegic migraine (SHM). Migraines typically cause intense, throbbing pain in one area of the head. Some people with migraines also experience nausea, vomiting, and sensitivity to light and sound [1, 2]. These recurrent headaches typically begin in childhood or adolescence and can be triggered by specific foods, emotional stress, and minor head trauma. Each headache may last from a few hours to a few days. Mutations in three different genes, two ion-channel genes and one encoding an ATP exchanger, calcium voltage-gated channel subunit alpha1 A *(CACNA1A)*, ATPase Na+/K+ transporting subunit alpha 2 *(ATP1A2)*, Sodium channel protein type 1 subunit alpha (*SCN1A)* are all responsible for the HM phenotype, thus indicating a genetic heterogeneity for this disorder [3, 4]. Recently, also proline rich transmembrane protein 2 (*PRRT2)* has been associated to HM [4]. *ATP1A2* is located on 1q23 (FHM2, MIM #182340) [5], and more than 60 mutations have been identified in association to the FHM phenotype. This gene, *ATP1A2*, encodes the alpha-2 catalytic subunit of a sodium-potassium-ATPases [5]. Mutations in *ATP1A2* are mainly missense; few deletions have been described [5] but so far no duplications in *ATP1A2* have been discovered [3]. In

* Correspondence: stella.gagliardi@mondino.it
†Equal contributors
[1]Genomic and Post-Genomic Center, "C. Mondino" National Neurological Institute, Mondino 2, 27100 Pavia, Italy
Full list of author information is available at the end of the article

this study, we describe, for the first time, a novel ATP1A2 exon duplication in an Italian patient with SHM phenotype.

Case presentation

We describe the case of a young woman who suffered from the age of 8 years of episodic weakness of the limbs, associated to other subjective and objective features.

The onset was with recurrent episodic fatigue, limb weakness with dysesthesias, paresthesias, hyperalgesias, pain triggered from febrile illness, arthralgias in all four limbs; furthermore she reported episodes of skin rash. The painful symptoms were categorized as a fibromyalgia and she underwent amitriptyline and ademetionine therapy without relief. Until the age of 25 years she was taken into care by rheumatologists and, given the concomitant presence of stomatitis, The Raynaud phenomenon, and episcleritis, a form of Behcet disease (HLA-B51 negative) was diagnosed, then disconfirmed, but meanwhile treated with steroids, azathioprine, colchicine. From year 2007, aged 25, she developed neurological symptoms, like dizziness, blurred vision and an MRI scan revealed aspecific peritrigonal white matter hyperintensities.

Aged 32 she suffered of right hemisomatic sudden-onset paresthesias, hypoesthesia and hyposthenia, confirmed on examination; this episode lasted 45 min and it was followed by headache, sleepness, diplopia. She was admitted on ED: a CT scan was negative; a mild antinuclear antibodies positivity (1:160) was found andan hemato-encephalic-barrier dysfunction on liquoral analysis, liquoral analysis showed an hemato-encephalic-barrier dysfunction with increased protein amount (57 mg/dl) without intratecal synthesis of IgG. CSF/serum albumin ratio (QAlb) = 9.43. A new MRI scan confirmed the previous result (Fig. 1). There were no abnormalities at the neurophysiological evaluation. The ophthalmologic evaluation revealed a bilateral hypovisus (7–8/10 in the right and 4–5/10 in the left), lax eyelid syndrome, bilateral posterior lenticonus, astigmatism, exothropia, monocular bilateral diplopia; OCT scan was normal. During hospitalization the patient suffered from episodic intense headache, with migrainous features.

The following year she suffered from another episode of right hemiparesis and hemi-hypoesthesia associated to sub-continuous diffuse arthromyalgia. After assumption of a tablet of triptane, she referred a severe crisis and between the crisis of migraine with motor aurea muscle pain and fatigue were present.

As the persistent headache, the patient started prophylactic long-term therapy with topiramate, with beneficial effects.

Due to the concomitant presence of recurrent hemiparesis associated or subsequent to migraine attacks, based on the headache classification criteria [6], the patient was genetically investigated for familial hemiplegic migraine (FHM); the familial history was negative for neurological disorders (Fig. 2), both parents and the twin sister never experienced migraine attack similar to the one of our patient.

Molecular analysis

DNA was extracted from peripheral blood cells using standard procedures. *ATP1A2* and *CACNA1A* exons were amplified by PCR using primers located in adjacent intronic regions. The amplicons were screened for sequence variations by direct sequencing using the Big-Dye Terminator v3.1 sequencing kit (Applied Biosystems, Milan, Italy) and ABI 3130 Genetic Analyser (Applied Biosystems, Milan, Italy). The alignment to reference sequence was performed using Sequencher 4.8 software. Primer sequences and PCR conditions are available upon request.

Search for CNVs was performed using MLPA assay using both the P348-A2 ATP1A2-CACNA1A probe mix and P279 CACNA1A probemix (SALSA MLPA Kit, MRC-Holland). Moreover also the second kit about migraine has been used for each sample (SALSA MLPA; MRC-Holland).

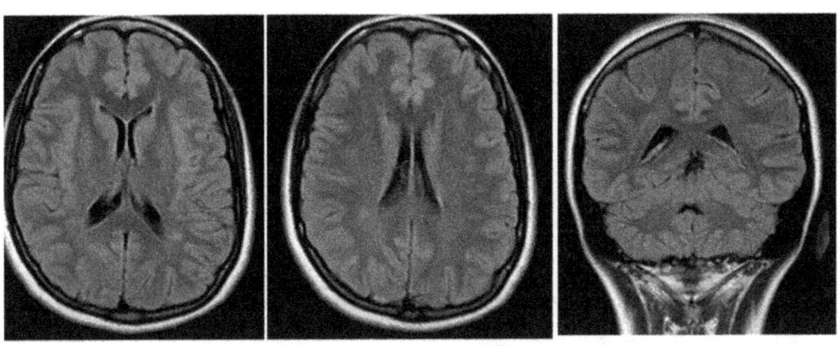

Fig. 1 MRI scan images revealing aspecific peritrigonal white matter hyperintensities. The control MRI was performed after 6 months and 1 year and confirmed the small focal peritrigonal white matter hyperintensities in T2/FLAIR. Hypertension, heart valvular disease and other vasculophaties were excluded. Transcranial doppler US no detected the micro-embolic signals. Another MRI was performed after 2 years and the picture is unvaried

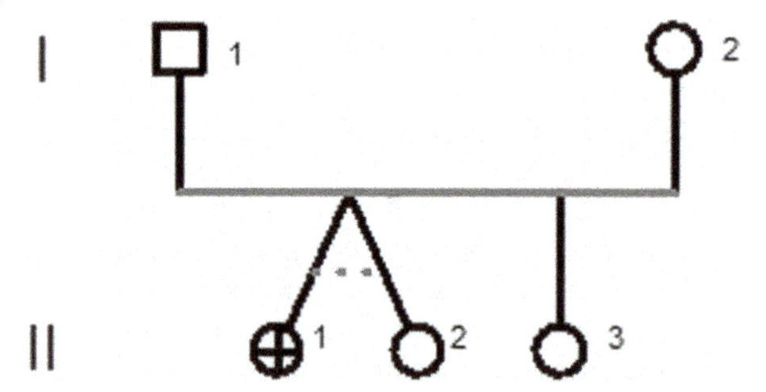

Fig. 2 Pedigree of the Italian family. Filled symbols represent affected individuals and open symbols non-affected individuals

Identified *ATP1A2* duplication was confirmed by Real Time PCR. All the experiments have been performed in triplicates.

Conclusion

We report here for the first time the identification of an exonic duplication in the *ATP1A2* associated with hemiplegic migraine. MLPA test identified a duplication involving the exon 21 of *ATP1A2* (plus 50% amplification in the signal) with multiple MLPA probes (Fig. 3a). ATP1A2 exonic duplication was not detected in 100 healthy subjects and 100 FHM patients. The identified exon 21 duplication resulted de novo at the segregation analysis in both patient's parents. Direct sequencing analysis was negative for small mutations both in *CACNA1A* and in *ATP1A2* exons.

Mutations of the genes encoding the Na/K-ATPase a-subunit (ATP1A2 and ATP1A3) have been described in three distinct human neurological disorders: familial hemiplegic migraine, rapid onset dystonia Parkinsonism, and alternating hemiplegia of childhood [3]. These neurological disorders are dominantly inherited and caused primarily by missense mutations, which are thought to confer a mild hypomorphic loss-of-function.

In the first two families in which FHM was associated to mutations in *ATP1A2* [7], six several affected individuals presented a history of seizures independent of

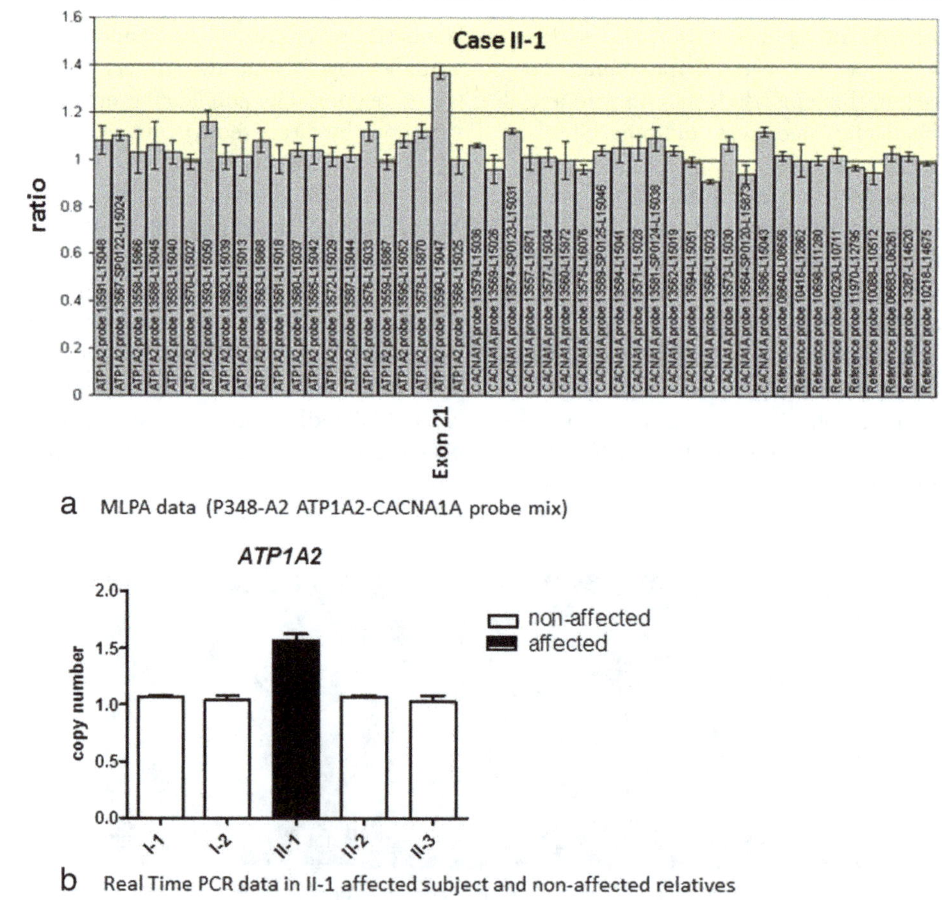

Fig. 3 **a** ATP1A2 duplication in SHM patient obtained by MLPA assay. For each probe, the ratio < 0.75 stands for deletion; and the ratio > 1.3 stands for duplication. **b** ATP1A2 quantification by Real Time PCR in patient and in unaffected relatives

hemiplegic migraine attacks; the penetrance of epilepsy is also incomplete in these families.

The clinical presentation in our patient is peculiar due to the fact that she experienced since childhood recurrent weakness with dysesthesias/paresthesias of limbs and pain triggered by fever, diagnosed firstly as fibromyalgia. From the age of 25, she developed more neurological symptoms, like dizziness, blurred vision and she suffered of hemisomatic sudden-onset paresthesias/hyposthenia, associated to severe headache. After assumption of a tablet of triptane, she referred a severe crisis and between the crisis of migraine with motor aurea muscle pain and fatigue were present.

Although the mutations in *ATP1A2* that cause hemiplegic migraine are not as well-studied, it is thought that they may impair the transport of sodium and potassium ions and prolonging the presence of neurotransmitters between neurons. The abnormal signalling resulting from these changes leads to the headaches and auras characteristic of the condition.

In fact, starting from hemiplegic migraine clinical features, these patients suffer from migraines with hemiplegia and partial paralysis during the aura phase and, in some cases, accompanied by seizures or cognitive dysfunction. Neuroimaging studies have shown that migraine aura is caused by cortical spreading depression (CSD) [8]. Inhibition of ATP1A2 leads to high levels of extracellular potassium, causing neurons to become depolarized which can cause CSD [9]. The penetrance of hemiplegic migraine is incomplete (about 65%), and mutation carriers may be affected by typical migraine with aura but not by hemi-plegic migraine [7].

To our knowledge, this report is the first to describe an exonic copy number change in *ATP1A2* associated to a clinical phenotype of hemiplegic migraine.

Several data support the possible pathogenic role of this variation; firstly the de novo nature of the variation itself, not inherited forms the healthy parents. Secondly, this copy number variation as not identified in 100 healthy controls neither in 100 hemiplegic migraine patients. Moreover, our hypothesis is supported by the guideline for variant interpretation of copy number variation [10] that suggests that if CNV is shown to represent a de novo mutation in the proband, this is generally taken as evidence supporting pathogenicity.

So far, the mechanism for the effects of ATP1A2 mutations is not clear. Moreover, point mutations in exon 21 or in flanking exons are reported as pathogenic in HM patients. These mutations result in a loss-of-function of the alpha(2) Na(+)/K(+)-ATPase with glutamate accumulation, alteration of synaptic function and neurotransmission. Also the duplication of exon 21 of *ATP1A2* is expected to alter the function of the alpha(2) subunit of the Na(+)/K(+) pump by the impairment of domain M9, where exon 21 is located.

The hypothesized mechanism for the effects of ATP1A2 duplication is that may cause an increase in extracellular potassium and intracellular sodium which increases intracellular calcium levels through the Na+/Ca2+ exchanger, resulting in glutamate release and a decrease in glutamate clearance which can also lead to CSD. This hypothesis results in making the brain more susceptible to CSD and therefore migraines with aura [11].

In conclusion, this work further strengthens the involvement of the *ATP1A2* in hemiplegic migraine and highlights the importance to complement analysis of direct sequencing with quantitative gene analysis to exactly describe the association between ATP1A2 variations and hemiplegic migraine.

Key findings bullet points

- Identification of novel mutation in ATP1A2 gene associated to Sporadic Hemiplegic Migraine
- Discovery of a duplication of exon 21 of ATP1A2 gene
- highlights the importance to complement analysis of direct sequencing with quantitative gene analysis

Acknowledgements
This study was supported by Ricerca Corrente 2013–2015 from the Italian Ministry of Health References.

Authors' contributions
SG She has made substantial contributions to conception and designs the experiments. She has also been involved in drafting the manuscript. GSG He has performed the experiments. FG She has been involved in revising the manuscript. MC She has made substantial contributions to analysis of data. EG She has made substantial contributions to interpretation of data. MV She has performed the experiments. NP He has given final approval of the version to be published. MN She has been involved in revising the manuscript. CC She has been involved in drafting the manuscript. All authors read and approved the final manuscript.

Competing interests
The authors declare that they have no competing interests.

Author details
[1]Genomic and Post-Genomic Center, "C. Mondino" National Neurological Institute, Mondino 2, 27100 Pavia, Italy. [2]Medical Genetics Unit, Department of Medical Sciences and Reproduction and Growth, University-Hospital S'Anna Ferrara, Ferrara, Italy. [3]Neurology Unit, Department of Neuroscience/Rehabilitation, University-Hospital S'Anna Ferrara, Ferrara, Italy. [4]Headache Science Center, C. Mondino National Neurological Institute, Pavia, Italy.

References

1. Thomsen LL, Eriksen MK, Roemer SF et al (2002) A population-based study of familial hemiplegic migraine suggests revised diagnostic criteria. Brain 125(Pt 6):1379–1391

2. Di Lorenzo C, Grieco GS, Santorelli FM (2012) Migraine headache: a review of the molecular genetics of a common disorder. J Headache Pain 13(7): 571–580 Review
3. Carreño O, Corominas R, Serra SA et al (2013) Screening of CACNA1A and ATP1A2 genes in hemiplegic migraine: clinical, genetic, and functional studies. Mol Genet Genomic Med 1(4):206–222
4. Riant F, Roze E, Barbance C et al (2012) PRRT2 mutations cause hemiplegic migraine. Neurology 79(21):2122–2124
5. de Vries B, Stam AH, Kirkpatrick M et al (2009) Familial hemiplegic migraine is associated with febrile seizures in an FHM2 family with a novel de novo ATP1A2 mutation. Epilepsia 50(11):2503–2504
6. Headache Classification Committee of the International Headache Society (IHS) (2013) The International classification of headache disorders, 3rd edition (beta version). Cephalalgia 33(9):629–808. doi:10.1177/0333102413485658
7. Thomsen LL, Kirchmann M, Bjornsson A et al (2007) The genetic spec-trum of a population-based sample of familial hemiplegic migraine. Brain 130:346e56
8. Headache Classification Committee of the International Headache Society (IHS), Costa C, Tozzi A, Rainero I et al (2013) Cortical spreading depression as a target for anti-migraine agents. J Headache Pain 14:62
9. Leo L, Gherardini L, Barone V et al (2011) Increased susceptibility to cortical spreading depression in the mouse model of familial hemiplegic migraine type 2. PLoS Genet 7(6):e1002129
10. Kearney HM, Thorland EC, Brown KK, Quintero-Rivera F, South ST. A Working Group of the American College of Medical Genetics (ACMG) Laboratory Quality Assurance Committee Genetics in Medicine. 2011;13(7):680–685. American College of Medical Genetics standards and guidelines for interpretation and reporting of postnatal constitutional copy number variants.
11. Gritz SM, Radcliffe RA (2013) Genetic effects of ATP1A2 in familial hemiplegic migraine type II and animal models. Hum Genom 7:8

15

Assessment of gray and white matter structural alterations in migraineurs without aura

Jilei Zhang[1†], Yi-Lan Wu[2,3†], Jingjing Su[2], Qian Yao[2], Mengxing Wang[1], Ge-Fei Li[2,3], Rong Zhao[2,3], Yan-Hui Shi[2,3], Ying Zhao[2], Qiting Zhang[2], Haifeng Lu[1], Shuai Xu[1], Zhaoxia Qin[1], Guo-Hong Cui[2,3], Jianqi Li[1], Jian-Ren Liu[2,3*] and Xiaoxia Du[1*]

Abstract

Background: Migraine constitute a disorder characterized by recurrent headaches, and have a high prevalence, a high socio-economic burden and severe effects on quality of life. Our previous fMRI study demonstrated that some brain regions are functional alterations in migraineurs. As the function of the human brain is related to its structure, we further investigated white and gray matter structural alterations in migraineurs.

Methods: In current study, we used surface-based morphometry, voxel-based morphometry and diffusion tensor imaging analyses to detect structural alterations of the white matter and gray matter in 32 migraineurs without aura compared with 32 age- and gender-matched healthy controls.

Results: We found that migraineurs without aura exhibited significantly increased gray matter volume in the bilateral cerebellar culmen, increased cortical thickness in the lateral occipital-temporal cortex, decreased cortical thickness in the right insula, increased gyrification index in left postcentral gyrus, superior parietal lobule and right lateral occipital cortex, and decreased gyrification index in the left rostral middle frontal gyrus compared with controls. No significant change in white matter microstructure was found in DTI analyses.

Conclusion: The significantly altered gray matter brain regions were known to be associated with sensory discrimination of pain, multi-sensory integration and nociceptive information processing and were consistent with our previous fMRI study, and may be involved in the pathological mechanism of migraine without aura.

Keywords: Migraine without aura, Voxel-based morphometry, Surface-based morphometry, Diffusion tensor imaging, Magnetic resonance imaging

Background

Migraine constitute a disorder characterized by recurrent headaches of moderate to severe intensity, pulsating quality, and unilateral location, that are aggravated by routine physical activity and associated with nausea, photophobia, and/or phonophobia [1]. It has been demonstrated that migraine have a high prevalence and a high social-economic burden, and they severely affect quality of life. In recent years, neuroimaging technology has provided more convenient methods for better understanding the pathological mechanism of migraine and identifying abnormal brain regions associated with migraine.

Several MRI studies have identified functional and structural changes between migraine patients and healthy controls, and have suggested that brain malfunctioning may be associated with migraine pathophysiology [2–7]. In addition, repeated and long-term migraine attacks may induce functional and structural plastic changes that may underlie the progression of the disorder [8, 9]. Voxel-based morphometry (VBM) and surface-based morphometry

* Correspondence: liujr021@vip.163.com; xxdu@phy.ecnu.edu.cn
†Equal contributors
[2]Department of Neurology and Jiuyuan Municipal Stroke Center, Shanghai Ninth People's Hospital, Shanghai Jiao Tong University School of Medicine, 639 Zhizaoju Road, 200011 Shanghai, People's Republic of China
[1]Shanghai Key Laboratory of Magnetic Resonance and Department of Physics, School of Physics and Materials Science, East China Normal University, 3663 North Zhong-Shan Road, 200062 Shanghai, People's Republic of China
Full list of author information is available at the end of the article

(SBM) are advantageous for evaluating structural alterations (such as gray matter volume, cortical thickness and gyrification index [GI]) of the gray matter due to their ability to localize abnormal brain regions in patients without a priori hypothesis [10–12]. Two previous meta-analyses aimed to locate concordant gray matter alterations in migraine patients and found concordant decreases in gray matter volume (GMV) in some brain regions involved in pain-related processes [13, 14]. The patient groups of previous VBM studies have been primarily migraineurs without aura, but other subtypes (such as migraineurs with aura, and patients with chronic migraine) were also included. Previous research has proposed that the different subtypes of migraine may present specific structural alterations [15, 16]. In addition, diffusion tensor imaging (DTI) has been extensively used to evaluate the microstructural changes in white matter based on the diffusion characteristics of water molecules in the brain [17]. Migraineurs exhibited several microstructural alterations in previous DTI studies [18–21]. Conversely, Need et al. did not identify microstructural white matter alterations in chronic and episodic migraine patients [22]. The results of structural studies of migraine patients seem contradictory and inconsistent, and the patients groups are characterized sample heterogeneity. Thus, structural alterations of the white matter and gray matter in migraineurs without aura should be further investigated.

Our previous studies detected dysfunction in various brain regions in migraineurs based on task functional magnetic resonance imaging (fMRI) and task-free fMRI [8, 23, 24]. We found activation in the visual cortex and anterior cerebellum lobe/culmen during presentation of negative emotion picture stimuli in migraineurs [23]. Furthermore, migraineurs without aura exhibited dysfunction in the default mode network and sensorimotor network during the task-free state [8, 24].It has been demonstrated that the function of the human brain is intimately related to its structure [25, 26]. Functional abnormalities in migraineurs may be caused by corresponding structural changes. Therefore, we used SBM, VBM and DTI analyses to detect structural alterations of the white matter and gray matter in 32 migraineurs without aura in current study. In addition, we hypothesized that migraine patients without aura may exhibit structural changes and that these changes may be consistent with the findings of previous fMRI studies and associated with the pathological mechanisms of migraine.

Methods

The East China Normal University Committee on Human Research (Project No. HR2016/03022) and the Independent Ethics Committee of Shanghai Ninth People's Hospital (Project No. [2016]01), Shanghai Jiao Tong University School of Medicine, approved the current study. All migraineurs without aura and healthy controls provided written informed consent using forms approved by the committee.

Subjects

Thirty-two migraineurs without aura (8 males, 24 females) were recruited from among the outpatients of the Department of Neurology at Shanghai Ninth People's Hospital. These patients were diagnosed with migraine by a neurologist based on the International Classification of Headache Disorders (ICHD-III beta, 2013) [1]. During the interview, the neurologist also obtained the migraineurs' demographic and clinical data, including age, sex, disease duration, attack frequency (times/month), and attack duration (hours), and their scores on the visual analogue scale (VAS), the Migraine Disability Assessment Scale (MIDAS) and the Headache Impact Test (HIT-6). Migraineurs reported that they had no headaches 48 h before MRI scans and did not suffer a migraine attack or discomfort during the MRI scans. In the current study, patients were excluded if they suffered chronic migraine or were taking preventive medication. Thirty-two age- and gender-matched healthy controls (8 males, 24 females) who had not experienced any headaches or chronic pain disorders in the past year and whose family members did not suffer from migraine or other headaches were recruited. All subjects reported right-handed and had no substance abuse, and all neurological and psychiatric diseases were excluded based on clinical examination and a structured interviews. The details are provided in Table 1.

MRI acquisition

DTI and high-resolution T_1-weighted MRI data were acquired using a 3.0 Tesla Siemens Trio Tim MRI scanner with a 12-channel head coil at the Shanghai Key Laboratory of Magnetic Resonance (East China Normal University, Shanghai, China). Custom-fit foam pads were used

Table 1 Demography and clinical scores of the migraine group and control group

	Migraine group (Mean ± SD)	Control group (Mean ± SD)
Male/Female	8/24	8/24
Age(years)	38.3 ± 10.16	38.8 ± 10.02
Disease duration(years)	9.5 ± 6.23	-
Attack duration (hours)	20.5 ± 20.02	-
Attack frequency (times/months)	3.36 ± 2.55	-
VAS	7.3 ± 2.04	-
MIDAS	13.2 ± 20.53	-
HIT-6	62.8 ± 10.04	-

Abbreviations: *VAS* visual analogue scale, *MIDAS* Migraine Disability Assessment Scale, *HIT-6* Headache Impact Test, – no data

to minimize head movement of the subjects. The parameters of the pulse sequence were as follows: 1) high-resolution T1-weighted 3-dimensional magnetization-prepared rapid-acquisition gradient-echo pulse sequence, repetition time = 2530 ms, echo time = 2.34 ms, inversion time = 1100 ms, flip angle = 7°, number of slices = 192, sagittal orientation, field of view = 256 × 256 mm^2, matrix size = 256 × 256, and slice thickness = 1 mm. 2) The DTI acquisition utilized a single-shot spin-echo echo planar imaging sequence in the contiguous axial plane, repetition time = 8900 ms, echo time = 86 ms, b-value = 0 and 1000 s/mm2, slice thickness = 2 mm, and 70 slices, matrix size = 128 × 128, field of view = 256 × 256 mm^2, diff direction = 64, and the resolution = 2 × 2 × 2 mm^3.

VBM and SBM analysis

The VBM and SBM analysis were conducted using the Computational Anatomy Toolbox (CAT12, http://dbm.neuro.uni-jena.de/cat/) that is an extension toolbox of Statistical Parametric Mapping software (SPM12, http://www.fil.ion.ucl.ac.uk/spm/software/spm12). We used the default settings that are described in detail in the manual of the CAT 12 toolbox (http://dbm.neuro.uni-jena.de/cat12/CAT12-Manual.pdf). The T1 images were spatially registered to the Montreal Neurological Institute (MNI) template. Then, the whole brain structural data were segmented into white matter, gray matter and cerebrospinal fluid. Bias correction was performed to remove intensity non-uniformities. Segmented images of the gray matter were preserved to assess the amount of volume changes based on spatial registration, and the modulated images of the gray matter could reflect the tissue volumes for using VBM analysis. The total intracranial volume (TIV) of each subject was calculated and used as a covariate for further statistical analyses. Finally, the normalized gray matter images were smoothed using a Gaussian filter (8 mm full-width half-maximum, FWHM).

CAT 12 provides a fully automated method to estimate cortical thickness and the central surface of hemispheres based on the projection-based thickness method [11]. The GI were extracted from central surface data based on the absolute mean curvature as previously described [12]. The cortical thickness and GI images of the left and right hemispheres were smoothed with a 15-mm FWHM Gaussian kernel.

DTI analyses

The analysis of DTI images was conducted using FSL v5.0 (http://fsl.fmrib.ox.ac.uk/fsl/fslwiki) and SPM 12 software. First, "eddy current correction" was implemented to correct for head motion artifacts and eddy current distortions. The brain was extracted using the Brian Extraction Tool (BET v2.1) in FSL. Then, FA and first, second and third eigenvalue (L1, L2, L3) maps were calculated in the individual space by fitting a diffusion model at each voxel using DTIFIT. The AD equals L1, and the RD equals the mean values of L2 and L3. Then, normalization and statistical analyses of the FA, RD and AD maps were performed using SPM 12. We co-registered the high-resolution T_1-weighted image to B_0 images. The T_1 images were then segmented into gray matter and white matter and generated bias-field corrected structural image and deformation fields. The FA, RD and AD maps were spatially normalized to the standard Montreal Neurological Institute (MNI) stereotaxic space and resampled to 2 × 2 × 2 mm^3. Finally, spatial smoothing was performed with an 8 mm FWHM Gaussian kernel.

Statistical analysis

The GMV was assessed by voxel-wise two-sample t-tests within the brain mask with TIV as a covariate to correct for different brain sizes among subjects. The cortical thickness and GI maps of the left and right hemispheres, and the FA, MD, AD and RD maps were separately statistically analyzed within a brain mask using voxel-wise two-sample t-tests. To address multiple comparisons, all statistical maps were assigned thresholds at $p < 0.005$ (voxel level), and the false discovery rate (FDR) was corrected to $p < 0.05$ at the cluster level. The surviving clusters were reported.

Results

Demographics

The demographic and clinical data of the migraine and control groups are presented in Table 1. The age and gender demographic factors did not significantly differ between the migraineurs without aura and controls.

VBM and SBM

Compared with controls, the migraineurs without aura exhibited significantly increased gray matter volume in bilateral cerebellar culmen (lobule I-IV and lobule V) extending to the lingual gyrus, thalamus, fusiform and parahippocampa gyrus (Fig. 1a). Cortical thickness was significantly thicker in the left inferior temporal and lateral occipital cortex, and significantly thinner in the right insula in migraineurs without aura than in the healthy controls (Fig. 1b). The GI were significantly increased in the left postcentral gyrus, the superior parietal lobule and the right lateral occipital cortex, and decreased in the left rostral middle frontal gyrus in the migraineurs (Fig. 1c).

DTI

There were not significant differences in FA, RD and AD between migraineurs without aura and healthy controls.

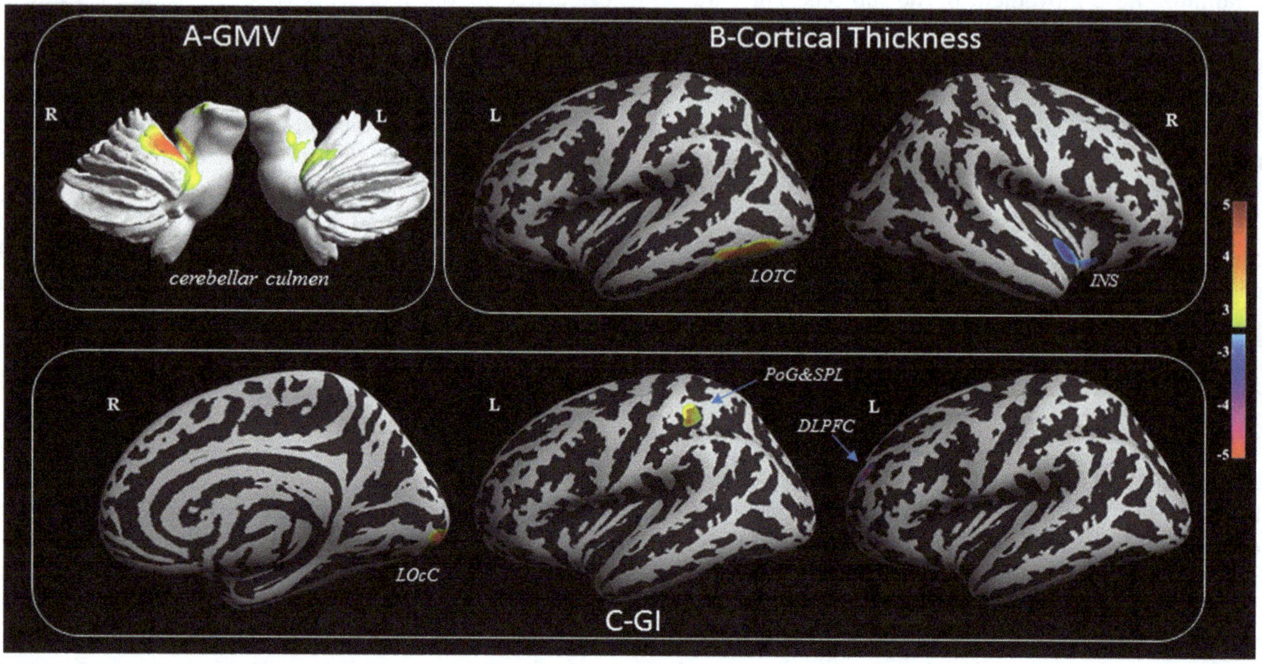

Fig. 1 The structural differences in gray matter between migraineurs without aura and healthy controls. a, compared with controls, the migraineurs without aura exhibited significantly increased gray matter volume in bilateral cerebellar culmen (lobule I-IV and lobule V). b, cortical thickness was significantly thicker in the left LOTC, and significantly thinner in the right INS in migraineurs without aura than in the healthy controls. c, the GI were significantly increased in the left POG, the SPL and the right LOcC, and decreased in the left DLPFC in the migraineurs. *LOTC* lateral occipital-temporal cortex, *INS* insula, *POG* postcentral gyrus, *SPL* superior parietal lobule, *LOcC* lateral occipital gyrus, *GI* gyrification index, *GMV* gray matter volume

Discussion

To the best of our knowledge, this is the first study to combine VBM, SBM and DTI analyses for evaluating structural and microstructural alterations of the gray matter and whiter matter in migraineurs without aura. We found that the significantly altered brain regions in migraine patients were primarily concentrated in the gray matter based on VBM and SBM analyses (Table 2, Fig. 1), whereas there were no significant microstructural changes in the white matter in DTI analyses.

Table 2 Significant inter-group differences in gray matter volume, cortical thickness and gyrification index between migraine patients without aura and healthy controls

Predominant regions in cluster	Cluster size	Peak T value	MNI coordinates		
			x	y	z
GMV increase in migraine group without aura					
Right cerebellar culmen extending to the right lingual gyrus, right thalamus and right parahippocampa gyrus	3742	5.77*	15	−38	−14
Left cerebellar culmen extending to left fusiform gyrus and left parahippocampal gyrus	1543	3.82	−21	−32	−15
Thickness increase in migraine group without aura					
Left inferior temporal gyrus and lateral occipital cortex	980	4.37	−48	−57	−10
		3.9	−41	−67	−7
Thickness decrease in migraine group without aura					
Right insula	653	-3.55	33	15	−13
GI increase in migraine group without aura					
Left postcentral gyrus and superior parietal lobule	601	3.67	−34	−35	40
Right lateral occipital cortex(pole occipital)	555	4.56	17	−99	−13
GI decrease in migraine group without aura					
left rostral middle frontal gyrus	308	-5.05*	−23	45	21

The results were thresholded at $p < 0.005$ (voxel level) and FDR corrected to $p < 0.05$ at the cluster level
'*' indicates that the peak T value passes the voxel-wise level FDR correction ($p < 0.05$). GI, gyrification index; GMV, gray matter volume

Compared with controls, migraineurs without aura exhibited significantly increased gray matter volume in the bilateral cerebellar culmen (lobule I-IV and lobule V) extending to the lingual gyrus, thalamus, fusiform and parahippocampal gyrus. The cerebellum has been recently proposed to be associated with cognitive, sensorimotor, pain and affective information processing [27–30], and to be involved in pathophysiological mechanism of migraine [31]. Moulton et al. found that the cerebellar activation areas overlapped with both unpleasant picture viewing and heat pain in healthy subjects and suggested that the cerebellum may have specific areas associated with encoding of generalized aversive processing [32]. In our previous task-fMRI study, we found that migraineurs exhibited hyperactivation in the anterior cerebellum lobe/culmen and visual cortex while viewing negative minus neutral affective pictures compared with healthy controls, and we proposed that migraine patients may have hypersensitivities to negative affective stimuli or that there is less inhibition in the cerebellum of migraineurs [23]. In addition, Mehnert J et al. demonstrated that the cerebellum, including lobules V and I-IV, is active during trigeminal nociceptive stimulation, and that the activity of the cerebellum is modulated by the perceived intensity of pain [33]. Nociceptive and negative emotion picture stimuli are parts of aversive stimuli and can active cerebellar responses. Thus, we propose that the increased GMV in the anterior cerebellum lobe (lobules V and I-IV) is consistent with our previous task-fMRI study and may be involved in the pathology mechanism of migraine.

Migraine patients exhibited increased cortical thickness in left inferior temporal gyrus and lateral occipital cortex and increased GI in the right lateral occipital cortex. It has been demonstrated that the lateral occipital-temporal cortex plays an important role in the multi-sensory integration of visual, auditory and tactile information [34, 35]. In line with our results, Messina et al. found that patients with migraine had an increased thickness of the left temporo-occipital incisure compared with control subjects [36]. The structural abnormalities of temporo-occipital cortex might be to explain the interictal deficits in visual motion processing described in migraineurs [37–39].

In our study, we found that migraineurs without aura exhibited decreased cortical thickness in the right insula, decreased GI in the left rostral middle frontal gyrus, and increased GI in the left postcentral gyrus and superior parietal lobule. In fact, it has been proposed that the postcentral gyrus, superior parietal lobule, insula and dorsolateral prefrontal cortex are involved in sensory discrimination of pain information [40–42]. Furthermore, Mehnert et al. observed increases in cerebellar-cortical connectivity in some brain regions, including insula and lingual gyrus [33], during trigeminal nociception stimuli. The postcentral gyrus and insula play important roles in the ascending trigemino-thalamo-cortical nociceptive pathway and have been implicated in the pathophysiology mechanism of migraine [3, 43]. Our previous study revealed that the bilateral postcentral gyrus is functional alterations in migraineurs without aura and that the postcentral gyrus has decreased functional connectivity with the contralateral insula, superior parietal lobule, prefrontal cortex and occipital cortex [8]. These findings suggest that structural alterations in the insula, postcentral gyrus, superior parietal lobule and rostral prefrontal cortex may disrupt the pathway used to discriminate sensory features of pain or the trigemino-thalamo-cortical pathway, and induce hypersensitivities to painful stimuli in migraineurs.

DTI analysis did not reveal any significant differences in migraineurs without aura comparing with healthy controls. Previous DTI studies in migraine patients detected several alterations, although the results of these studies are contradictory and inconsistent [18–21]. Liu et al. did not find that the migraineurs without aura exhibited significant microstructural alterations of white matter at a 1-year follow-up evaluation [44]. In line with our results, Need et al. demonstrated no microstructural white matter changes in episodic and chronic migraine patients based on Tract-based spatial statistics (TBSS) analysis [22].

Conclusions

In the current study, we evaluated the structural alterations of white matter and gray matter in migraine patients without aura using VBM, SBM and DTI analyses. Gray matter structural alterations in migraine patients were detected in the bilateral cerebellar culmen, lateral occipital-temporal cortex, right insula, left prefrontal cortex, left postcentral gyrus and superior parietal lobule. No significant changes in white matter regions were found in the DTI analyses. Our findings are consistent with previous fMRI studies, and we propose that the significant alterations in the gray matter, which are associated with sensory discrimination of pain, multi-sensory integration and nociceptive information processing, and may be involved in the pathological mechanism of migraine without aura.

Abbreviations

AD: Axial diffusivity; DTI: Diffusion tensor imaging; FA: Fractional anisotropy; fMRI: Functional magnetic resonance imaging; FWHM: Full-width half-maximum; GI: Gyrification index; GMV: Gray matter volume; HIT-6: Headache Impact Test; MIDAS: Migraine Disability Assessment Scale; RD: Radial diffusivity; SBM: Surface based morphometry; TIV: Total intracranial volume; VAS: Visual analogue scale; VBM: Voxel based morphometry

Funding

This research was supported by grants from the National Natural Science Foundation of China (Nos. 81571658 and 81201082 to X.X. Du, Nos. 31400838 to G.H. Cui, 81271302 to J.R. Liu), research innovation project from

Shanghai municipal science and technology commission [No. 14JC1404300, to J.R. Liu], the "prevention and control of chronic diseases project" of Shanghai Hospital Development Center [No. SHDC12015310, to J.R. Liu], project from SHSMU-ION Research Center for Brain Disorders [No. 2015NKX006, to J.R. Liu], project from Shanghai Municipal Education Commission—Gaofeng Clinical Medicine Grant Support [No. 20161422 to J.R. Liu], Clinical Research
Project from Shanghai Jiao Tong University School of Medicine [No. DLY201614 to J.R. Liu], and Biomedicine Key program from Shanghai Municipal Science and Technology Commission [No. 16411953100 to J.R. Liu].

Authors' contributions

XD and JL designed the study. JZ, YW, JS, QY, MW, GL, RZ, YS, QZ, YZ, HL, SX, ZQ and GC performed the experiments. JZ, YW and JL analysed the data. XD, JL and JZ prepared the manuscript. All authors read and approved the final manuscript.

Competing interests

The authors declare that they have no competing interests.

Author details

[1]Shanghai Key Laboratory of Magnetic Resonance and Department of Physics, School of Physics and Materials Science, East China Normal University, 3663 North Zhong-Shan Road, 200062 Shanghai, People's Republic of China. [2]Department of Neurology and Jiuyuan Municipal Stroke Center, Shanghai Ninth People's Hospital, Shanghai Jiao Tong University School of Medicine, 639 Zhizaoju Road, 200011 Shanghai, People's Republic of China. [3]Clinical Research Center, Shanghai Jiao Tong University School of Medicine, Shanghai 200011, China.

References

1. Headache Classification Committee of the International Headache S (2013) The international classification of headache disorders, 3rd edition (beta version). Cephalalgia 33(9):629–808. doi:10.1177/0333102413485658
2. Maleki N, Gollub RL (2016) What have we learned from brain functional connectivity studies in migraine headache? Headache 56(3):453–461. doi:10.1111/head.12756
3. Goadsby PJ, Holland PR, Martins-Oliveira M, Hoffmann J, Schankin C, Akerman S (2017) Pathophysiology of migraine: a disorder of sensory processing. Physiol Rev 97(2):553–622. doi:10.1152/physrev.00034.2015
4. Chen Z, Chen X, Liu M, Liu S, Ma L, Yu S (2017) Texture features of periaqueductal gray in the patients with medication-overuse headache. J Headache Pain 18(1):14. doi:10.1186/s10194-017-0727-0
5. Iwasaki A, Suzuki K, Takekawa H, Takashima R, Suzuki A, Suzuki S, Hirata K (2017) The relationship between right-to-left shunt and brain white matter lesions in Japanese patients with migraine: a single center study. J Headache Pain 18(1):3. doi:10.1186/s10194-016-0714-x
6. Chen Z, Chen X, Liu M, Liu S, Ma L, Yu S (2017) Disrupted functional connectivity of periaqueductal gray subregions in episodic migraine. J Headache Pain 18(1):36. doi:10.1186/s10194-017-0747-9
7. Chen Z, Chen X, Liu M, Dong Z, Ma L, Yu S (2017) Altered functional connectivity architecture of the brain in medication overuse headache using resting state fMRI. J Headache Pain 18(1):25. doi:10.1186/s10194-017-0735-0
8. Zhang J, Su J, Wang M, Zhao Y, Zhang QT, Yao Q, Lu H, Zhang H, Li GF, Wu YL, Liu YS, Liu FD, Zhuang MT, Shi YH, Hou TY, Zhao R, Qiao Y, Li J, Liu JR, Du X (2017) The sensorimotor network dysfunction in migraineurs without aura: a resting-state fMRI study. J Neurol doi:10.1007/s00415-017-8404-4
9. Neeb L, Bastian K, Villringer K, Israel H, Reuter U, Fiebach JB (2017) Structural gray matter alterations in chronic migraine: implications for a progressive disease? Headache 57(3):400–416. doi:10.1111/head.13012
10. Ashburner J, Friston KJ (2005) Unified segmentation. NeuroImage 26(3):839–851. doi:10.1016/j.neuroimage.2005.02.018
11. Dahnke R, Yotter RA, Gaser C (2013) Cortical thickness and central surface estimation. NeuroImage 65:336–348. doi:10.1016/j.neuroimage.2012.09.050
12. Luders E, Thompson PM, Narr KL, Toga AW, Jancke L, Gaser C (2006) A curvature-based approach to estimate local gyrification on the cortical surface. NeuroImage 29(4):1224–1230. doi:10.1016/j.neuroimage.2005.08.049
13. Hu W, Guo J, Chen N, Guo J, He L (2015) A meta-analysis of voxel-based morphometric studies on migraine. Int J Clin Exp 8(3):4311–4319
14. Jia Z, Yu S (2017) Grey matter alterations in migraine: a systematic review and meta-analysis. NeuroImage Clin 14:130–140. doi:10.1016/j.nicl.2017.01.019
15. Tedeschi G, Russo A, Conte F, Corbo D, Caiazzo G, Giordano A, Conforti R, Esposito F, Tessitore A (2016) Increased interictal visual network connectivity in patients with migraine with aura. Cephalalgia 36(2):139–147. doi:10.1177/0333102415584360
16. Tessitore A, Russo A, Conte F, Giordano A, De Stefano M, Lavorgna L, Corbo D, Caiazzo G, Esposito F, Tedeschi G (2015) Abnormal connectivity within executive resting-state network in migraine with Aura. Headache 55(6):794–805. doi:10.1111/head.12587
17. Alexander AL, Lee JE, Lazar M, Field AS (2007) Diffusion tensor imaging of the brain. Neurotherapeutics 4(3):316–329. doi:10.1016/j.nurt.2007.05.011
18. Schmitz N, Admiraal-Behloul F, Arkink EB, Kruit MC, Schoonman GG, Ferrari MD, van Buchem MA (2008) Attack frequency and disease duration as indicators for brain damage in migraine. Headache 48(7):1044–1055. doi:10.1111/j.1526-4610.2008.01133.x
19. Yuan K, Qin W, Liu P, Zhao L, Yu D, Zhao L, Dong M, Liu J, Yang X, von Deneen KM, Liang F, Tian J (2012) Reduced fractional anisotropy of corpus callosum modulates inter-hemispheric resting state functional connectivity in migraine patients without aura. PLoS One 7(9):e45476. doi:10.1371/journal.pone.0045476
20. Yu D, Yuan K, Qin W, Zhao L, Dong M, Liu P, Yang X, Liu J, Sun J, Zhou G, von Deneen KM, Tian J (2013) Axonal loss of white matter in migraine without aura: a tract-based spatial statistics study. Cephalalgia 33(1):34–42. doi:10.1177/0333102412466964
21. Yu D, Yuan K, Zhao L, Dong M, Liu P, Yang X, Liu J, Sun J, Zhou G, Xue T, Zhao L, Cheng P, Dong T, von Deneen KM, Qin W, Tian J (2013) White matter integrity affected by depressive symptoms in migraine without aura: a tract-based spatial statistics study. NMR Biomed 26(9):1103–1112. doi:10.1002/nbm.2924
22. Neeb L, Bastian K, Villringer K, Gits HC, Israel H, Reuter U, Fiebach JB (2015) No microstructural white matter alterations in chronic and episodic migraineurs: a case-control diffusion tensor magnetic resonance imaging study. Headache 55(2):241–251. doi:10.1111/head.12496
23. Wang M, Su J, Zhang J, Zhao Y, Yao Q, Zhang Q, Zhang H, Wang S, Li GF, Liu JR, Du X (2017) Visual cortex and cerebellum hyperactivation during negative emotion picture stimuli in migraine patients. Sci Rep 7:41919. doi:10.1038/srep41919
24. Zhang J, Su J, Wang M, Zhao Y, Yao Q, Zhang Q, Lu H, Zhang H, Wang S, Li GF, Wu YL, Liu FD, Shi YH, Li J, Liu JR, Du X (2016) Increased default mode network connectivity and increased regional homogeneity in migraineurs without aura. J Headache Pain 17(1):98. doi:10.1186/s10194-016-0692-z
25. Greicius MD, Supekar K, Menon V, Dougherty RF (2009) Resting-state functional connectivity reflects structural connectivity in the default mode network. Cereb Cortex 19(1):72–78. doi:10.1093/cercor/bhn059
26. Bullmore E, Sporns O (2009) Complex brain networks: graph theoretical analysis of structural and functional systems. Nat Rev Neurosci 10(3):186–198. doi:10.1038/nrn2575
27. Timmann D, Drepper J, Frings M, Maschke M, Richter S, Gerwig M, Kolb FP (2010) The human cerebellum contributes to motor, emotional and cognitive associative learning. A review. Cortex 46(7):845–857. doi:10.1016/j.cortex.2009.06.009
28. Stoodley CJ, Schmahmann JD (2010) Evidence for topographic organization in the cerebellum of motor control versus cognitive and affective processing. Cortex 46(7):831–844. doi:10.1016/j.cortex.2009.11.008
29. Stoodley CJ, Schmahmann JD (2009) Functional topography in the human cerebellum: a meta-analysis of neuroimaging studies. NeuroImage 44(2):489–501. doi:10.1016/j.neuroimage.2008.08.039
30. Coombes SA, Misra G (2016) Pain and motor processing in the human cerebellum. Pain 157(1):117–127. doi:10.1097/j.pain.0000000000000337
31. Vincent M, Hadjikhani N (2007) The cerebellum and migraine. Headache 47(6):820–833. doi:10.1111/j.1526-4610.2006.00715.x
32. Moulton EA, Elman I, Pendse G, Schmahmann J, Becerra L, Borsook D (2011) Aversion-related circuitry in the cerebellum: responses to noxious heat and

unpleasant images. J Neurosci 31(10):3795–3804. doi:10.1523/JNEUROSCI.6709-10.2011

33. Mehnert J, Schulte L, Timmann D, May A (2017) Activity and connectivity of the cerebellum in trigeminal nociception. NeuroImage 150:112–118. doi:10.1016/j.neuroimage.2017.02.023
34. Beauchamp MS (2005) See me, hear me, touch me: multisensory integration in lateral occipital-temporal cortex. Curr Opin Neurobiol 15(2):145–153. doi:10.1016/j.conb.2005.03.011
35. Amedi A, Stern WM, Camprodon JA, Bermpohl F, Merabet L, Rotman S, Hemond C, Meijer P, Pascual-Leone A (2007) Shape conveyed by visual-to-auditory sensory substitution activates the lateral occipital complex. Nat Neurosci 10(6):687–689. doi:10.1038/nn1912
36. Messina R, Rocca MA, Colombo B, Valsasina P, Horsfield MA, Copetti M, Falini A, Comi G, Filippi M (2013) Cortical abnormalities in patients with migraine: a surface-based analysis. Radiology 268(1):170–180. doi:10.1148/radiol.13122004
37. Granziera C, DaSilva AF, Snyder J, Tuch DS, Hadjikhani N (2006) Anatomical alterations of the visual motion processing network in migraine with and without aura. PLoS Med 3(10):e402. doi:10.1371/journal.pmed.0030402
38. McKendrick AM, Badcock DR (2004) Motion processing deficits in migraine. Cephalalgia 24(5):363–372. doi:10.1111/j.1468-2982.2004.00679.x
39. Ditchfield JA, McKendrick AM, Badcock DR (2006) Processing of global form and motion in migraineurs. Vis Res 46(1–2):141–148. doi:10.1016/j.visres.2005.09.014
40. Oshiro Y, Quevedo AS, McHaffie JG, Kraft RA, Coghill RC (2009) Brain mechanisms supporting discrimination of sensory features of pain: a new model. J Neurosci 29(47):14924–14931. doi:10.1523/JNEUROSCI.5538-08.2009
41. Oshiro Y, Quevedo AS, McHaffie JG, Kraft RA, Coghill RC (2007) Brain mechanisms supporting spatial discrimination of pain. J Neurosci 27(13):3388–3394. doi:10.1523/JNEUROSCI.5128-06.2007
42. Hofbauer RK, Rainville P, Duncan GH, Bushnell MC (2001) Cortical representation of the sensory dimension of pain. J Neurophysiol 86(1):402–411
43. Burstein R, Noseda R, Borsook D (2015) Migraine: multiple processes, complex pathophysiology. J Neurosci 35(17):6619–6629. doi:10.1523/JNEUROSCI.0373-15.2015
44. Liu J, Lan L, Li G, Yan X, Nan J, Xiong S, Yin Q, von Deneen KM, Gong Q, Liang F, Qin W, Tian J (2013) Migraine-related gray matter and white matter changes at a 1-year follow-up evaluation. J Pain 14(12):1703–1708. doi:10.1016/j.jpain.2013.08.013

16

Fluctuations in episodic and chronic migraine status over the course of 1 year: implications for diagnosis, treatment and clinical trial design

Daniel Serrano[1*], Richard B. Lipton[2,3*], Ann I. Scher[4], Michael L. Reed[5], Walter (Buzz) F. Stewart[6], Aubrey Manack Adams[7] and Dawn C. Buse[8]

Abstract

Background: Relatively little is known about the stability of a diagnosis of episodic migraine (EM) or chronic migraine (CM) over time. This study examines natural fluctuations in self-reported headache frequency as well as the stability and variation in migraine type among individuals meeting criteria for EM and CM at baseline.

Methods: The Chronic Migraine Epidemiology and Outcomes (CaMEO) Study was a longitudinal survey of US adults with EM and CM identified by a web-questionnaire. A validated questionnaire was used to classify respondents with EM (<15 headache days/month) or CM (≥15 headache days/month) every three months for a total of five assessments. We described longitudinal persistence of baseline EM and CM classifications. In addition, we modelled longitudinal variation in headache day frequency per month using negative binomial repeated measures regression models (NBRMR).

Results: Among the 5464 respondents with EM at baseline providing four or five waves of data, 5048 (92.4%) had EM in all waves and 416 (7.6%) had CM in at least one wave. Among 526 respondents with CM at baseline providing four or five waves of data, 140 (26.6%) had CM in every wave and 386 (73.4%) had EM for at least one wave. Individual plots revealed striking within-person variations in headache days per month. The NBRMR model revealed that the rate of headache days increased across waves of observation 19% more per wave for CM compared to EM (rate ratio [RR], 1.19; 95% CI, 1.13–1.26). After adjustment for covariates, the relative difference changed to a 26% increase per wave (RR, 1.26; 95% CI, 1.2–1.33).

Conclusions: Follow-up at three-month intervals reveals a high level of short-term variability in headache days per month. As a consequence, many individuals cross the CM diagnostic boundary of ≥15 headache days per month. Nearly three quarters of persons with CM at baseline drop below this diagnostic boundary at least once over the course of a year. These findings are of interest in the consideration of headache classification and diagnosis, the design and interpretation of epidemiologic and clinical studies, and clinical management.

Keywords: Migraine, Chronic migraine, Episodic migraine, Longitudinal, Remission

* Correspondence: daniel.serrano@endpointoutcomes.com; Richard.Lipton@einstein.yu.edu
Daniel Serrano and Richard B. Lipton are co-first authors.
[1]Endpoint Outcomes, Boston, MA, USA
[2]The Saul R. Korey Department of Neurology, Albert Einstein College of Medicine, Bronx, NY, USA
Full list of author information is available at the end of the article

The Enrico Greppi 2017 Selection Committee is:
Messoud Ashina, Anne Ducros, Antoinette Maassen van den Brink, Paolo Martelletti, Francesco Pierelli, Massimiliano Valeriani

Background

Episodic migraine (EM) and chronic migraine (CM) are primarily differentiated by monthly headache days, with EM having fewer than 15 headache days per month and CM having 15 or more headache days per month for at least three months [1]. The epidemiologic profiles of people with EM and CM are well characterized [2–5], as are annual rates of CM remission and CM onset from 1 year to the next [6]. However, relatively little is known about the longitudinal within-person variation in self-reported headache frequency when assessed repeatedly over the course of 1 year.

Migraine can be characterized as a chronic disorder with episodic attacks [7]. Within-person variation in headache days per month logically influences the epidemiologic estimates of EM and CM incidence and persistence reported in the literature [2–5], as well as the assessment of treatment response. However, epidemiology studies, for the most part, have evaluated incidence, persistence, remission, and disease progression by examining only two adjacent points in time. Furthermore, typically, only group mean data are reported. The natural within-person variation in headache day frequency, which is the fundamental driver of the instability in diagnostic classification for EM and CM reported in the literature, has been studied inadequately, if at all. Understanding of this natural history has been obscured in epidemiologic studies because of infrequent repeated measures and the emphasis on aggregated rather than within-person data.

To better characterize within-person change in headache days we analyzed longitudinal data from the Chronic Migraine Epidemiology and Outcomes (CaMEO) Study [8]. We examined transitions from EM to CM and from CM to EM. Of primary importance, we modelled natural history of self-reported headache day variation in quarterly assessments across the span of 15 months. Natural history of headache frequency was modeled accounting for both within-person and between-person changes in headache days per month. These findings have implications for classification and diagnosis, the design and conduct of observational studies, and for the design, management, and interpretation of randomized controlled trials (RCTs).

Methods

CaMEO study design and baseline survey

The CaMEO Study used a web-based panel (Research Now) constructed to be demographically representative of the US population, as previously detailed [8]. The baseline survey, e-mailed to participants, assessed headache symptoms and severity, headache frequency, headache-related disability, healthcare consulting and utilization, medication use for headache, comorbid medical and psychiatric conditions, and family-related burden associated with headache (Fig. 1).

Ethics, consent and permissions

Independent ethics committee approval was obtained before initiation of the CaMEO Study. Given that participation by individuals in the web-based survey was voluntary and that survey research does not expose respondents to known health risks, informed consent was not requested. No person-level identifiable data are included in this study report.

Study classifications of EM and CM

Respondents were identified as having migraine if they met modified International Classification of Headache Disorders Third edition (beta version) (ICHD-3 [beta]) criteria [1]. Among those with migraine, respondents were classified as having CM if they reported ≥15 headache days per month averaged over the preceding 90 days (i.e., the Silberstein-Lipton approach [9]), otherwise they were classified as having EM. This definition of CM differs from standard ICHD-3 (beta) criteria by not requiring that headaches on eight of the 15 headache days per month be migraine (Criterion C).

Questionnaire

Of the 58,418 respondents to the baseline survey, 16,789 met criteria for EM or CM and received follow-up surveys at three-month intervals from September 2012 to November 2013. The baseline and four quarterly follow-up assessments constituted the five quarterly waves of data collection in the CaMEO Study, as previously described [8].

Headache frequency was assessed in all five waves using a question from the MIDAS questionnaire about the number of headache days over the last three months [10]. The three-month estimate was rescaled to a monthly estimate by dividing by three, paralleling the approach taken in the American Migraine Prevalence and Prevention (AMPP) study [3]. A diagnosis of EM or CM was assigned at each quarterly assessment. In addition, a continuous measure of headache days per month was retained to model variation in headache days within- and between-persons.

Sociodemographic covariates assessed at baseline included sex (female vs. male), employment status (full-time/part-time employment vs. other), education (college graduate or higher vs. less than college), race (Caucasian vs. non-Caucasian), Hispanic ethnicity (Hispanic vs. not), health insurance status (having health insurance vs. not), household income at or above the national median, and personal income at or above the national median. The two income variables were coded based on median income estimates obtained from the

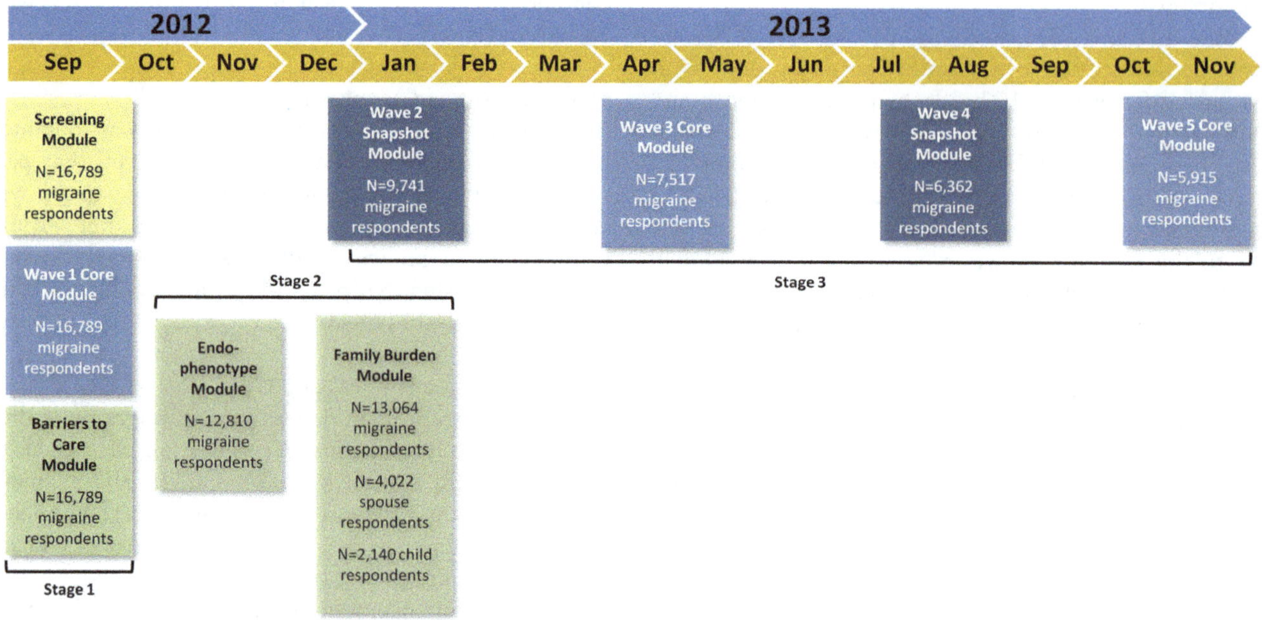

Fig. 1 CaMEO study design, reprinted from Manack Adams A, et al. *Cephalalgia* 2015;35:563–578. [8]

2012 American Community Survey conducted by the National Census Bureau [11].

In addition, the Migraine Disability Assessment questionnaire (MIDAS) categories were used as a disability covariate, with categories of zero to five indicating no disability (Grade I), six to 10 indicating mild disability (Grade II), 11–20 indicating moderate disability (Grade III), 21–40 indicating severe disability (Grade IV-A), and ≥41 indicating very severe disability (Grade IV-B) [4]. A count of the self-report of physician diagnosis of comorbid conditions was used to generate a comorbidity index; included conditions were asthma, diabetes, high blood pressure, overactive bladder, shingles or herpes zoster, and post-herpetic neuropathy, with a count range of zero (no comorbidities) to six (all comorbidities). Lastly, age at migraine onset reported at baseline and migraine duration (age at baseline minus reported age at migraine onset) were included as disease duration covariates.

The longitudinal wave-specific participation rates for the total sample and stratified by baseline EM and CM status have been presented previously [8]; rates of participation were nearly identical between baseline EM and CM over time.

Analyses

Analysis first measured longitudinal persistence of baseline EM and CM classification, while accounting for attrition patterns in participation [8]. Analysis was also completed to model variation in average monthly headache days using the longitudinal negative binomial mixed effect models. Orthogonal polynomial terms were used to characterize the longitudinal variation in repeated measures trends and random effects were employed to account for subject-level variance in repeated measures. Technical details of the model building process are available in a separate document. Interested readers may request this document from the first author.

After determining the best-fitting mixed-effect polynomial parameterization, two primary models were fit. The first was an unadjusted model that included only the repeated measures trend terms and main effects and interactions between the repeated measures trend terms and EM/CM status (with EM as reference). The second model adjusted the first with the incorporation of demographic characteristics as well as MIDAS disability, comorbidity count, and disease duration covariates. For the adjusted models, EM and CM status varied over time while all other covariates were entered as predictors based on their baseline status. The GLIMMIX procedure as implemented in SAS (Version 9.2) was used to estimate negative binomial models. All available data were used. Respondents with baseline data only contributed to the estimation of the intercept only. Respondents with more than a single wave of data contributed to estimates of longitudinal trends.

Results

Previously presented data [8] on the sampling design and participation rates will be reviewed to contextualize our findings. Sampling response, attrition, and cleaning rates have been published previously (see Table 2 in Manack et al. 2015) [8]. Of the 16,789 respondents with

EM or CM at baseline, (wave one), 10,023 (59.7%) responded and 9741 provided clean and useable returns (58.0% of the baseline sample) at wave two. For subsequent waves, data are available for 7517 participants at wave three, 6363 participants for wave four and 5915 participants at wave five (Fig. 2). The attrition rate decreased with increasing follow-up.

The stability in headache diagnosis was examined descriptively by evaluating the proportion of individuals whose headache diagnosis was maintained across all waves (Table 1). The variation in headache diagnosis was examined by evaluating the proportion of individuals who had at least one wave with the alternative diagnosis. Among the 5464 respondents with EM at baseline providing four or five waves of data, 5048 (92.4%) had EM at all waves and 416 (7.6%) had CM in at least one wave. Among 526 respondents with CM at baseline providing four or five waves of data, 140 had CM at every wave (26.6%) and 386 (73.4%) had EM for at least one wave.

We modeled headache days per month at three-month intervals using linear, quadratic and cubic polynomial trends for time as well as measures of headache status. In these models, each individual subject is a random effect while the fixed effects represent average trends. As seen in Table 2, relatively large random-effect variances were observed for the polynomial trend terms, including the intercept (0.82), linear trend (0.17), and quadratic trend (0.09), as well as the negative binomial scaling variance parameter (0.09). These random effects reflect the substantial individual variation in monthly headache days. Plots of headache days at an individual-level revealed substantial subject-specific differences and striking curvatures (Additional file 1: Figure. S1). In addition, many fixed-effect estimates were statistically significant. The significant linear trend by headache status interaction indicated that headache days per wave changed differently for those with EM vs CM. Headache days per wave decreased slightly in the EM group and increased slightly in the CM group. This difference in change resulted in a rate of headache day increase of 19% more per wave for CM compared to EM (rate ratio [RR], 1.19; 95% CI 1.13–1.26).

In Table 3, we augmented the unadjusted model with a set of covariates which diminished the random-effect variance estimates compared with the unadjusted model, particularly the baseline variance (intercept random effect). After adjustment, the random effect variance estimates for the intercept was 0.52, with limited or no reductions in the linear trend variance (0.15), quadratic trend variance (0.09), and the negative binomial scaling variance (0.08) (Table 3). Nearly all fixed effects were statistically significant in the final model. After adjustment, the headache status by linear trend interactions revealed that headache days per month increased 26% more per wave for CM compared to EM (RR, 1.26; 95% CI, 1.20–1.33). Figure 3 demonstrates how closely predicted values reproduced observed variation and oscillation for subjects. Although the predicted values

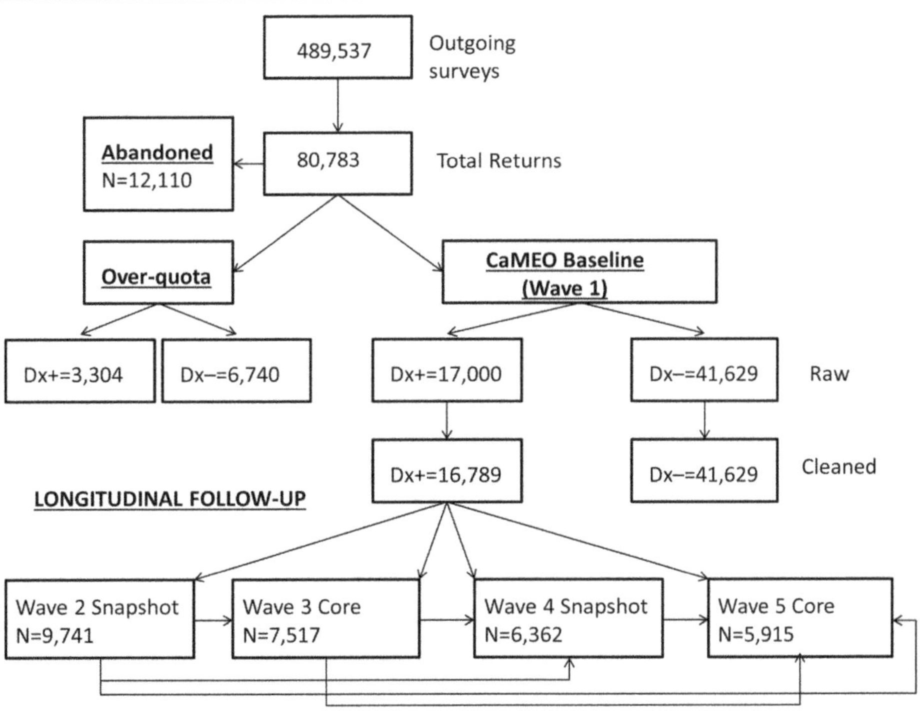

Fig. 2 Longitudinal study sample flow

Table 1 Baseline headache status stability stratified on waves of study participation

Waves participated	Number of waves baseline headache status maintained	EM at Baseline, n (%)[a]; n = 15,313	CM at Baseline, n (%)[a]; n = 1476
Respondents participating in 1 wave only (EM, n = 4801; CM, n = 474)			
1	1	4801 (100)	474 (100)
Respondents participating in any 2 waves (EM, n = 2839; CM, n = 270)			
2	1	99 (3.5)	159 (58.9)
2	2	2740 (96.5)	111 (41.1)
Respondents participating in any 3 waves (EM, n = 2209; CM, n = 206)			
3	1	29 (1.3)	98 (47.6)
3	2	98 (4.4)	53 (25.7)
3	3	2082 (94.3)	55 (26.7)
Respondents participating in any 4 waves (EM, n = 2161; CM, n = 206)			
4	1	12 (0.6)	87 (42.9)
4	2	31 (1.4)	34 (16.7)
4	3	106 (4.9)	34 (16.7)
4	4	2012 (93.1)	48 (23.6)
Respondents participating all 5 waves (EM, n = 3303; CM, n = 323)			
5	1	21 (0.6)	101 (31.3)
5	2	35 (1.1)	43 (13.3)
5	3	46 (1.4)	32 (9.9)
5	4	165 (5)	55 (17)
5	5	3036 (91.9)	92 (28.5)

CM chronic migraine, *EM* episodic migraine
[a]Percentages are the percentages of the respondents participating in the identified number of waves

Table 2 Unadjusted model for headache days per month for persons with EM and CM

Random-effect variance parameter estimates				
	Estimate	**Standard Error**		
Intercept	0.82	0.01		
Linear trend	0.17	0.01		
Quadratic trend	0.09	0.01		
Scale	0.09	0.005		
Fixed Effects				
Label	**RR (95% CI)[a]**	**DF**	**t**	***P* value**
Intercept	**3.98 (3.82–4.15)**	16,788	66.53	<0.0001
Linear trend	**0.73 (0.72–0.75)**	29,528	−28.49	<0.0001
Quadratic trend	**1.09 (1.06–1.11)**	29,528	7.90	<0.0001
Cubic trend	0.98 (0.97–1.00)	29,528	−1.51	0.1318
Headache status: CM vs. EM	**4.45 (4.3–4.59)**	29,528	89.36	<0.0001
Headache status by linear trend interaction	**1.19 (1.13–1.26)**	29,528	6.67	<0.0001
Headache status by quadratic trend interaction	1.03 (0.98–1.08)	29,528	1.26	0.2075
Headache status by cubic trend interaction	0.99 (0.95–1.03)	29,528	−0.72	0.4710

CM chronic migraine, *DF* degrees of freedom, *EM* episodic migraine, *RR* rate ratio, *t* t-statistic
[a]Statistically significant RRs are bolded

Table 3 Final adjusted and trimmed model for headache days per month[a]

Random-Effect Variance Parameter Estimates

	Estimate	**Standard Error**
Intercept	0.52	0.01
Linear trend	0.15	0.01
Quadratic trend	0.09	0.01
Scale	0.08	0.005

Fixed Effects[b]

Label	**RR (95% CI)**[c]	**DF**	**t**	***P* value**
Intercept	**1.16 (1.02–1.32)**	16,650	2.28	0.0224
Sex: male vs. female	**0.9 (0.87–0.93)**	16,650	−6.62	<0.0001
Education: college graduate vs. non-college graduate	**0.96 (0.93–0.99)**	16,650	−2.92	0.0035
Race: Caucasian vs. nonwhite	**1.19 (1.14–1.23)**	16,650	8.78	<0.0001
Household income: at or above national median vs. those below	**0.96 (0.94–0.99)**	16,650	−2.42	0.0155
Comorbid count	**1.07 (1.05–1.09)**	16,650	8.06	<0.0001
Disability: MIDAS category TIC	**1.47 (1.46–1.49)**	16,650	73.56	<0.0001
Age at onset, y	**0.998 (0.997–0.999)**	16,650	−3.20	0.0014
Duration of illness	1.00 (1.00–1.00)	16,650	0.83	0.4090
Linear trend	**0.74 (0.73–0.76)**	29,304	−28.63	<0.0001
Quadratic trend	**1.09 (1.07–1.11)**	29,304	8.35	<0.0001
Cubic trend	0.99 (0.97–1.01)	29,304	−1.34	0.1797
Headache status: CM vs. EM	**3.95 (3.84–4.07)**	29,304	90.71	<0.0001
Headache status by linear trend interaction	**1.26 (1.2–1.33)**	29,304	9.34	<0.0001
Headache status by quadratic trend interaction	0.99 (0.94–1.03)	29,304	−0.51	0.6434
Headache status by cubic trend interaction	1.00 (0.96–1.04)	29,304	−0.17	0.8627

CM chronic migraine, *DF* degrees of freedom, *EM* episodic migraine, *MIDAS* Migraine Disability Assessment questionnaire, *RR* rate ratio, *t* t-statistic; *TIC* time invariant covariate, *TVC* time-varying covariate

[a]In persons with EM and CM and adjusting for demographic variables, headache related disability and comorbidity

[b]All covariates were specified as TICs, though TVCs could have been specified for several including MIDAS and comorbidity count, which may not have been constant over time

[c]Statistically significant RR are bolded

are shrunken toward the mean relative to the observed values, they recover the observed value oscillations quite well. Figure 4 presents a plot of the EM- and CM-specific longitudinal trajectories characterizing this interaction. One can see that headache frequency for EM diminishes over time. In contrast, headache frequency oscillates for CM, but the overall trend is one of subtle increase. The reported rate ratios of 1.19 and 1.26 (adjusted) arise from this difference between headache frequency decreasing over time for EM while increasing over time for CM.

Discussion

This study demonstrates that in persons with migraine assessed at three-month intervals, there are frequent transitions between CM and EM with substantial within-person variation in the number of headache days per month over the course of 15 months. Random-effect variance estimates demonstrated that there was significant temporal variability in headache days, both within and between the EM and CM populations. We observed statistically significant increases in headache frequency for CM relative to EM over time, both before and after adjustment for potential confounders. The high rates of transition between EM and CM have implications for headache classification and diagnosis, epidemiologic studies and clinical trial design.

Implications for headache classification, diagnosis, and clinical practice

We found that 73.4% of people with CM at baseline and four or five follow-up waves of data had at least 1 three-month period when they did not meet the 15 or more headache day per month criteria for CM. Among persons with EM at baseline and four or five waves of follow-up, 7.6% had at least one period when they met the headache frequency criteria for CM. These findings suggest that over the course of 15 months, transitions

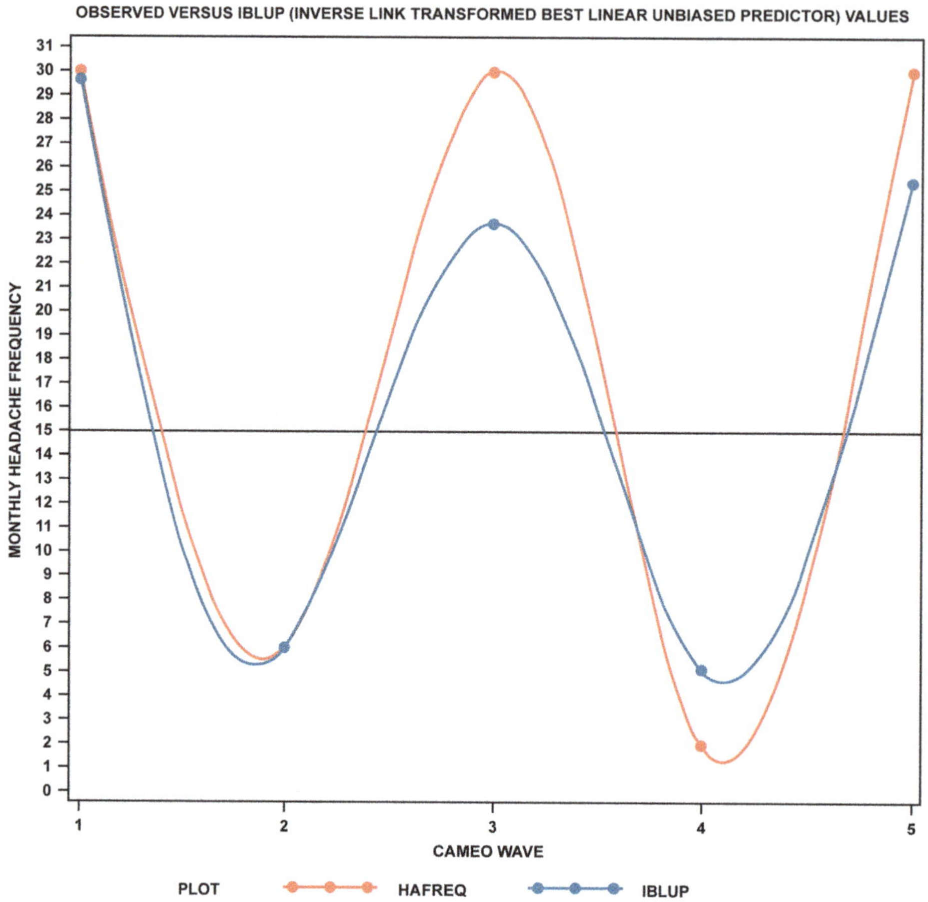

Fig. 3 Observed monthly headache frequency over 15 months compared with that predicted using IBLUP = approach HAFREQ = observed monthly headache frequency: IBLUP = inverse link function best linear unbiased predictor

between EM and CM are very common. In clinical practice, headache diagnosis is often assumed to be relatively stable for an individual, and yet we have found headache frequency changes substantially over time, potentially moving individuals between diagnostic categories (i.e., between EM and CM). When a person transitions from 16 headache days per month to 14 headache days per month, their ICHD-3 (beta) diagnostic label may change but the biology of their disorder most likely does not. The finding that headache day frequency within an individual changes substantially over time poses a considerable challenge to headache classification, diagnosis and subsequently clinical management. As diagnosis is intended to reflect a relatively stable set of clinical features and is used to predict treatment response and clinical course, this level of diagnostic instability is disconcerting. Perhaps headache days alone are not sufficiently stable to be the basis for distinguishing two related nosological entities such as EM and CM. We believe that there are more severe and less severe migraine biological subtypes of migraine, imperfectly differentiated by headache days criteria as EM and CM. Future work could focus on identifying trait predictors of biotype, rather than time-varying features such as headache days per month.

When it comes to interpreting the effects of preventive treatment in practice, we often rely on a short-term reduction in headache days per month. The present findings suggest that at least part of the improvements we attribute to our treatments in practice may represent variation in headache days unrelated to treatment. This hypothesis requires further exploration by examining changes in headache days associated with stable treatment and with changes in treatment.

Implications for epidemiologic studies

Among people with EM at baseline, when assessed every three months, 7.6% of individuals met headache day criteria for CM at least once over a 15-month period. This is much larger than the 2.5% rate of CM onset in persons with EM we reported after 1 year of follow-up in the AMPP study [12]. This apparent three-fold increased rate of CM onset in persons with EM with more frequent assessments, when coupled with the evidence of

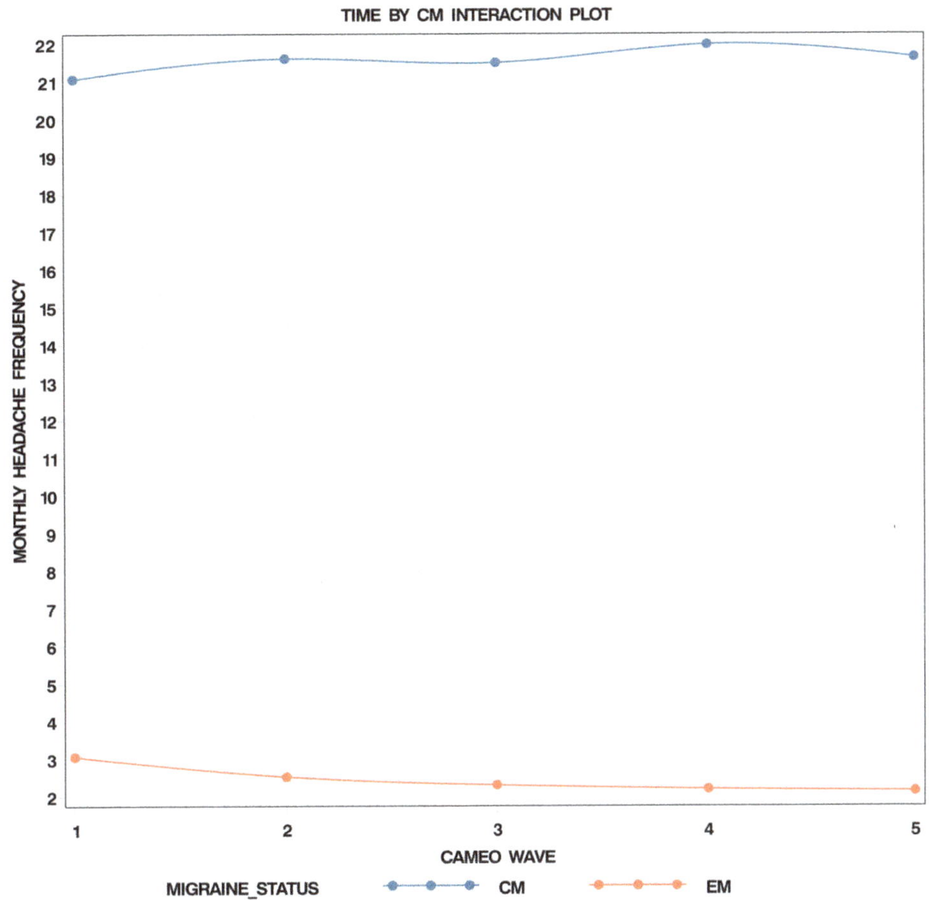

Fig. 4 Episodic- and chronic migraine-specific longitudinal trajectories. Time by chronic migraine interaction plot

transition from CM to EM, suggests that in studies using annual assessments, persons whose CM developed and remitted over the course of the year may be missed. Prior studies have also examined risk factors for CM [3, 13–16] and rates and risk factors for the remission of CM [12, 17, 18]. Previously reported factors associated with an increased risk of CM onset include headache features (such as cutaneous allodynia) [19], a broad array of comorbidities (including depression, allergic rhinitis, and asthma) [15] and poor acute treatment optimization among others [12]. Given the observed relative fluid and repeated movement across the "boundary" of 15 headache days per month in this systematically recruited sample of persons with migraine, the underlying framing of these studies may need to be reconsidered. The defining feature of CM, the number of headache days per month over three months in a person with migraine, may reflect a process of continuous change within a single classification of migraine and not a change in the classification of disease as implied by the previous framing. It is likely that more frequent sampling will identify both higher rates of CM onset and stronger associations between risk factors and this outcome.

Implications for clinical trial design

Studies of CM use symptom profiles and headache day frequency to determine participation eligibility [20]. In preventive treatment trials of CM, individuals judged by a clinician to have CM typically enter into a four-week diary study prior to study enrollment. If individuals have <15 headache days per month they are deemed ineligible for enrollment into the study. If they have ≥15 headache days per month they are likely to be eligible and offered enrollment into the study. The primary endpoint in prevention trials is typically the change from baseline in the number of headache days per 28-day period on active drug vs. placebo or an active comparator [20]. Change in headache day frequency is typically assessed across two periods (from baseline to follow-up). The spontaneous and rarely measured variation in headache days provides a backdrop for interpreting treatment effects in individuals. There is a substantial probability that persons with CM at baseline will experience reductions unrelated to treatment in headache days as illustrated by the data reported here. Enrolling people with headache days above a threshold may lead to regression to the mean and high "placebo rates" [20]. This in turn can lead to modest therapeutic gains when active drug and placebo are compared [21]. We suggest that the high rate of spontaneous reduction in headache day frequency in RCTs may have contributed to what is widely regarded as an inescapably large placebo effect. This high presumed placebo effect observed in several studies may simply reflect the cyclic nature of CM [22–25].

When the results of our analysis (Fig. 3) are considered, one would expect that a majority of subjects selected at any high monthly headache-frequency value would, within three months, have a period of low headache-frequency suggesting that the high placebo rate may be, at least in part, an artifact of inclusion criteria interacting with the natural history of headache frequency. To empirically evaluate this point, we took the data from the CaMEO Study analyzed here, and looked at two waves of data. In the next three paragraphs we demonstrate that by selecting two waves of data and computing change in headache frequency between the two waves, headache frequency decreases for CM in a context where models fit to all waves demonstrated that frequency actually increased for CM. This calls into question the interpretability of two time-point change computations for headache frequency outcomes in both epidemiology studies and clinical trials.

Change in one-month recall of headache frequency was compared across two pairs of complete data from the CaMEO Study waves. The first pair was composed of waves one and two, which, with three months between them, directly mimics the assessment interval for the placebo arm in many prophylaxis trials. The second pair assessed longer-term change and was composed of waves one and five. Two variables were considered: (1) raw headache frequency and (2) change in headache frequency (headache frequency reported in the follow-up wave minus that reported in wave one). The effect of interest was whether change in headache frequency across the waves was different for EM and CM. Descriptive statistics, including wave EM- and CM-specific sample sizes and means for these three variables are given in Table 4. For the wave-specific headache frequency variables, a repeated measures negative binomial model was parameterized to calculate the difference between waves and estimate the difference in this difference between EM and CM through a time-by-headache status interaction term. The resulting time-by-headache status interaction RR emerging from this model along with the corresponding 95% CI and P values are reported in Table 4. This model was employed because it matches the modeling framework for the other models reported in this paper. For the variable in which change from baseline was calculated, a simple one-way analysis of variance (ANOVA) was conducted in which the only effect was baseline headache status. This model estimated the mean difference in change in headache frequency between baseline and follow-up between EM and CM, treating EM as the reference group. The resulting mean difference and corresponding 95% CI and P values are reported in Table 4.

In both cases (wave one and two pairing or wave one and five pairing), the results were identical. It appears that no matter what pairing of waves is used, headache frequency significantly decreases for CM, while headache frequency for EM remains mostly constant. The change in headache frequency for CM was so great that at follow-up the average headache frequency would have resulted in the average population being classified as having achieved CM remission in both wave pairings through the natural history of the condition alone. The reported RRs for the time-by-baseline headache status interaction and the ANOVA mean difference support this conclusion and indicate that the CM reduction in headache frequency between wave pairings was statistically significantly greater than that of EM.

Results presented here suggest that when subject selection is made on the basis of high frequency of headache days at baseline, as a direct consequence of the cyclical nature of monthly headache day frequency, there is a nontrivial probability that within a short period of time, headache frequency will organically fall to lower levels. However, and most importantly, headache day frequency does not remain low, and for a sizeable number of people, headache frequency values return to even higher levels. This appears as a fundamental paradox: in the full data headache frequency for CM increases over time while comparisons between pairs of waves suggest that headache frequency decreases for CM. This paradox is related to a variant of the Yule-Simpson effect [26], where conclusions are distorted by specific binning or grouping of the data that is not representative of the true global trend in the phenomenon. Results presented in this manuscript would suggest that variation in headache frequency is substantial. Moreover, the practice in RCTs of restricting attention to a baseline period obtained through selection based on a high frequency of headache days in the baseline period coupled with examination of only a single subsequent follow-up period leads to the frequently observed placebo effect for CM prophylaxis trials. The use of more sensitive and sophisticated designs and analyses may enable more accurate characterization of longitudinal headache epidemiology and determine with greater certainty the efficacy of treatment.

Strengths and limitations

This study has a number of strengths and limitations. Strengths include the large sample size with inclusion of large numbers of persons with migraine, the three-month

Table 4 Approximation of placebo-arm findings in RCTs as a result of "natural" remission of CM

Time Contrast	EM				CM				Negative Binomial Mixed-Model for Change From Baseline to Follow-Up[e]			1-Way ANOVA for Headache Frequency Change Score From Baseline to Follow-Up	
		Baseline	Follow-Up[b]	Change Score		Baseline	Follow-Up[b]	Change Score	Baseline Headache Status by Time Interaction Random-Effect Model-Based			Baseline Headache Status ANOVA Effect	
	Sample size[a]	μ_1	μ_2^d	μ_Δ	n	μ_1	μ_2^d	μ_Δ	Raw[f]	RR	*P* value	Mean Difference[c]	*P* value
Wave 1 vs. Wave 2	7759	3.98	4.14	0.16	829	19.77	14.61	−5.16	0.71	0.67 (0.64 to 0.71)	<0.0001	−5.32 (−5.69 to −4.95)	<0.0001
Wave 1 vs. Wave 5	4407	4.05	4.09	0.05	502	19.80	13.69	−6.12	0.68	0.64 (0.59 to 0.69)	<0.0001	−6.17 (−6.69 to −5.64)	<0.0001

ANOVA analysis of variance, *CM* chronic migraine, *EM* episodic migraine, *HA* headache, *RCT* randomized controlled trial, *RR* rate ratio, *SAS* statistical analysis system

[a]Sample sizes were based on complete case data, and are therefore lower for the second time contrast than the first because less subjects chose to respond to the survey by wave 5 than wave 2. The combined sample sizes are less than the wave 2 or wave 5 sample sizes respectively (i.e., 4407 + 502 = 4909, which is <5915) because the complete case data restriction also required the same subjects contribute data on the past month HA frequency variable at both the baseline and follow-up assessments

[b]Baseline Headache status by time interaction estimation: $(CM\_ \mu_2 / CM\_ \mu_1)/(EM\_ \mu_2 / EM\_ \mu_1)$

[c]Baseline Headache status ANOVA mean difference: $CM\_ \mu_\Delta - EM\_ \mu_\Delta$

[d]Random-effect model-based estimate parameterized with a random subject-specific intercept, fixed intercept, main effect for headache status (EM vs. CM, EM reference), main effect for time contrast (baseline vs. follow-up, baseline reference), and the interaction between headache status and time

[e]Random-effect negative binomial models were fit in SAS' GLIMMIX procedure. The model estimation was identical to the primary models presented in this manuscript and described in the methods section with adaptive Gauss-Hermite quadrature based on 13 quadrature points and 9 pseudo-likelihood initial iterations for start values, with no generalized linear model–based iterations

[f]Raw means, raw RRs, and random-effect model-based rate ratios indicate that HA frequency for CM declines over time while HA frequency for EM remains stable. Moreover, CM declines more as the amount of time between assessments increases (2 waves vs. 5). Specifically, with only three months between assessment, HA frequency declines 33% more for CM than EM (100*[1–0.67]), while HA frequency declines 36% more for CM than EM (100*[1–0.64]) when the time between assessments is 12 months

follow-up interval over a period of 15 months and our well-accepted modeling strategy. Limitations include the modest participation rate and the relatively high drop-out rate from wave to wave. The modest participation rate is offset in part by the evidence that results from the CaMEO Study are largely comparable to those from the larger AMPP study [6] and the non-responder study that did not provide any suggestion of participation bias [8]. As headache frequency varies over longer periods, modeling headache days using control theory–based models may provide better long-term characterization of the natural history of migraine across multiple intervals. Furthermore, the dynamic nature of migraine (transitioning between EM and CM) needs to be considered when a categorical description (i.e., EM or CM) is captured at baseline or individual time points. For example, a person categorized as having EM at baseline may have been classified with CM previously.

In addition, this study used modified ICHD-3 criteria which did not confirm ≥ five lifetime migraine events (criterion A) or duration of attack untreated from four to 72 h (criterion B). Likewise, the definition of CM did not include criterion C which states that migraine occurred ≥ 8 days per month. Confirmation of these parameters is difficult to evaluate via self-report retrospective surveys and requires data collection via diary cards and physician interview to verify.

Conclusions

Results confirm that there is substantial variation in headache day frequency in people with EM and CM followed at three-month intervals. Transitions from EM to CM are more common (7.6%) than previously observed when sampled less frequently; in addition, nearly 75% of people with CM will remit to EM at some point during a 12-month period. More research is required to more fully understand the implications of these findings. Importantly, this natural variation should be considered when designing epidemiologic and clinical trials and when clinicians diagnose, treat and study CM.

Abbreviations

AMPP: American Migraine Prevalence and Prevention; ANOVA: Analysis of variance; CM: Chronic migraine; EM: Episodic migraine; IBLUP: Inverse link function best linear unbiased predictor; ICHD-3 (beta): International Classification of Headache Disorders Third edition (beta version); MIDAS: Migraine Disability Assessment questionnaire; RCT: Randomized controlled trial; RR: Rate ratio; SAS: Statistical analysis system

Acknowledgments

This study was sponsored by Allergan plc (Dublin, Ireland). Editorial assistance was provided to the authors by Lee B. Hohaia, Pharm D, and Gerard P. Johnson, PhD, of Complete Healthcare Communications, LLC (Chadds Ford, PA, USA), a CHC Group company, and funded by Allergan plc (Dublin, Ireland). All authors met the ICMJE authorship criteria. Neither honoraria nor payments were made for authorship.

Funding

Allergan plc (Dublin, Ireland) provided funding for this study. An individual employee from Allergan, who is acknowledged as an author, was involved in the conception and design, interpretation of data, and revising the manuscript critically for important intellectual input; giving final approval for publication of manuscript.

Authors' contributions

DS made substantial contributions to conception and design, and analysis and interpretation of data, drafting of manuscript and revising critically for important intellectual input; giving final approval for publication of manuscript; and agrees to be accountable for all aspects of the work. RBL made substantial contributions to conception and design, acquisition of data, and interpretation of data, drafting of manuscript and revising critically for important intellectual input; giving final approval for publication of manuscript; and agrees to be accountable for all aspects of the work. AIS made substantial contributions to acquisition of data and interpretation of data, revising critically for important intellectual input; giving final approval for publication of manuscript; and agrees to be accountable for appropriate portions of the work. MLR made substantial contributions to conception and design, analysis and interpretation of data, revising critically for important intellectual input; giving final approval for publication of manuscript; and agrees to be accountable for appropriate portions of the work. WFS made substantial contributions to acquisition of data and interpretation of data, revising critically for important intellectual input; giving final approval for publication of manuscript; and agrees to be accountable for appropriate portions of the work. AMA made substantial contributions to conception and design, acquisition of data, and interpretation of data, revising critically for important intellectual input; giving final approval for publication of manuscript; and agrees to be accountable for appropriate portions of the work. DCB made substantial contributions to conception and design, acquisition of data, and interpretation of data, revising critically for important intellectual input; giving final approval for publication of manuscript; and agrees to be accountable for appropriate portions of the work.

Competing interests

Daniel Serrano is an employee of Endpoint Outcomes. This work was initiated while he was serving as a consultant for Vedanta Research and completed while Associate Director of Psychometrics at Endpoint Outcomes. He has received support funded by Allergan plc, CoLucid, Endo Pharmaceuticals, GlaxoSmithKline, MAP Pharmaceuticals, Merck & Co., Inc., NuPathe, Novartis, and Ortho-McNeil, via grants to the National Headache Foundation. In addition, he has received funding from Allergan plc, Astellas, Genenteck, Lumena, Neurocrine, Shire and Supernus. Richard B. Lipton serves on the editorial board of *Neurology* and as senior advisor to *Headache*. He has received research support from the NIH. He also receives support from the Migraine Research Foundation and the National Headache Foundation. He has reviewed for the NIA and NINDS, serves as consultant, advisory board member, or has received honoraria from: Alder, Allergan, Amgen, Autonomic Technologies, Avanir, Boston Scientific, Colucid, Dr. Reddy's, Electrocore, Eli Lilly, eNeura Therapeutics, GlaxoSmithKline, Merck, Pfizer, Teva, and Vedanta. He receives royalties from Wolff's Headache, 8th Edition, Oxford University Press, 2009 and Informa. He holds stock options in eNeura Therapeutics and Biohaven. Ann I Scher, in the past 12 months has received honoraria from and is an advisory board member for Allergan, Inc., receives grant support from CDMRP and CNRM, and is on the editorial boards of *Cephalalgia* and *Pain Medicine*. The Views expressed are those of the author (s) and do not necessarily reflect the official views of the Uniformed Services University of the Health Sciences or the Department of Defense. Michael Reed is Managing Director of Vedanta Research, which has received research funding from Allergan, Amgen, CoLucid, Dr. Reddy's Laboratories, Endo Pharmaceuticals, GlaxoSmithKline, Merck & Co., Inc., NuPathe, Novartis, and Ortho-McNeil, via grants to the National Headache Foundation. Vedanta Research has received funding directly from Allergan for work on the CaMEO Study. Walter (Buzz) F. Stewart consulted for Amgen and received support for research from Astra-Zeneca. Aubrey Manack Adams is a full-time employee of Allergan plc and owns stock in the company. Dawn C. Buse in the past 12 months, has received grant support and honoraria from Allergan, Avanir, Amgen, and Dr. Reddy's Laboratories. She has served as a consultant for Eli Lilly. She is an employee of Montefiore Medical Center, which in the past 12 months, has received research support funded by Allergan, Alder, Avanir, CoLucid, Dr. Reddy's Laboratories, and

Labrys via grants to the National Headache Foundation and/or Montefiore Medical Center. She is on the editorial board of *Current Pain and Headache Reports*, the *Journal of Headache and Pain, Pain Medicine News*, and *Pain Pathways* magazine.

Author details

[1]Endpoint Outcomes, Boston, MA, USA. [2]The Saul R. Korey Department of Neurology, Albert Einstein College of Medicine, Bronx, NY, USA. [3]Montefiore Headache Center; Department of Neurology and Department of Epidemiology and Population Health, Albert Einstein College of Medicine, Bronx, NY, USA. [4]Department of Preventive Medicine and Biometrics, Uniformed Services University of the Health Sciences, Bethesda, MD, USA. [5]Vedanta Research, Chapel Hill, NC, USA. [6]Sutter Health, Walnut Creek, CA, USA. [7]Allergan plc, Irvine, CA, USA. [8]Montefiore Medical Center, Department of Neurology, Albert Einstein College of Medicine, Bronx, NY, USA.

References

1. Headache Classification Committee of the International Headache Society (2013) The International Classification of Headache Disorders, 3rd edition (beta version). Cephalalgia 33:629–808. doi:10.1177/0333102413485658
2. Lipton RB, Stewart WF, Diamond S, Diamond ML, Reed M (2001) Prevalence and burden of migraine in the United States: data from the American Migraine Study II. Headache 41:646–657
3. Buse DC, Manack AN, Fanning KM, Serrano D, Reed ML, Turkel CC, Lipton RB (2012) Chronic migraine prevalence, disability, and sociodemographic factors: results from the American Migraine Prevalence and Prevention Study. Headache 52:1456–1470. doi:10.1111/j.1526-4610.2012.02223.x
4. Blumenfeld AM, Varon SF, Wilcox TK, Buse DC, Kawata AK, Manack A, Goadsby PJ, Lipton RB (2011) Disability, HRQoL and resource use among chronic and episodic migraineurs: results from the International Burden of Migraine Study (IBMS). Cephalalgia 31:301–315. doi:10.1177/0333102410381145
5. Payne KA, Varon SF, Kawata AK, Yeomans K, Wilcox TK, Manack A, Buse DC, Lipton RB, Goadsby PJ, Blumenfeld AM (2011) The International Burden of Migraine Study (IBMS): study design, methodology, and baseline cohort characteristics. Cephalalgia 31:1116–1130. doi:10.1177/0333102411410610
6. Lipton RB, Manack Adams A, Buse DC, Fanning KM, Reed ML (2016) A comparison of the Chronic Migraine Epidemiology and Outcomes (CaMEO) Study and American Migraine Prevalence and Prevention (AMPP) Study: demographics and headache-related disability. Headache 56:1280–1289
7. Bigal ME, Lipton RB (2008) Concepts and mechanisms of migraine chronification. Headache 48:7–15
8. Manack Adams A, Serrano D, Buse DC, Reed ML, Marske V, Fanning KM, Lipton RB (2015) The impact of chronic migraine: the Chronic Migraine Epidemiology and Outcomes (CaMEO) Study methods and baseline results. Cephalalgia 35:563–578. doi:10.1177/0333102414552532
9. Silberstein SD, Lipton RB, Sliwinski M (1996) Classification of daily and near-daily headaches: field trial of revised IHS criteria. Neurology 47:871–875
10. Buse DC, Manack AN, Serrano D, Reed ML, Varon S, Turkel CC, Lipton RB (2012) Headache impact of chronic and episodic migraine: results from the American Migraine Prevalence and Prevention study. Headache 52:3-17. doi:10.1111/j.1526-4610.2011.02046.x
11. National Census Bureau (2012) 2012 American Community Survey. US Census Bureau. https://www.census.gov/programs-surveys/acs/data/pums.html. Accessed 9 Feb 2017
12. Bigal ME, Serrano D, Buse D, Scher A, Stewart WF, Lipton RB (2008) Acute migraine medications and evolution from episodic to chronic migraine: a longitudinal population-based study. Headache 48:1157–1168. doi:10.1111/j.1526-4610.2008.01217.x
13. Aamodt AH, Stovner LJ, Langhammer A, Hagen K, Zwart JA (2007) Is headache related to asthma, hay fever, and chronic bronchitis? The Head-HUNT Study. Headache 47:204–212
14. Linde M, Stovner LJ, Zwart JA, Hagen K (2011) Time trends in the prevalence of headache disorders. The Nord-Trondelag Health Studies (HUNT 2 and HUNT 3). Cephalalgia. doi:10.1177/0333102410391488
15. Wang SJ, Fuh JL, Lu SR, Juang KD (2007) Outcomes and predictors of chronic daily headache in adolescents: a 2-year longitudinal study. Neurology 68:591–596. doi:10.1212/01.wnl.0000252800.82704.62
16. Scher AI, Stewart WF, Liberman J, Lipton RB (1998) Prevalence of frequent headache in a population sample. Headache 38:497–506. doi:10.1046/j.1526-4610.1998.3807497.x
17. Stewart WF, Wood GC, Bruce C, Buse DC, Runken MC, Lipton RB (2011) Longitudinal change in migraine headache-days and indirect cost consequences. J Occup Environ Med 53:478–487
18. Lipton RB (2009) Tracing transformation: chronic migraine classification, progression, and epidemiology. Neurology 72:S3–S7
19. Manack A, Buse DC, Serrano D, Turkel CC, Lipton RB (2011) Rates, predictors, and consequences of remission from chronic migraine to episodic migraine. Neurology 76:711-718. doi:10.1212/WNL.0b013e31820d8af2
20. Silberstein S, Tfelt-Hansen P, Dodick DW, Limmroth V, Lipton RB, Pascual J, Wang SJ (2008) Guidelines for controlled trials of prophylactic treatment of chronic migraine in adults. Cephalalgia 28:484-495. doi:10.1111/j.1468-2982.2008.01555.x
21. Aurora SK, Dodick DW, Turkel CC, DeGryse RE, Silberstein SD, Lipton RB, Diener HC, Brin MF (2010) OnabotulinumtoxinA for treatment of chronic migraine: results from the double-blind, randomized, placebo-controlled phase of the PREEMPT 1 trial. Cephalalgia 30:793–803. doi:10.1177/0333102410364676
22. Bigal ME, Edvinsson L, Rapoport AM, Lipton RB, Spierings EL, Diener HC, Burstein R, Loupe PS, Ma Y, Yang R, Silberstein SD (2015) Safety, tolerability, and efficacy of TEV-48125 for preventive treatment of chronic migraine: a multicentre, randomised, double-blind, placebo-controlled, phase 2b study. Lancet Neurol 14:1091–1100
23. Dodick DW, Turkel CC, DeGryse RE, Aurora SK, Silberstein SD, Lipton RB, Diener HC, Brin MF (2010) OnabotulinumtoxinA for treatment of chronic migraine: pooled results from the double-blind, randomized, placebo-controlled phases of the PREEMPT clinical program. Headache 50:921-936. doi:10.1111/j.1526-4610.2010.01678.x
24. Silberstein S, Lipton R, Dodick D, Freitag F, Mathew N, Brandes J, Bigal M, Ascher S, Morein J, Wright P, Greenberg S, Hulihan J (2009) Topiramate treatment of chronic migraine: a randomized, placebo-controlled trial of quality of life and other efficacy measures. Headache 49:1153–1162. doi:10.1111/j.1526-4610.2009.01508.x
25. Stovner LJ, Linde M, Gravdahl GB, Tronvik E, Aamodt AH, Sand T, Hagen K (2014) A comparative study of candesartan versus propranolol for migraine prophylaxis: a randomised, triple-blind, placebo-controlled, double cross-over study. Cephalalgia 34:523–532
26. Blyth CR (1972) On Simpson's paradox and the sure-thing principle. J Am Stat Assoc 67:364–366. doi:10.2307/2284382

My Migraine Voice survey: a global study of disease burden among individuals with migraine for whom preventive treatments have failed

Paolo Martelletti[1,2], Todd J. Schwedt[3*], Michel Lanteri-Minet[4], Rebeca Quintana[5], Veruska Carboni[6], Hans-Christoph Diener[7], Elena Ruiz de la Torre [8], Audrey Craven[9], Annette Vangaa Rasmussen[10], Simon Evans[11], Annik K. Laflamme[12], Rachel Fink[12], Donna Walsh[13], Paula Dumas[14] and Pamela Vo[12]

Abstract

Background: Migraine is associated with many debilitating symptoms that affect daily functioning. *My Migraine Voice* is a large global cross-sectional study aimed at understanding the full burden and impact of migraine directly from patients suffering from ≥4 monthly migraine days (MMDs) with a history of prophylactic treatment failure.

Methods: This study was conducted worldwide (31 countries across North and South Americas, Europe, the Middle East and Northern Africa, and the Asia-Pacific region) using an online survey administered to adults with migraine who reported ≥4 MMDs in the 3 months preceding survey administration, with pre-specified criteria of 90% having used preventive migraine treatment (80% with history of ≥1 treatment failure). Prophylactic treatment failure was defined as a reported change in preventive medication by individuals with migraine for any reason, at least once.

Results: In total, 11,266 individuals participated in the survey. Seventy-four percent of the participants reported spending time in darkness/isolation due to migraine (average: 19 h/month). While 85% of all respondents reported negative aspects of living with migraine (feeling helpless, depressed, not understood), sleeping difficulties (83%), and fear of the next attack (55%), 57% shared ≥1 positive aspect (learning to cope, becoming a stronger person). Forty-nine percent reported feeling limited in daily activities throughout all migraine phases. Migraine impact on professional, private, or social domains was reported by 87% of respondents (51% in all domains). In the previous 12 months, 38% of respondents had visited the emergency department (average: 3.3 visits), whereas 23% stayed in hospital overnight (average: 3.2 nights) due to migraine.

Conclusions: The burden of migraine is substantial among this cohort of individuals with at least 4 migraine days per month and for whom at least 1 preventive migraine treatment had failed. Interestingly, respondents reported some positive aspects in their migraine journey; the greater resilience and strength brought on by coping with migraine suggests that if future treatments could address existing unmet needs, these individuals with migraine will be able to maximize their contribution to society.

Keywords: Migraine, Burden, Global survey, Work productivity, Migraine experience

* Correspondence: Schwedt.Todd@mayo.edu
[3]Department of Neurology, Mayo Clinic, 5777 East Mayo Boulevard, Phoenix, AZ 85054, USA
Full list of author information is available at the end of the article

Background

Migraine is a painful, debilitating neurological disease, which consistently ranks among the top 10 leading causes of years lived with disability (YLD) worldwide [1, 2]. It is currently the first-leading cause of YLD among individuals under 50 years old [3].

The impact of migraine on all domains of life contributes to the complexity of adequately capturing its true wide-ranging burden from the perspective of people with migraine, particularly those experiencing a relatively high frequency of migraine attacks and with unmet treatment needs. Multiple previous studies and surveys described various manifestations of the burden of migraine, such as the American Migraine Prevalence and Prevention (AMPP) study, the International Burden of Migraine Study (IBMS), the Chronic Migraine Epidemiology and Outcomes (CaMEO) study, the Eurolight project, and the Global Burden of Disease (GBD) study [4–10]. However, the current understanding of migraine burden among individuals with the highest unmet needs, specifically those experiencing ≥4 monthly migraine days (MMDs) and prior prophylaxis failure, is limited. This particular subgroup is of interest since new preventive migraine therapies have demonstrated efficacy and safety in this population. Furthermore, understanding the burden of disease in individuals with ≥4 MMDs is very important to enable physicians and/or others involved in migraine management to make well-informed decisions on appropriate preventive migraine care for these people. Specifically, no detailed assessment of the current treatment pathway, impact on work productivity, or burden associated with premonitory and postdromal phases of migraine is available in individuals experiencing ≥4 MMDs who have had previous prophylactic treatments that failed and continue to experience frequent migraines.

A qualitative study was conducted using online bulletin boards (OBBs) to identify the key issues experienced by people living with migraine prior to the present global study [11, 12]. OBBs are a qualitative data collection method that allow anonymous participation across varied geographic locations, customization of questions, and interactions and answers in local languages to facilitate and enhance data quality; qualitative data from OBBs were used to inform the *My Migraine Voice* study. The OBB study highlighted the challenges and important impacts of migraine on many aspects of the daily lives of individuals with migraine. This permitted the substantial functional and emotional burden associated with migraine to be described by affected individuals in their own words [11, 12]. People with migraine reported facing significant challenges in pursuing daily activities or work and difficulties with coping mechanisms. The negative impact of migraine also extended to caregivers, most of them being torn between commitment, self-sacrifice, and resentment in relation to their responsibilities toward the person with migraine for whom they were providing care [11, 12].

Building on this first initiative, the quantitative *My Migraine Voice* study was undertaken on a much larger and comprehensive scale via an online survey to further understand views of people with migraine and its worldwide impact across 31 countries. The objectives of *My Migraine Voice* were to assess migraine characteristics and describe the current real-world burden and impact of living with migraine from clinical, personal, and economic perspectives among adults with migraine experiencing ≥4 MMDs.

Methods

Study design and participants

This was a large, cross-sectional, multi-country online survey of adult participants (≥18 years of age) with migraine. Screening questions to determine eligibility included a description of migraine based on the International Classification of Headache Disorders 3rd edition (ICHD-3) criteria followed by a series of migraine symptom and characteristic questions to qualify that participants were experiencing migraine. Participants could also record whether they had received a medical diagnosis of migraine, although this was not part of the inclusion criteria. Further, only those who self-reported experiencing ≥4 MMDs each month for the previous 3 months were eligible for inclusion in the survey.

Prespecified quotas were applied to people reporting a history of taking a prophylactic medication to prevent their migraine: 90% of participants reported current or previous use of preventive migraine medication, of which 80% switched preventive treatment, and the remaining 10% were preventive treatment-naïve. Individuals with migraine who reported changing their preventive medication for any reason at least once were defined to have had a preventive treatment failure (TF). The applied quotas were required to ensure that the occurrence of TF was adequately represented among study participants, with a substantive proportion of individuals that had a history of ≥2 TFs.

Participants were recruited by means of existing online panels (GfK Health) and support organizations for people with migraine. Participants' consent was obtained prior to participation in the survey and those who completed the survey were compensated with an incentive in the form of a voucher and aligned with local standards. Data were collected via Confirmit, an online platform, and internet surveys were completed independently by respondents. Data were handled confidentially and anonymity of respondents was maintained throughout the study. As such, and due to its research format, this study was exempted from ethics committee review.

Survey design and outcomes

The survey drew upon the previous OBB study results. Details on the methods of the OBB study are published elsewhere [11, 12]. A steering committee composed of migraine specialists, a specialized nurse, and patient support group leaders also informed the methodology and additional topics of importance. The final survey comprised 88 questions and included country-specific questions tailored to reflect differences in healthcare systems and available treatments.

Table 1 presents the outcome parameters assessed in the survey relating to sociodemographic factors, health and medical history, health-related quality of life, impact on daily activities, treatment patterns and participants' treatment experience, and healthcare utilization.

Table 1 Parameters Collected in the Survey

Domain	Items
Sociodemographic characteristics	• Age • Gender • Income • Place of living • Occupation status • Family status
Health/medical history	• Monthly migraine days • Monthly headache days • Characteristics of migraine (eg, symptoms, pain, nausea, aura, duration) • Medication history • Migraine history (eg, time affected by migraine, diagnosis, time since diagnosis, engagement with HCPs) • Family history of migraine and headache (parents, siblings, children) • Comorbidities (chronic conditions)
QoL	• QoL • Experience of living with migraine (eg, fear of migraine attack, ability to focus, fatigue, feelings of frustration/hopelessness)
Healthcare utilization	• Healthcare utilization (eg, hospitalizations, ED visits, outpatient visits, general practitioners, neurologists, headache centers, brain scans) • Treatments for relief of headache/migraine • Treatments for prevention of headache/migraine • Non-pharmacological management
Impact on daily life	• Work status (including changes in employment due to migraine) • Daily activities and household activities • Work productivity using WPAI-Migraine
Treatment patterns/ participants' treatment experience	• Time on treatment • Treatment satisfaction • Reason for switching (if any)

ED Emergency department; *HCP* Healthcare provider; *QoL* Quality of life; *WPAI* Work Productivity and Activity Impairment

Because of limited published information on the burden before and after the migraine attack, the survey included questions on the migraine phases. Descriptions of migraine phases were provided to participants (Table 2).

In addition, a validated questionnaire was included in the survey to assess the impact of migraine on work productivity and daily activities among employed respondents. The impact of migraine on work productivity and regular activities during the past 7 days was evaluated using the Work Productivity and Activity Impairment (WPAI) questionnaire and was compared among treatment -naive, no prior TF, 1 TF, and ≥ 2 TF patient subgroups.

Data analysis

Data analysis was conducted using IBM SPSS Statistics (version 24) to generate summary statistics on country and aggregate levels, and Qlikview software was used for charting. Quality assessment of the data was performed and included an evaluation of response patterns and inconsistencies and an analysis of answers to open-ended questions. Comparisons of different subset of participants were completed using frequencies, means, medians, and standard deviations. The reported *P*-values are from the T-student test when testing differences between averages, and from the Chi-square test when testing differences between percentages or proportions.

Results

Worldwide recruitment occurred from September 2017 to February 2018 across 31 countries in North America (n = 1689) and South America (n = 1438), Europe (n = 6156), the Middle East and Northern Africa (n = 1111), and the Asia-Pacific region (n = 872), resulting in the participation of a total of 11,266 individuals with migraine in *My Migraine Voice* (Fig. 1). Per the predefined inclusion criteria, approximately 90% of participants (n = 9856) had taken preventive medication (past or present) for migraine, and ≥ 80% of these (n = 7678) had experienced at least 1 or more TF, which represents 68% of the total survey population (Fig. 1). The majority of participants with a previous treatment failure were those who had ≥2 TFs (n = 6717; 87% of those with any TF).

The characteristics of the study participants are summarized in Table 3. Of the total 11,266 participants, a majority were female, had children, and had a family history of migraine. The majority of participants were in either full- (47%) or part-time (12%) paid

Table 2 Description of Migraine Phases

Premonitory Phase (Before the Attack)		Headache Phase (The Attack)	Postdromal Phase (After the Attack)	
Warning phase *Might occur days or hours before* • Concentration problems • Irritability • Repetitive yawning • Sleep issues • Food cravings • Tiredness	Aura • Sensory disturbances • Speech disturbances • Visual disturbances • Symptoms last up to one hour	The attack *(and accompanying symptoms)* • Throbbing one-sided headache • Sickness, nausea • Sensitive to light, sound	Resolution • Sleep helps • Fatigue • Food intolerance • Altered mood • Impaired concentration • Less intense pain	Recovery • Hangover feeling • Weak • Need rest

employment or self-employment (7%) or were students (7%). On average, participants had migraine for 11.6 years, but over one-quarter (27%) had it for more than 20 years. The majority of participants (86%) also reported currently having a healthcare professional for their migraine, most frequently a neurologist or headache specialist (41%) or general practitioner (42%).

Seventy-six percent of survey participants reported taking medications for acute treatment, which increased to 81% among those with ≥2 TFs. Of the participants taking medications for acute treatment, 83% took these based on a doctor's prescription and 51% also took over-the-counter (OTC) medications, indicating that a substantive proportion of respondents were taking both doctor-prescribed and OTC medications. Notably, among respondents taking acute treatments, 20% reported using opioids for their migraine. Overall, study respondents reported having 3.3 other chronic conditions on average, with anxiety, insomnia/sleep disorders, and depression being most commonly reported in all participants, irrespective of whether they had experienced previous preventive TF.

Migraine characteristics

Considering all phases of the migraine attack, survey participants had on average 9.8 days/month affected by migraine over the last 3 months. For 44% of respondents, migraine episodes lasted 1 to 2 days or more, and 19% reported episodes lasting longer than 3 days. A headache phase duration longer than 1 day was reported by 27% of respondents without any TF compared with 38% of respondents who had ≥2 TFs ($P < 0.05$) (Table 4). Almost half of respondents (49%) reported feeling limited in completing daily activities throughout the 3 migraine attack phases (feeling limited over a total of 10.5 days/month on average). Peak of limitations occurred during the headache phase as reported by 71% of respondents vs 75% for those with ≥2 TFs ($P < 0.05$) who felt very to extremely limited during the phase. About one-third of respondents also felt this level of limitation in the premonitory and postdromal phases (Table 4). Very few respondents reported feeling "no limitation" in each of the migraine phases (4%, 1%, and 5% in the premonitory, headache, and postdromal phases, respectively).

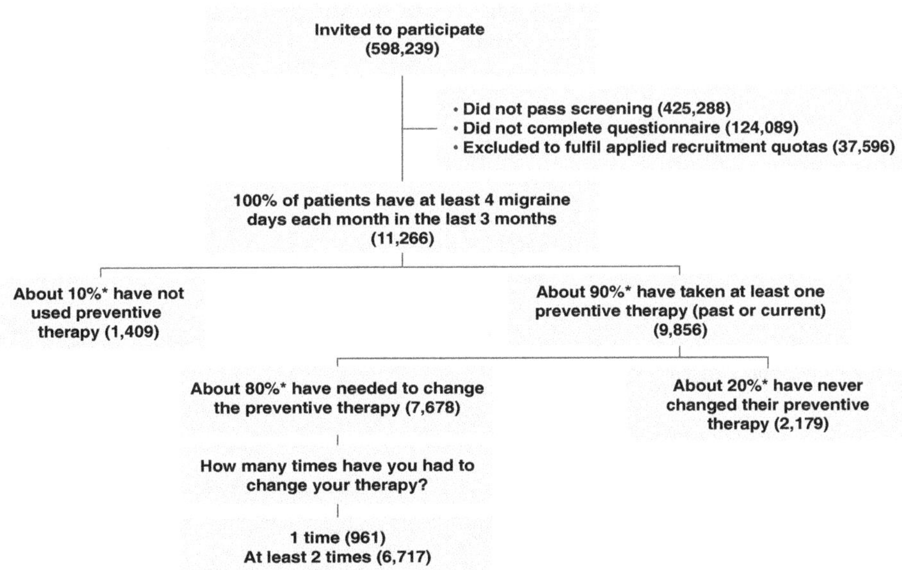

Fig. 1 The *My Migraine Voice* Study Population Accrued per Applied Criteria. *Predetermined quotas

Table 3 Baseline Characteristics of the *My Migraine Voice* Population

	Total Population (n = 11,266)	Migraine Individuals With 1 TF (*n* = 961)	Migraine Individuals With ≥2 TFs (n = 6717)
Gender			
Female	75% (8396)	77% (735)	73% (1859)
Male	25% (2689)	24% (226)	27% (652)
Age (mean)	39.4 years	39 years	40.2 years
With children (yes)	63% (7098)	58% (557)	67% (4500)
Employed (full time or part-time)	58% (6534)	57% (548)	59% (3963)
Family history of migraine (yes)	54% (6083)	53% (509)	56% (3761)
Time being affected by migraine (mean)	11.6 years	10.9 years	12.2 years
< 1 year	4% (423)	5% (49)	2% (150)
1–5 years	26% (2929)	29% (281)	23% (1537)
6–10 years	21% (2381)	21% (199)	22% (1492)
11–15 years	12% (1350)	10% (96)	13% (852)
16–20 years	10% (1149)	9% (84)	11% (717)
21 years or more	27% (3034)	26% (252)	29% (1969)
Taking acute migraine medications	76% (8562)	75% (721)	81% (5440)
Average number of self-reported chronic conditions	3.3	3.1	3.4
First most commonly reported: anxiety	27% (3042)	25% (240)	28% (1881)
Second most commonly reported: insomnia/ sleep disorder	24% (2704)	21% (202)	26% (1746)
Third most commonly reported: depression	23% (2591)	22% (211)	25% (1679)

TF Treatment failure

Living with migraine

Although the main symptom of migraine reported by 86% of respondents was a long-lasting headache (from 4 to 72 h), other symptoms such as severe pain either on one side of the head (75%) or throbbing pain (78%), light sensitivity (80%), sound sensitivity (75%), and nausea (74%) were also reported by 74% to 80% of participants. On a scale from 0 to 10 (highest level), the severity of pain experienced during the last month by respondents was 7.4 on average, including 57% of respondents with a higher than average pain severity (8–10). Notably, overall, 74% of respondents (78% of those with ≥2 TFs) reported spending long periods of time in darkness and isolation—an average of 19 h per month and increasing to 21 h per month in those with ≥2 TFs. Migraine was also reported to cause

Table 4 Characteristics of Migraine Phases

	Premonitory Phase, % (N)	Headache Phase, % (N)	Postdromal Phase, % (N)
Duration of phase			
< 4 h	50% (5676)	20% (2280)	30% (3419)
4–24 h	30% (3312)	45% (5067)	40% (4516)
> 24 h	14% (1622)	34% (3835)	27% (3006)
Not experiencing this phase	6% (656)	1% (84)	3% (325)
Proportion of individuals in each preventive treatment group reporting the duration of this migraine attack phase > 24 h:			
- No failure to migraine preventive treatment	11% (250)	27% (599)	20% (436)
- 1 TF of migraine preventive treatment	11% (103)	29% (282)	23% (218)
- ≥2 TFs of migraine preventive treatment	17% (1114)	38% (2539)	31% (2048)
- *P*-value: ≥2 failures vs no failure of migraine preventative treatment	< 0.05	< 0.05	< 0.05
Feeling very to extremely limited during the phase	29% (3047)	71% (8023)	30% (3291)

TF Treatment failure

sleeplessness by 83% of all respondents on average (86% for those with ≥2 TFs).

Table 5 summarizes the range of circumstances and ways in which respondents reported that over the previous 1 month, migraine had negatively affected their daily functioning. Notably, in each case, a higher proportion of respondents with ≥2 TFs reported a negative impact on daily functioning compared with the overall participant population. Four out of 5 respondents reported having to cancel plans due to migraine. When asked how they felt about living with migraine, overall 85% of respondents (88% of those with ≥2 TFs) reported at least 1 negative aspect of living with migraine. The most mentioned aspect was the feeling of being misunderstood by people (48%), followed by depression (41%) and feelings related to hating their own life (39%), feeling helpless (39%), and feeling that migraine controls and dictates their lives (39%). An average of 27% of all respondents were either very or extremely fearful of experiencing another episode of migraine (average of 32% among those with ≥2 TFs). Despite all the negative aspects, 57% of respondents mentioned at least 1 positive aspect of living with migraine, mainly related to gaining resilience and strength: 'I have learnt to cope with the disease' (40%), 'I am responsible for my migraine' (13%), and 'It has made me stronger' (11%).

Impact on private, social, and professional life

Impact of migraine on professional, private, or social domains was reported by 87% of respondents (51% in all domains). Sixty-four percent of respondents reported that migraine had affected their private life (70% of respondents with ≥2 TFs), including relationships with friends, relatives, and partners. On average each respondent mentioned 4 negative impacts related to missing important events (birthdays, weddings) (52%), avoiding making commitments (50%), effect on sex life (49%), and feeling guilty about the impact migraine has on their family life (44%).

Social activities were also affected for 78% of respondents (82% in the ≥2 TFs subgroup). On average each respondent mentioned 3 negative impacts with the most mentioned being not participating in all activities/hobbies they used to (59%), being stopped from going to social events (57%), and being stopped from engaging in sports activities or exercise (34%).

Over the previous 3 months, 61% had relied on external support from family friends or someone else to cope with daily tasks (64% in the ≥2 TFs subgroup). In the 3 months before answering the survey, assistance was required for 12.8 days on average for physical (eg, cooking, cleaning, shopping), emotional (eg, support, comfort, understanding), and medical (eg, taking/providing medication, transport to doctor, buying medication at pharmacy) aspects of life by 86%, 66%, and 49% of respondents, respectively. In the same time period, respondents with ≥2 TFs required more support (13.6 days on average), and 54% of respondents with ≥2 TFs required help with medical aspects compared with 49% of all respondents with migraine.

Impact of migraine on work productivity

Of all survey respondents, 70% reported that migraine has affected their professional life, which rose to 75% in the ≥2 TFs subgroup and was significantly higher than those with no TF (60%) ($P < 0.05$). The top 3 impacts of migraine on work reported by the respondents were inability to concentrate on work (52%), missing too many days of work (32%), and lack of understanding among colleagues about their condition or taking it seriously (27%). Out of the 58% of respondents who were in full- or part-time paid employment, 63% reported that their employers were aware of their

Table 5 Functional and Emotional Impact of Migraine

Impact	Total Population (n = 11,266)	Migraine Individuals With 1 TF (n = 961)	Migraine Individuals With ≥2 TFs (n = 6717)	P-value (≥2 TFs vs 1 TF)
Severity of pain (range from 0 to 10; mean reported)	7.4	7.3	7.5	< 0.05
Ever cancelled plans due to migraine	80% (9013)	75% (721)	83% (5575)	< 0.05
Often or always feeling frustrated by migraine	56% (6309)	55% (529)	59% (3963)	< 0.05
Migraine often or always interfering with ability to think clearly or to focus on daily life activities and tasks	52% (5838)	52% (500)	56% (3762)	< 0.05
Level of migraine interference with daily activities ("a lot" or "constantly")	51% (5746)	48% (461)	57% (3829)	< 0.05
Often or always lacking the energy to complete daily living or felt fatigued	50% (5633)	48% (461)	54% (3627)	< 0.05
Level of impairment in daily activity due to migraine (needing to stop and rest "a lot" or "always")	45% (5070)	42% (404)	49% (3291)	< 0.05
Often or always feeling hopeless or helpless by migraine	43% (4844)	38% (365)	47% (3157)	< 0.05

TF Treatment failure

migraine (68% in the ≥2 TFs subgroup), whereas only 18% reported receiving any support from their employer. Of all respondents, 9% (12% of those with ≥2 TFs) reported receiving a disability-related allowance because of their migraine.

A majority of respondents in employment (60%) reported missing ≥1 day of work in the last month due to migraine, with an average of 4.6 working days being missed in the last month, which is consistent with the average of 4.5 working days missed due to migraine (absenteeism) measured by the WPAI questionnaire. Notably, the ≥2 TFs subgroup missed an average of 5 working days due to migraine, which was significantly higher vs 3.8 days missed by those with 1 TF ($P < 0.05$). However, paid sick days reported by respondents in employment in the last month were on average 2.4 days: 2.7 days in the ≥2 TFs subgroup vs 1.7 days in those with 1 TF ($P < 0.05$).

Of the 7339 (65%) respondents who reported being currently employed, 6606 reported having worked in the last 7 days. These study participants reported that migraine led to a reduction of 13% in their working time (absenteeism) and 48% in productivity while working (presenteeism); 52% reported impairment in both overall work productivity (absenteeism and presenteeism combined) and daily activities due to migraine. Subgroup analysis according to prior treatment failure showed that impairment in all WPAI scores (absenteeism, presenteeism, and impairment in overall work productivity and daily activities) was highest in respondents with ≥2 TFs, followed by the 1 TF, no TF, and treatment-naïve subgroups.

Healthcare resource utilization

In the previous 6 months, the majority of respondents reported visiting a general practitioner (GP) (53%), whereas smaller but notable proportions also visited a neurologist (40%), pharmacist (19%), headache specialist (15%), dentist (12%), physiotherapist (11%), and psychologist or psychiatrist (10%). A majority of respondents (58%) reported having had a brain scan (average of 2.1 scans); by comparison, 68% of respondents in the ≥2 TFs subgroup had undergone an average of 2.3 brain scans over time (Table 6), which was significantly higher than the 29% of treatment-naïve respondents who had undergone an average of 1.7 brain scans ($P < 0.05$).

In the previous 12 months, more than a third of respondents had visited the emergency department (ED) because of their migraine and had on average 3.3 visits in the last year, whereas nearly a quarter stayed in hospital overnight (3.2 nights on average) (Table 6).

Table 6 Resource Utilization by Number of Previously Used Migraine Preventive Treatments

	Total Population (n = 11,266)	Persons With Migraine With 1 TF (n = 961)	Persons With Migraine With ≥2 TFs (n = 6717)
Brain scan			
Proportion of respondents	58% (6534)	56% (538)	68% (4568)
Average number of scans	2.1	1.7	2.3
ED visits in past 12 months			
Proportion of respondents	38% (4281)	28% (269)	46% (3090)
Average number of visits	3.3	2.7	3.5
Overnight hospital stay in past 12 months			
Proportion of respondents	23% (2591)	15% (144)	29% (1948)
Average nights of stay	3.2	2.3	3.4

ED Emergency department; *TF* Treatment failure

Discussion

This large worldwide study of 11,266 participants constitutes the largest survey to date conducted in individuals with migraine suffering from ≥4 MMDs and focused mostly on those who previously experienced failure of migraine prevention treatments. The size and granularity of this study have created a rich data source to describe the impact of migraine in this economically active population, with personal, social, and professional commitments and high healthcare use in unprecedented detail.

The study data reveal that individuals with migraine, especially those with a history of previous preventive treatment failures, have higher levels of unmet needs. This study describes the personal, social, humanistic, and economic burden of migraine in detail, and for the first time, it allows quantifying the burden during different phases of the migraine attack for individuals suffering from ≥4 MMDs with a history of prophylactic treatment. Although the headache phase itself caused the highest degree of impairment, the findings demonstrate that the burden of migraine extends beyond the headache phase itself and is higher for individuals who had at least one previous preventive treatment failure.

Respondents that had ≥4 MMDs reported a high rate of ED visits and overnight stays in the hospital due to migraine. Also, those with a history of failed preventive treatments for migraine had even higher utilization of healthcare resources. This trend suggests that treatment failure in migraine may be an important driver of increased healthcare utilization. These findings are consistent with the results of the IBMS study, which found that for each of the five European countries studied, chronic migraine (per ICHD-2 criteria, persons with ≥15 MMDs) was associated with additional healthcare costs attributable to an increased use of medical services and associated cost [6]. However, unlike the IBMS study, the *My Migraine Voice* participants cover a larger range of migraine individuals (≥4 MMDs), therefore providing a more comprehensive appraisal of burden and healthcare utilization.

In addition to the direct economic burden, results of this study highlight the substantial indirect economic burden imposed by migraine. Loss in work productivity and activity impairment due to migraine is higher in individuals with previously failed preventive treatments, further establishing the need for more effective treatment options in this particular population to ensure that these affected persons can fully contribute to the productive workforce and society.

The present study has some limitations for consideration. The recruitment of participants aimed to select migraine individuals with ≥4 MMDs. While the sample does not entirely mirror the overall general population of people with migraine, it allowed selecting a representative and generalizable sample of individuals with severe disease. Recruitment bias may affect the estimates where differences are present between survey participants and the population from each country. For example, individuals with 1 to 3 MMDs are not included as part of this study, nor are people with migraine without ready access to the internet or those who are not part of the catchment group contacted to participate in this survey. Pooling data from different countries may also introduce some variability in the dataset, unless country-specific nuances can be accounted for. Another limitation of this study is the use of self-reported data because diagnosis of migraine and other relevant diagnoses (eg, those used in the comorbidity index) and reporting of healthcare visits and other variables of interest cannot be clinically confirmed. However, there is no substantial reason why one would not believe a self-reported migraine diagnosis if that individual can identify what type and when the physician diagnosed him/her with migraine. The magnitude of migraine impact is likely affected by the frequency, severity, and duration of migraine, which may also be susceptible to impact from reporting and recall biases. Moreover, *My Migraine Voice* has been completed and currently no follow-ups are planned. Therefore, although it is the largest cross-sectional study specifically reporting the burden of disease in individuals with severe migraine to date, it does not benefit from the additional insights that a longitudinal study in the same population might reveal about the time evolution of migraine and its multifaceted burden.

Despite the limitations above, this study strikes a balance between the sample size needed to obtain a higher-resolution description about the burden of migraine imposed on affected individuals with the highest unmet need (≥4 MMDs) and potential caveats in generalizing its findings to all people with migraine (irrespective of disease severity) resulting from the above-mentioned limitations. The impact of migraine on the lives of affected individuals was also measured by some patient-reported outcome measures. A web-based approach appears to be an appropriate method to capture cross-sectional or longitudinal data and grants access to a population that would typically not be found in clinical settings, allowing a determination of the global burden of migraine [5, 13]. A follow-up study, IBMS-II, was conducted [14] with the objective to characterize patterns of preventive medication use in persons with migraine; it concluded that persons experiencing a higher frequency of migraine days tried more medications than those with a lower number of MMDs. *My Migraine Voice* adds to the existing literature since it includes a large number of countries, involves people with migraine meeting the ICHD-3 criteria, and assesses migraine burden during premonitory, headache, and postdrome phases of the migraine attack, thereby allowing for a comprehensive and truly global assessment of migraine burden.

Conclusions

This study demonstrates that the burden of migraine is significant and poses several challenges among those with ≥4 MMDs and a history of prophylactic treatment failure. However, despite challenges posed by migraine, only 9% reported receiving disability allowance due to their migraine. Interestingly, the data show that individuals with migraine report some positive aspects in their migraine journey, which relate to developing a positive outlook on personal growth that is likely triggered by learning to cope with the disease. The greater resilience and strength brought on by coping with migraine suggests that if future treatments could address their existing unmet needs, these individuals with migraine will be able to maximize their contribution to society.

Abbreviations

AMPP: American Migraine Prevalence and Prevention; CaMEO: Chronic Migraine Epidemiology and Outcomes; ED: Emergency department; GBD: Global Burden of Disease; GP: General practitioner; IBMS: International Burden of Migraine Study; ICHD-3: International Classification of Headache Disorders 3rd edition; MMD: Monthly migraine day; OBB: Online bulletin board; OTC: Over-the-counter; TF: Treatment failure; WPAI: Work Productivity and Activity Impairment; YLD: Years lived with disability

Acknowledgements

The authors thank Vishwas Agashe from Xcenda for his assistance with medical writing for this manuscript and all study participants for their generous contribution to the *My Migraine Voice* initiative. The authors wish to thank Angela Fiorin and Stephanie Ribbe from Novartis for their assistance with this study.

Funding
This study was sponsored by Novartis Pharma AG; Novartis supported the design of the study, data collection, the data analysis, the manuscript development and submission.

Authors' contributions
Design of the study (all authors): PM, TS, MLM, RQ, VC, H-CD, ERT, AC, AVR, SE, AKL, RF, DW, PD, and PV. Data collection: RQ, VC. Data analysis and interpretation (all authors): PM, TS, MLM, RQ, VC, H-CD, ERT, AC, AVR, SE, AKL, RF, DW, PD, and PV. Manuscript development and review (all authors): PM, TS, MLM, RQ, VC, H-CD, ERT, AC, AVR, SE, AKL, RF, DW, PD, and PV. All authors read and approved the final manuscript.

Competing interests

- Todd Schwedt receives research funding from the National Institutes of Health, the U.S. Department of Defense, the Patient Centered Outcomes Research Institute, the American Migraine Foundation, Arizona State University, and the Mayo Clinic. He serves as a consultant or on advisory boards for Alder, Allergan, Amgen, ATI, Aural Analytics, Avanir, Eli Lilly, the International Concussion Society, Ipsen Bioscience, Nocira, Novartis, Promius Pharma, Second Opinion, Teva. He is on the Board of Directors for the American Headache Society and the International Headache Society.
- Michel Lanteri-Minet receives research funding from the Direction Générale de la Santé, the Agence Nationale de Sécurité des Médicaments, the Société Française de la Douleur, the Fondation Apicil, the Migraine Foundation. He serves as a consultant or on advisory boards for Allergan, Amgen, Astellas, ATI, BMS, Boehringer, Boston Scientific, CoLucid, Convergence, Glaxo-SmithKline, Grunenthal, Lilly, Medtronic, Menarini, MSD, Novartis, Pfizer, ReckittBenckiser, Saint-Jude, Sanofi-Aventis, Teva, UCB, Zambon.
- Rebeca Quintana and Veruska Carboni are employees of GfK Health
- Hans-Christoph Diener received honoraria for participation in clinical rials, contribution to advisory boards or oral presentations from: Addex Pharma, Alder, Allergan, Almirall, Amgen, Autonomic Technology, AstraZeneca, Bayer Vital, Berlin Chemie, Böhringer Ingelheim, Bristol-Myers Squibb, Chordate, Coherex, CoLucid, Electrocore, GlaxoSmithKline, Grünenthal, Ipsen, Janssen-Cilag, Labrys Biologicals, Lilly, La Roche, 3 M Medica, Medtronic, Menerini, Minster, MSD, Neuroscore, Novartis, Johnson & Johnson, Pierre Fabre, Pfizer, Schaper and Brümmer, Sanofi, St. Jude, Teva and Weber & Weber. Financial support for research projects was provided by Allergan, Almirall, AstraZeneca, Bayer, Electrocore, GSK, Janssen-Cilag, MSD and Pfizer. Headache research at the Department of Neurology in Essen is supported by the German Research Council (DFG), the German Ministry of Education and Research (BMBF) and the European Union. H.C. Diener has no ownership interest and does not own stocks of any pharmaceutical company. HCD serves on the editorial boards of Cephalalgia and Lancet Neurology. HCD chairs the Clinical Guidelines Committee of the German Society of Neurology and is member of the Clinical Trials Committee of the IHS.
- Paolo Martelletti received funds for research, education, advisory boards and editorial activity from ACRAF Angelini, Allergan, Amgen, Electrocore, Novartis, Teva, Springer HealthCare, SpringerNature. He received travel reimbursement from SpringerNature, European Medicine Agency and royalties from Springer. He is President of European Headache Federation and serves as Editor-in-Chief of The Journal of Headache and Pain, Section Editor, Medicine of SpringerNature Comprehensive Clinical Medicine, Editorial Board Member of Internal and Emergency Medicine and of International Journal of Environmental Research and Public Health. He has no ownership interest and does not own stocks of any drug company.
- Elena Ruiz de la Torre is President of the European Headache Alliance.
- Audrey Craven is President of the Migraine Association of Ireland
- Annette Vangaa Rasmussen is a member of the Novartis Advisory Board
- Simon Evans is Chief Executive of Migraine Action which receives funding from Allergan, Novartis, RB, electroCore, BHR Pharmaceuticals, MAC Clinical Research, Norville Group
- Donna Walsh is Executive Director of the European Federation of Neurological Associations which receives grants from a consortia of pharmaceutical companies. In 2017, EFNA funding was provided by the following companies: MSD, Merck, Genzyme, Teva, Biogen, UCB, Pfizer, Grunenthal, Janssen, European Academy of Neurology. In a personal capacity, she has been reimbursed for participation on advisory/steering committees organized by Pfizer and Novartis
- Paula K. Dumas is on the Board of the American Migraine Foundation and the Steering Committee of Coalition of Headache and Migraine Patients. She has an equity interest in Migraine Again LLC and Migraine Health Ventures
- Annik K. Laflamme, Rachel Fink, and Pamela Vo are Novartis employees.

Author details
[1]European Headache Federation, Rome, Italy. [2]Department of Clinical and Molecular Medicine, Sapienza University of Rome, Rome, Italy. [3]Department of Neurology, Mayo Clinic, 5777 East Mayo Boulevard, Phoenix, AZ 85054, USA. [4]Département d'Evaluation et Traitement de la Douleur CHU Nice, FHU InovPain, Université Côte Azur, Nice, France. [5]GfK EMER, Madrid, Spain. [6]IPSOS Switzerland (formerly GfK Health), Basel, Switzerland. [7]Department of Neurology and Headache Center, University of Duisburg-Essen, Duisburg, Germany. [8]European Migraine and Headache Alliance (EMHA), Brussels, Belgium. [9]Migraine Association of Ireland (MAI), Dublin, Ireland. [10]Danish Headache Center, Rigshospitalet Glostrup, Copenhagen, Denmark. [11]Migraine Action, Leicester, UK. [12]Novartis Pharma AG, Basel, Switzerland. [13]European Federation of Neurological Associations, Brussels, Belgium. [14]Migraine Again, Irvine, USA.

References

1. Vos T, Allen C, Arora M, Barber RM, Bhutta ZA, Brown A et al (2016) Global, regional, and national incidence, prevalence, and years lived with disability for 310 diseases and injuries, 1990–2015: a systematic analysis for the global burden of disease study 2015. Lancet 388:1545–1602
2. World Health Organization. Headache disorders. Fact sheet N°277. 2016. http://www.who.int/mediacentre/factsheets/fs277/en/. Accessed 01 Oct 2018
3. Steiner TJ, Sovner LJ, Vos T, Jensen R, Katsarava Z (2018) Migraine is first cause of disability in under 50s: will health politicians now take notice? J Headache Pain 19:17
4. Buse DC, Manack AN, Fanning KM et al (2012) Chronic migraine prevalence, disability, and sociodemographic factors: results from the American migraine prevalence and prevention study. Headache 52(10):1456–1470
5. Payne KA, Varon SF, Kawata AK et al (2011) The international burden of migraine study (IBMS): study design, methodology, and baseline cohort characteristics. Cephalalgia 31(10):1116–1130
6. Bloudek LM, Stokes M, Buse DC et al (2012) Cost of healthcare for patients with migraine in five European countries: results from the international burden of migraine study (IBMS). J Headache Pain. 13:361–378
7. Blumenfeld A, Varon SF, Wilcox TK et al (2011) 2011. Disability, HRQoL and resource use among chronic and episodic migraineurs: results from the international burden of migraine study. Cephalalgia 31(3):301–305
8. Adams AM, Serrano D, Buse DC et al (2015) The impact of chronic migraine: the chronic migraine epidemiology and outcomes (CaMEO) study methods and baseline results. Cephalalgia 35(7):563–578
9. Andrée C, Stovner LJ, Steiner TJ et al (2011) The Eurolight project: the impact of primary headache disorders in Europe. Description of methods. J Headache Pain 12:541–549
10. GBD 2015 Disease and Injury Incidence and Prevalence Collaborators (2016) Global, regional, and national incidence, prevalence, and years lived with disability for 310 diseases and injuries, 1990–2015: a systematic analysis for the Global Burden of Disease Study 2015. Lancet 388:1545–1602
11. Ruiz de la Torre E, Martelletti P, Craven A et al (2017) Real-world patient perspective on the burden and impact of migraine. Presented at: Congress of the International Headache Society, Vancouver; September 7–10, [Poster #PO-02-184]
12. Ruiz de la Torre E, Martelletti P, Craven A et al (2017) Burden and impact of migraine: a caregiver's perspective. Presented at: Congress of the International Headache Society, Vancouver September 7–10, [Poster #PO-02-185]

18

Habituation of laser-evoked potentials by migraine phase

Martin Uglem[1,4*], Petter Moe Omland[1,2], Marit Stjern[1,2], Gøril Bruvik Gravdahl[3] and Trond Sand[1,2]

Abstract

Background: Migraineurs seem to have cyclic variations in cortical excitability in several neurophysiological modalities. Laser-evoked potentials (LEP) are of particular interest in migraine because LEP specifically targets pain pathways, and studies have reported different LEP-changes both between and during headaches. Our primary aim was to explore potential cyclic variations in LEP amplitude and habituation in more detail with a blinded longitudinal study design.

Methods: We compared N1 and N2P2 amplitudes and habituation between two blocks of laser stimulations to the dorsal hand, obtained from 49 migraineurs with four sessions each. We used migraine diaries to categorize sessions as interictal (> one day from previous and to next attack), preictal (< one day before the attack), ictal or postictal (< one day after the attack). Also, we compared 29 interictal recordings from the first session to 30 controls.

Results: N1 and N2P2 amplitudes and habituation did not differ between preictal, interictal and postictal phase sessions, except for a post hoc contrast that showed deficient ictal habituation of N1. Habituation is present and similar in migraineurs in the interictal phase and controls.

Conclusions: Hand-evoked LEP amplitudes and habituation were mainly invariable between migraine phases, but this matter needs further study. Because hand-evoked LEP-habituation was similar in migraineurs and controls, the present findings contradict several previous LEP studies. Pain-evoked cerebral responses are normal and show normal habituation in migraine.

Keywords: Headache, Migraine cycle, Pain, Pathophysiology, Preictal, Ictal, Premonitory, Laser evoked potential, Habituation, LEP

Background

Migraine is a cyclic disorder as evidenced by subjective symptoms and imaging and neurophysiological studies [1–7]. Therefore, it is preferable to investigate migraine physiology repeatedly during the different phases, i.e., between, before, during and after attacks (interictal, preictal, ictal and postictal phase, respectively) [8, 9].

Laser-evoked potentials (LEP) are well suited to study the cortical response to noxious input since brief laser pulses mainly evoke cortical responses with a latency corresponding to the conduction velocity of Aδ fibers [10–14]. Aδ fiber activation yields a middle-latency component over the contralateral temporal lobe (N1) and a late biphasic vertex response (N2P2). The operculo-insular cortex and possibly the primary somatosensory cortex largely contributes to N1 [11, 15, 16], while the anterior cingulate cortex contributes to N2P2 [11]. Hence, LEP may reflect both pain-specific activation of the primary sensory cortex and cognitive and inhibitory "top-down control" aspects of pain physiology in migraine.

LEPs in migraineurs have mainly been studied by an Italian collaboration [17–24]. The results are not entirely coherent, but deficient N2P2-habituation has been observed in the interictal phase [17–19, 21, 22], a deficit that seems to persist during attacks [21]. Deficient LEP-

* Correspondence: martin.uglem@ntnu.no; https://www.ntnu.edu/inb
[1]Department of Neuromedicine and Movement Science, NTNU, Norwegian University of Science and Technology, Trondheim, Norway
[4]NTNU, Faculty of Medicine and Health Sciences, P.B. 8905, N-7491 Trondheim, Norway
Full list of author information is available at the end of the article

habituation has also been observed in painful radiculopathy [25], fibromyalgia [26] and cardiac syndrome X [27]. The apparently reduced LEP-habituation in migraineurs do not differ systematically between stimulation sites [17, 18, 20–22], and whether the N1 or N2P2-potential are best suited to demonstrate an alteration is not clear [17, 20]. Accordingly, these results for LEP N2P2 should be independently confirmed [28]. N1-habituation should also be studied further in migraine as only two studies have recorded this early LEP-component [17, 20].

LEPs or other pain evoked potentials have, as far as we know, not been investigated previously in the preictal or postictal phases. In the interictal phase, lack of habituation of the nociceptive blink reflex and pain scores to repeated noxious stimuli has been shown [29, 30], with a tendency towards normalization during the migraine attack [30, 31]. However, several studies have measured evoked responses to repeated non-nociceptive stimuli in migraineurs. The results are conflicting regarding visual evoked potentials (VEP) as some studies show reduced habituation in migraineurs between attacks while others do not [9, 32, 33]. Most migraine-studies of evoked potentials habituation have focused on the interictal phase, but some have also investigated cyclic changes. One such study showed normal habituation of the standard blink reflex interictally and decreased habituation in the preictal phase [34]. However, several studies have shown an opposite effect with deficient habituation of VEP, visual evoked magnetic fields, somatosensory evoked potentials, and contingent negative variation between attacks that normalizes right before or during the attack [35–44]. One study has shown increasing loss of habituation of VEP during the interictal interval with a normalization within the migraine attack [45], while other longitudinal studies did not find VEP or brainstem auditory-evoked potential habituation differences related to the migraine cycle [4, 5]. It is accordingly of interest to extend the knowledge about general phase-related neurophysiological changes in migraine to the cortical pain-processing network.

The primary aim of the present blinded longitudinal study was to investigate generalized "third order neuron" pain network excitability in migraineurs by LEP amplitude and habituation during different stages of the migraine cycle. We examined 50 migraineurs four times to investigate intraindividual changes at both the interictal, preictal, ictal and postictal phases. We test the main working hypothesis that LEP amplitude and habituation, and subjective pain scores to laser stimulation, differs between phases. The secondary aims were to confirm previously reported deficient LEP habituation in migraineurs in the interictal phase compared to controls, and to test the effect of aura, headache laterality, years lived with migraine, and subjective pain scores on habituation and habituation-differences between phases.

Methods

We measured LEPs and pain scores once a week for four weeks in migraineurs (mean ± SD: 6.7 ± 1.9 days between sessions) in the second half of 2012. The four sessions in one migraineur were at the same time each day for almost all subjects, but for a few subjects, it was necessary to reschedule one or two sessions. Mean variation between the latest and the earliest of the four sessions were 23 ± 28 min, and the variation was no more than an hour in 41 of 49 subjects. At most, one subject had to postpone two sessions by 3.5 h. The migraineurs completed a headache diary for four weeks before, during and four weeks after the examinations to determine how the examinations were related to the migraine attacks (i.e., interictal, preictal, ictal or postictal). We measured LEPs and pain scores once in headache-free controls. Investigators were blinded to diagnosis on subjects' first visit and migraine phase on the subsequent visits. Co-workers performed the inclusion and follow-up, and participating subjects were specifically told not to reveal their diagnosis to the investigators.

Subjects

Seventy-four migraineurs and 40 controls responded to an advertisement in the local newspaper, on the local hospital's web page [46] and the Intranet within our university [47]. We screened both groups over telephone and migraineurs were evaluated by neurologists per the ICHD-II criteria for migraine with or without aura [48]. Controls could not have a headache more than once a month. If they occasionally had a headache, we asked if they had consulted a physician regarding the headache, if they experienced the headache as painful and if they used abortive medication for their headache. We excluded controls if they confirmed more than one of these three questions. Included migraineurs had an attack frequency between two and six per month and had no more than ten days with migraine attacks per month. They could use symptomatic, but not prophylactic migraine treatment. Exclusion criteria were: coexisting tension-type headache seven days or more per week in migraineurs, neurological or psychiatric diseases, sleep disorders, active infectious diseases, connective tissue diseases, metabolic, endocrine or neuromuscular diseases, other clinically relevant painful conditions including recent injuries, malignancy, previous craniotomy or cervical spine surgery, heart disease, cardiopulmonary or cerebrovascular diseases, pregnancy, medication for acute or chronic pain, antipsychotics, antidepressants, anticonvulsants or other drugs that may influence neuronal, vascular or muscular function, substance abuse, ferromagnetic implants and prophylactic allergy treatment.

Fifty migraineurs and 31 controls participated in the study. One migraineur withdrew consent after the first examination and was not included in the analysis. Three migraineurs attended only once, twice and three out of four times respectively. We excluded one control because we were unable to obtain reliable LEPs as most trials were rejected. Thus, 49 migraineurs completed a total of 190 examinations, and 30 controls completed one examination each. Table 1 shows demographic and clinical data. We report details of exclusions and dropouts in Additional file 1: Table S1.

The Regional Committees for Medical and Health Research Ethics approved the protocol, and all subjects gave their written informed consent. Migraineurs and controls received an equivalent of $ 125 and $ 30 respectively to cover expenses.

Procedure

Painful heat stimuli were generated by a pulsed solid-state (Nd:YAP) laser (STIMUL 1340, DEKA M.E.L.A. SRL, Calenzano (FI), Italy) with a wavelength of 1340 nm. The laser stimulator settings were the same as in a previous study at our lab [49]: The pulse duration was 6 ms, a relatively short stimulus duration to maximize the N1-amplitude [50]. We set the laser beam diameter to 8 mm (area ≈ 50 mm^2) with an energy ranging from 2 to 6.5 J (4.0–12.9 J/cm^2). The diameter and durations are comparable to other researchers using the same type of laser [51, 52]. A diode laser aiming beam visualized the stimulation site. We recorded LEPs with a Viking Select system (Nicolet Biomedical Inc., Madison, WI, USA). The recording silver disc electrodes were placed at the Fz, Cz, Pz, T3, T4, A1 and A2 sites of the 10–20 system. The impedance was kept below 5 kΩ. The two most important analysis channels, Cz referred to the nose, and T3 referred to Fz, were preselected as recommended by the international IFCN-guidelines [53]. We used the other channels as back up to account for interindividual variation in field topography and to improve detectability of waves. For control of artifacts, we monitored the electrooculogram from a left infraorbital electrode referred to T4. The onset of stimuli triggered the recording system. The sampling rate was 1000 Hz, the sweep time was 750 ms and the filter setting was 0.2–100 Hz. Rejection level was set to ±225 μV, and total rejection rate after exclusions was 3 %. We applied online averaging [49, 54] since rejection effectively canceled artifacts and eye movements also were included in a separate channel.

Subjects lay comfortably on an examination table with laser safety glasses and acoustic earmuffs to avoid any acoustical interference at the time of stimulation [53, 55]. We delivered laser stimuli to the dorsum of the right hand between the carpal bones, metacarpophalangeal joints and second and fourth metacarpal bone. The laser beam was moved randomly within this area to avoid skin lesions and nociceptor fatigue or sensitization [56]. We measured skin temperature before the test. Because we previously observed that the recommend fixed intensity (equal to twice the mean pin-prick threshold [12]) did not always elicit pain and LEP in every healthy subject [49], we used stimulus intensities based on *intraindividual* thresholds [51, 57, 58]. First, the individual thresholds for pinprick pain were identified, starting at 2 J and increasing with 0.5 J steps [49]. The subject had to differentiate between burning pain and pinprick pain. Subjects scored pinprick pain on a verbal, numerical rating scale (NRS) with range 0 = "no pain" to 10 = "unbearable pain." We measured the threshold twice, and we defined the pinprick threshold as

Table 1 Demographic and clinical data after exclusions

	Migraineurs (n = 49)	Controls (n = 30)
Age	40 ± 10 [19–62]	38 ± 11 [21–59]
BMI	26 ± 3	25 ± 3
Women	*41* (84%)	*25* (83%)
Days since 1st day of last menstruation	17 ± 12	19 ± 10
MwoA, MA + MwoA, MA	*27* (55%), *18* (37%), *4* (8%)	NA
Years with headache	21 ± 9 [1–40]	NA
Migraine days/month[a]	1:*14*, 2:*30*, 3:*5*, 4:*0*	NA
Migraine intensity[b]	1:*2*, 2:*20*, 3:*27*, 4:*0*	NA
Headache duration[c]	16 ± 21 [0.5–72]	NA
Energy level (J) used in LEP test	4.3 ± 0.5	4.4 ± 0.4
Thresholds (J) for pinprick pain	3.7 ± 0.6	3.7 ± 0.7

[a]Migraine days/month: 0: < 1/month, 1: 1–3/month, 2: 4–7/month, 3: 8–14/month, 4: > 14/month
[b]Migraine intensity: 1: Mild, 2: Moderate, 3: Severe, 4: Extreme
[c]Average duration (hours) of an attack with or without use of symptomatic medication
Data displayed as mean ± SD [range] or n (%). MwoA: migraine without aura. MA + MwoA: some attacks with and some without aura (both diagnoses according to ICHD-3 Beta [88]. MA: migraine with aura (in 100% of attacks). NA: not applicable

the lowest intensity inducing pain in at least one of the two trials at that intensity. A tolerable intensity was 4.5 J (9.0 J/cm^2), in most subjects, corresponding to about two times the pinprick threshold. However, 4.5 J generated too much pain in 22 subjects, and too little pain in five subjects and the energy had to be adjusted up or down (range: 3–5.5 J ≈ 6.0–10.9 J/cm^2). The chosen intensity did generally elicit reliable N2P2 potentials [59]. We recorded two blocks of 21 stimulations with six to ten seconds between each stimulation since six seconds was recommended as the minimum interval to avoid peripheral nociceptor habituation [53]. The between-block interval was also short, between 6 and 10 s, to prevent recovery of central habituation. Subjects kept their eyes open and rated perceived pain verbally (NRS 0–10) after each stimulation to prevent LEP-amplitude decrease by distraction and drowsiness [12, 60, 61]. We stored pain scores for analysis. We used identical energy levels for all sessions within subjects. However, we did not tell participants that the energy was constant.

Data analysis and statistics

Examinations were classified by the headache diary as interictal (more than one day before attack onset or one day after the attack ended), preictal (less than one day before attack onset), ictal (a migraine headache during the examination) and postictal (less than one day after the attack ended). We applied this definition in previous studies of pain physiology related to migraine phase [6, 62]. Eleven of the 190 examinations were unclassifiable and excluded from data analysis, mainly because they had migraines both the day before and the day after examination.

We analyzed in LabChart® (Version 7 pro, ADInstruments, Dunedin, New Zealand). A random number identified each LEP session and we randomized the order of the two blocks within each session. Thus, the investigator who analyzed the LEPs was blinded to diagnosis, migraine phase and order of the two blocks. The N1 and the N2P2 components were assessed, N1 at the contralateral temporal electrode (T3) against Fz (best bipolar derivation to show N1 [63]) and N2P2 at Cz against nose [53]. We measured the N1-amplitude from baseline (start of N1) to the N1 peak and the N2P2-amplitude from the most negative to the most positive peak. We had to discard some LEPs due to unrecognizable responses, too much noise/artifacts or latencies far from normal values [53]. The N1-amplitude may have a low signal-to-noise ratio, and it was not detectable in 15% of LEPs in migraineurs and 22% of LEPs in controls. These responses were included in the analysis as interval censored responses [64, 65] by setting the lower bound to zero and the upper bound to the maximal negative noise peak within the N1-time window. The exact N1-amplitude was then unknown, but we presumed that it was between zero and the largest noise peak, and we included the amplitude as an interval, a rough estimate, instead of a point estimate. We discarded recordings with technical errors, 17 of 358 in total in migraineurs. We present the grand average of all recordings by phase (Fig. 1) and by group (Fig. 2).

We analyzed data with STATA version 13.1 (StataCorp LP). We applied separate multilevel models [66] for the response variables N1, N2P2 and pain scores. The first set compared the within-subject change in migraineurs and the second set compared interictal recordings from the first exam and controls. The interaction effects were the main outcomes. For the first set, interactions-of-interest reflect differences between phases. For the second set, interactions-of-interest reflect differences between migraine and healthy subjects. We have included full model specifications in the Additional file 1.

We added explorative post hoc contrasts that tested if the slopes (i.e., habituation) at each phase, and in all phases combined, were different from zero. Also, based on the main results, we performed data-driven explorative post hoc contrasts comparing the first-block amplitudes and habituation slope of N1 between the preictal and ictal phases. We used diagnosis as a fixed factor to compare migraineurs in the interictal phase and controls. Only interictal recordings from the first exam were compared to controls because the investigator was blinded to diagnosis only on the first session, and to avoid possible long-term habituation/sensitization effects in subsequent exams. N1 and N2P2 in both sets were square rooted to improve normality.

We analyzed phase and group differences in pain scores with pain scores from both blocks combined consecutively into one continuous time variable which was interacted with phase or group, respectively. The time variable was centered at its mean and divided by 10. Thus, the regression constant shows the average pain score and the habituation coefficient the change in pain score per ten stimulations. We tested group differences in pain thresholds and laser intensity with independent samples Student's t-test and present results as 95% confidence intervals (CI). Thus we consider intervals not containing zero to be significant at a level of $p < 0.05$. We have back transformed the data and tabulate result-parameters in the original scale. However, results are presented as transformed units in the Additional file 1.

We extended the original models to test the effect of additional variables. We specified four separate models that estimated the phase-differences in habituation for 1) migraineurs with and without aura, 2) sessions differentiated by headache laterality, 3) by years lived with migraine, and 4) by pain scores. Headache laterality was classified by the related attack if the phase was preictal, ictal or postictal. Interictal recordings were classified by

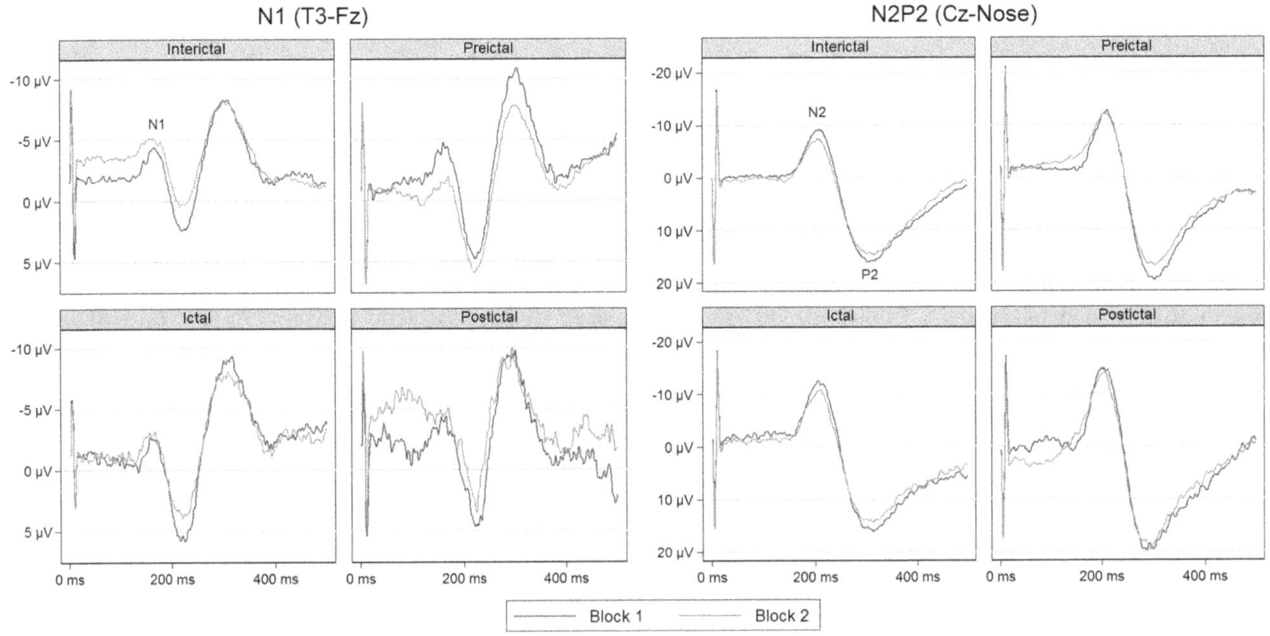

Fig. 1 Grand average of the LEP-traces by phase. Habituation was present in all phases at both LEP-components but ictal and postictal N1, and postictal N2P2. The amplitudes in the figures are smaller than those presented in Table 2 due to slightly different LEP-latencies between participants

the side the subject most commonly experienced headache, either left, right or bilateral. Sixteen interictal recordings had an equal amount of left and right-sided unilateral migraine and were not included in the laterality-analysis. We included age, migraine intensity, and migraine frequency as control variables (not included in the interactions) in the extended model 3 that estimated the effect of years lived with migraine.

We conducted three additional analyses to explore the relationship between habituation and number of days to next attack. We conducted these analyses in two steps, first with interictal phase only and then with both interictal and preictal phases included. We interpret the interaction effects in the latter analyses as the interictal-preictal day-to-day change in habituation towards the next migraine attack. Also, we performed a secondary set of analyses with a three-day limit to test if postictal phase-related LEP-changes last longer than 24 h after the attack.

With 30 controls and 50 migraineurs, the statistical power to detect a low medium-sized effect equal to 0.65 SD [67] based on a two-sample Student's t-test is 80%. As we estimated to have approximately 20 pairs for intraindividual phase-related comparisons, power (based on paired Student's t-tests) to detect a similar medium-sized effect (0.65 SD) was calculated to 83%.

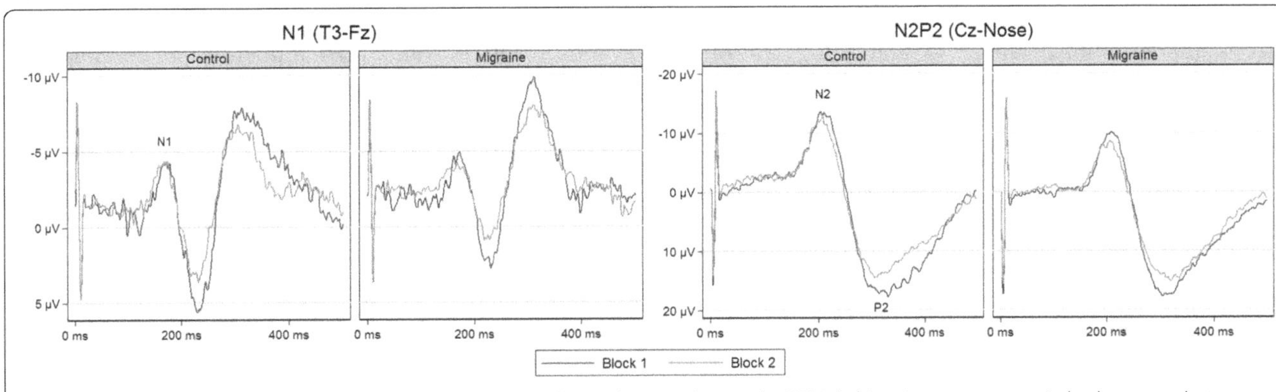

Fig. 2 Grand average of the LEP-traces in first session interictal recordings and controls. N2P2-habituation was present in both groups, but we found no significant N1-habituation. The amplitudes in the figures are smaller than those presented in Table 4 due to slightly different LEP-latencies between participants

Results

Analyses by phase

Table 2 shows means and standard deviations of N1 and N2P2-amplitudes, and pain scores by phase.

N1-habituation was significant in the interictal phase as shown by the negative coefficient of block (Fig. 3 and Table 3). The degree of habituation was not different between the interictal phase and the preictal, ictal and postictal phases respectively (interaction effects in Table 3). However, post hoc contrasts showed significant habituation in the preictal phase (95% CI [−2.71, −0.33] μV/block), but not in the ictal and postictal phases (95% CI [−1.29, 0.57] and [−3.44, 0.00] μV/block, respectively). The habituation in all phases combined was significant (95% CI [−1.40, −0.38] μV/block). The contrast of the difference in habituation between the preictal and ictal phase was not significant (95% CI [−0.54, 2.86] μV/block). Neither the first-block amplitudes nor the combined first and second-block amplitudes differed between phases, but the post hoc contrast that compared first-block amplitudes between the preictal and ictal phases showed a tendency towards lower first-block amplitudes in the ictal phase (95% CI [−3.20, 0.04] μV).

The N2P2-amplitude change from the first to the second block was significant in the interictal phase, and none of the interactions were significant (Fig. 3 and Table 3), interpreted as interictal habituation with no differences between phases. Post-hoc contrasts showed significant habituation in both the preictal and ictal phases (95% CI [−6.66, −1.58] and [−7.38, −0.77] μV/block, respectively), but not in the postictal phase (95% CI [−7.01, 1.22] μV/block). The habituation in all phases combined was significant (95% CI [−4.90, −2.55] μV/block). N2P2-amplitude sizes did not differ between phases.

Pain scores increased linearly in the interictal phase (95% CI [0.11, 0.33] NRS-change/10 stimuli, Table 3). The linear increase, i.e., sensitization of pain scores, was not different between phases. Mean pain scores did not differ between phases.

We present complete results from the secondary analyses in the Additional file 1. N1 and N2P2 first-block amplitudes and habituation did not differ between migraineurs with and without aura as none of the three-way or two-way interactions were significant. Amplitudes and habituation did not differ between a left and right-sided migraine. Subjects with a bilateral migraine had reduced N2P2-habituation (more positive slope) in the postictal phase compared to the interictal phase (95% CI [0.07, 25.3] μV/block), and the same tendency was present in the ictal phase (95% CI [−0.01, 19.8] μV/block). The more years lived with migraine; the less was the N2P2-habituation in the preictal phase compared to the interictal phase (95% CI [0.11, 0.82] μV/block/year adjusted for age). No other interaction effects were significant.

Both N1 and N2P2 interictal first-block amplitudes correlated with pain scores (95% CI [0.08, 0.93] and [1.74, 3.65] μV/unit pain score for N1 and N2P2, respectively). The interactions between phase and pain score were not significant, that is, the correlations were not different between phases. Habituation of N1 and N2P2-amplitudes did not correlate with a change in pain scores from the first to the second block.

The analyses that explored the relationship between habituation and number of days to next attack showed no significant interactions. Thus, there was no interictal day-to-day linear change in habituation towards the next migraine attack. Changing the definition of the postictal phase from a one-day limit to a three-day limit did not alter the interpretation of LEP-habituation. Habituation of pain scores did not change by changing the definitions of the phases, although the mean pain score was significantly increased in the postictal compared to the interictal phase (95% CI [0.11, 1.28] unit pain score).

Analyses by diagnosis

Table 4 shows means and standard deviations of N1 and N2P2-amplitudes, and pain scores by group.

Controls did not show habituation of the N1 amplitude, and habituation did not differ between migraineurs and controls (Fig. 4 and Table 5). Post-hoc contrasts showed no habituation in the groups combined (95% CI [−1.32, 0.30] μV) and no habituation in the migraine group (95% CI [−1.77, 0.49] μV). Neither the first-block

Table 2 N1 and N2P2-amplitudes, and pain scores by phase and block

			N1 (μV)		N2P2 (μV)		Pain scores	
	N	*n*	Block 1	Block 2	Block 1	Block 2	Block 1	Block 2
Interictal	44	99	6.6 (3.5)	5.9 (2.6)	40.2 (16.6)	35.2 (13.8)	4.2 (1.9)	4.3 (2.0)
Preictal	26	36	7.9 (5.0)	6.3 (3.6)	42.3 (13.4)	37.3 (11.2)	4.1 (1.9)	4.4 (2.0)
Ictal	19	21	5.7 (2.2)	5.0 (2.2)	39.6 (12.8)	34.6 (10.1)	4.4 (1.7)	4.7 (1.9)
Postictal	13	15	6.8 (3.0)	4.9 (3.7)	45.7 (13.7)	43.2 (12.5)	5.4 (2.6)	5.7 (2.7)

Mean (SD) N1 and N2P2-amplitudes, and pain scores. The means were calculated in two steps; first, phase-specific means for each subject (most subjects had two or more measurements classified within the same phase), before phase-specific means in all subjects combined. Because some N1-amplitudes were interval censored, i.e., defined only by a minimum and maximum with the actual value somewhere in between, the interval midpoints were used as approximate estimates to calculate the means. *N:* number of subjects with at least one recording at the respective phase. *n*: total number of recordings at the respective phase

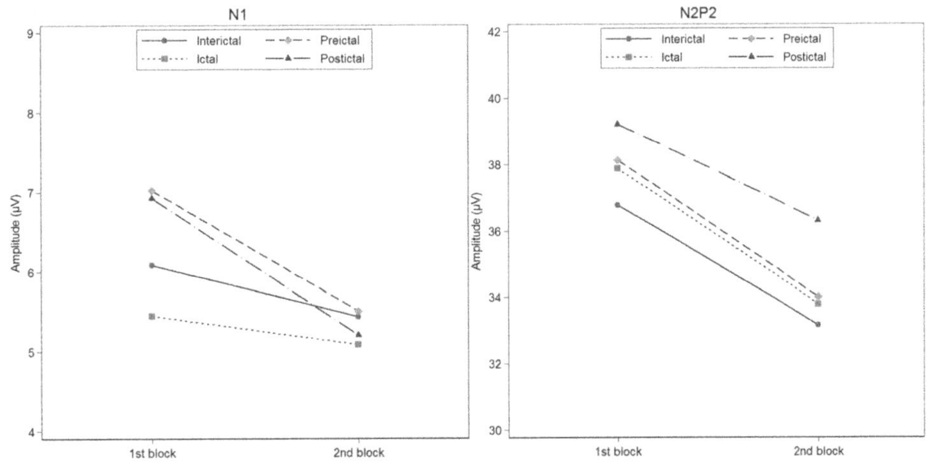

Fig. 3 Estimates of N1 (left) and N2P2-amplitude (right) habituation by phase

amplitudes nor the combined first and second-block amplitudes differed between migraineurs and controls.

The N2P2-amplitude decreased from the first to the second block in controls, and the decrease was not different between controls and migraineurs (Fig. 4 and Table 5). Post-hoc contrasts confirmed a significant habituation in migraineurs (95% CI [−8.07, −2.48] µV). Overall amplitudes were not different between groups (95% CI [−9.87, 5.11] µV).

The linear change in pain scores was not significantly different from zero in controls (95% CI [−0.06, 0.27] NRS-change/10 stimuli) and did not differ between migraineurs and controls (95% CI [−0.09, 0.35] NRS-change/10 stimuli, Table 5). Pain thresholds and stimulation intensities were not different between groups (Student's t-test 95% CI [−0.37, 0.34] and [−0.04, 0.44], respectively).

Discussion

As far as we know, this is the first study to measure cyclic changes of LEP N1-habituation in migraine. Our results show habituation of both N1 and N2P2 amplitudes in all phases combined. In line with the overall responses, both interictal and preictal N1 and N2P2 habituated. Habituation of N2P2 was present in the ictal phase as well. The deficient ictal habituation of N1 was only present in the post hoc contrasts, not in the main analysis, and the number of ictal recordings was relatively small (n = 21). Thus, we interpret the finding of

Table 3 Estimated magnitudes and habituation of N1, N2P2 and pain scores by phase

	N1 (µV)		N2P2 (µV)		Pain scores	
	Coef.	95% CI	Coef.	95% CI	Coef.	95% CI
Main effects						
Preictal	0.939	[−0.476, 2.353]	1.342	[−1.993, 4.677]	−0.01	[−0.36, 0.34]
Ictal	−0.641	[−1.753, 0.470]	1.088	[−2.862, 5.039]	0.23	[−0.28, 0.74]
Postictal	0.839	[−0.487, 2.166]	2.426	[−2.419, 7.272]	0.37	[−0.35, 1.10]
Habituation	−0.653*	[−1.315, −0.001]	−3.623***	[−5.147, −2.098]	0.21***	[0.09, 0.33]
Interaction effects						
Preictal × Habituation	−0.868	[−2.283, 0.547]	−0.497	[−3.445, 2.451]	0.07	[−0.10, 0.24]
Ictal × Habituation	0.293	[−0.746, 1.331]	−0.455	[−4.086, 3.176]	0.06	[−0.18, 0.31]
Postictal × Habituation	−1.070	[−2.890, 0.749]	0.726	[−3.657, 5.108]	0.12	[−0.17, 0.41]
Constant	6.088	[5.186, 6.989]	36.783	[33.002, 40.565]	4.11	[3.56, 4.67]

The constant represents interictal first-block or mean pain score responses, the first three main effects are first-block amplitude or pain score differences from the interictal phase and the fourth "Habituation" main effect is the difference between first and second block, or the linear change of pain scores, in the interictal phase. The interaction effects represent habituation differences between the interictal phase and the preictal, ictal and postictal phases, respectively. Thus, the significant coefficients are interpreted as decreased second-block N1 and N2P2-amplitudes, and linear increase in pain scores, in the interictal phase, i.e. interictal N1 and N2P2 habituation and subjective pain sensitization. Lack of significant interaction effects are interpreted as no habituation differences between the interictal phase and the other phases. Random effects estimates are shown in Supplementary Table 2. * $p < 0.05$, ** $p < 0.01$, *** $p < 0.001$

Table 4 N1 and N2P2-amplitudes, and pain scores in migraineurs in the interictal phase and controls

		N1 (μV)		N2P2 (μV)		Pain scores	
	N	Block 1	Block 2	Block 1	Block 2	Block 1	Block 2
Migraineur	29	7.0 (4.0)	6.1 (3.1)	38.7 (17.5)	33.5 (14.5)	4.2 (2.0)	4.1 (2.3)
Control	30	8.5 (8.6)	7.8 (7.5)	41.1 (16.9)	35.2 (15.3)	3.6 (1.6)	3.5 (1.6)

Mean (SD) N1 and N2P2-amplitudes, and pain scores. The migraine group consists of interictal recordings from the first session. The means and SD of N1-amplitudes are calculated with the interval midpoints of interval censored responses. *N*: number of subjects with a recording of at least one block

deficient ictal N1 habituation with caution, and we believe that it needs to be replicated.

It has been suggested that lack of habituation and normal or slightly decreased first-block amplitudes are functional properties of migraine between attacks [33]. These properties seem to normalize during the attack, at least for non-noxious evoked potentials [9]. The reduced habituation may be due to thalamocortical "dysrhythmia" [9], as suggested by both high-frequency [68] and low-frequency oscillations [69]. This proposed dysrhythmia may reduce thalamic control of the sensory cortices and render the pre-activation level low [33]. Thalamocortical dysrhythmia has been suggested in several diseases, e.g., tinnitus [70], neuropsychiatric disorders [71, 72] and chronic pain [73, 74]. However, in the present study, we found normal interictal LEP-habituation, although we observed deficient habituation and a tendency towards lower first-block amplitude of N1 during attacks, i.e., no tendency towards "normalization." Our present findings do not support the concept of a generally reduced interictal habituation in migraine.

On the other hand, the discrepancy between a preserved ictal N2P2-habituation, as opposed to a subtle deficient N1-habituation, suggests a centrally mediated ictal alteration [75]. The N1-component likely reflects the sensory-discriminative component of pain whereas the N2P2-component reflects the motivational and cognitive component of pain [59]. Thus, migraine pain seems to primarily affect sensory processes rather than cognitive, in contrast to the effects of sleep deprivation shown in one study [76].

In the present study, we could not reproduce altered N2P2-habituation or amplitude during attacks. This result contradicts the findings of other smaller studies. One study has shown reduced hand and face N2P2-habituation in interictal recordings (n = 14) compared to controls (n = 10) and a similar habituation deficit during attacks (n = 8) [21]. Two studies (n = 10 and 18) have demonstrated an increased N2P2-amplitude during compared to between attacks [23, 24]. Two of the studies included subjects with mean migraine frequency close to chronic migraine (we had none), and this could have contributed to the discrepancy between their and our results [21, 24].

The post hoc contrasts showing a lack of habituation of both N1 and N2P2-amplitudes in the postictal phase should be interpreted with caution as the number of postictal measurements were lower than for the other phases. Accordingly, this negative finding may be a result of rather low statistical power. Importantly, the main analyses showed no significant differences between habituation slopes, and Fig. 3 indicates that habituation is present in the postictal phase as well.

Pain scores increased linearly throughout the stimulation, in contrast to the decrease in N1 and N2P2-amplitudes. However, the negative correlations between

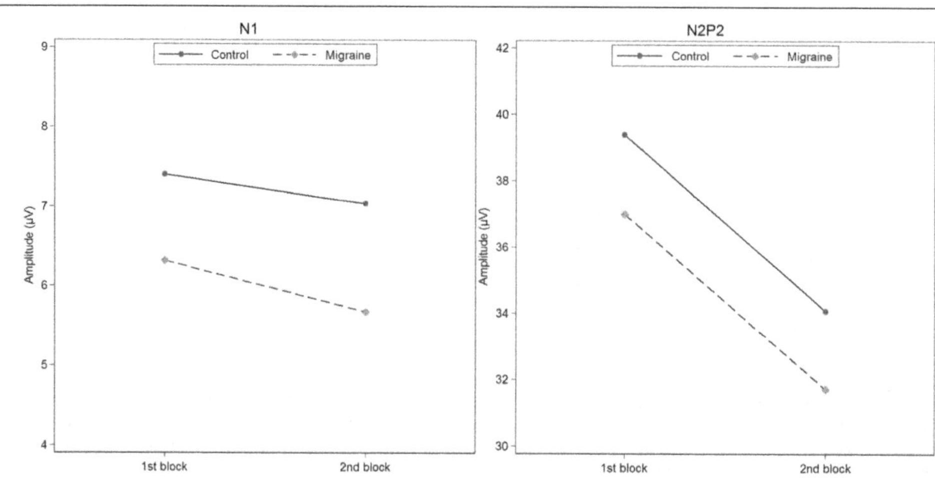

Fig. 4 Estimates of N1 (left) and N2P2-amplitude (right) habituation in interictal recordings and controls

Table 5 Estimated magnitudes and habituation in migraineurs in the interictal phase and controls

	N1 (μV)		N2P2 (μV)		Pain scores	
	Coef.	95% CI	Coef.	95% CI	Coef.	95% CI
Main effects						
Migraine	−1.014	[−3.767, 1.739]	−2.395	[−10.707, 5.917]	0.60	[−0.32, 1.52]
Habituation	−0.374	[−1.527, 0.778]	−5.307***	[−9.232, −1.383]	0.10	[−0.06, 0.26]
Interaction effect						
Migraine × Habituation	−0.268	[−1.875, 1.339]	−0.036	[−4.781, 4.854]	0.13	[−0.09, 0.35]
Constant	7.365	[5.070, 9.660]	39.382	[33.531, 45.234]	3.54	[3.01, 4.07]

The constant represents first-block amplitude or pain score responses in controls. The main effect of migraine represents the first-block amplitude or pain score difference between groups. The main effect of habituation represents the difference between first and second block amplitudes, or linear change in pain scores, in the control group. The interaction effect represents the habituation-difference between groups. Thus, the significant coefficient is interpreted as N2P2 habituation in the control group. The corresponding interaction effect is not significant, indicating no difference in habituation between controls and migraineurs in the interictal phase. Random effects estimates are shown in Supplementary Table 3. * $p < 0.05$, ** $p < 0.01$, *** $p < 0.001$

pain score and amplitudes were not significant. Mean pain scores and linear change of pain scores were not different between phases. Previous studies have shown reduced laser-pain thresholds during the attack [23, 24], and one study has shown increased pain scores during compared to between attacks by stimulation on both sides of the face but not the hands [21].

Habituation did not differ between migraineurs with and without aura. This finding cannot be compared to previous studies of LEP-habituation as they only included migraineurs without aura [17–22]. The positive correlation between pain scores and LEP amplitudes fits with earlier migraine studies [18–21, 24]. Interestingly, subjects with a bilateral headache had deficient postictal habituation compared to lateralized headache. We speculate if bilaterality represents excessive headache load, but a similar habituation deficiency was not observed for the load-parameter "years lived with migraine" (controlled for age, intensity, and frequency). However, *preictal* habituation was less pronounced in subjects with more migraine-years. Thus, there is some evidence of subtle changes of habituation by clinical features in proximity to attack, but the subgroups are small (e.g., only ten interictal and seven postictal sessions were associated with a bilateral headache), and the analyses many, hence it may be a random type 1 error.

Migraineurs in the interictal phase and controls showed no group differences. The amplitudes and pain scores were similar, and both groups had no significant N1-habituation but significant N2P2-habituation, and no linear change in pain scores. These findings are in contrast with some of the previously published results. The group differences in amplitude have varied considerably between studies. Group differences in N1 or N2P2-amplitudes after hand or face stimulation have only been reported in small studies (n = 9–14 in each group) [18–20]. There were no amplitude differences between groups in a larger study (n = 24 and 28) [17], including the present study (n = 29 and 30). In contrast to our results, one small study has reported habituation of N1-amplitudes in controls after hand stimulation compared to no habituation in migraineurs [20]. The same study showed no habituation in controls after face stimulation, but an extreme amplitude *potentiation* of more than 90% in migraineurs [20]. Valeriani et al. [17] showed N1-habituation after hand stimulation in controls (but not in migraineurs) and no habituation in either group after face stimulation. However, it is unclear if the migraine group had significantly reduced amplitude habituation compared to the control group because the authors did not compare the degree of habituation between groups statistically.

N2P2-habituation was reduced in migraineurs compared to controls after face [17–19, 21, 22] and hand [17, 18, 21, 22] stimulation in most previous studies, although one study showed no differences [20]. The reliability of significant effects in small studies is low even in the absence of other biases [77]. Independent replications are thus necessary to increase the reliability of the estimated effects. Based on the results of the present larger and blinded study, it seems reasonable to conclude that habituation and amplitudes after hand stimulation are not different in migraineurs compared to non-headache control subjects, or if they are different, the differences are small. It has been argued that deficient habituation is a neurophysiological hallmark of migraine [78, 79]. However, as for VEP [32], the contradictory findings of LEP studies do not support that hypothesis.

Pain score changes by stimulus repetitions did not differ between migraineurs and controls in the present study. Previous studies have demonstrated similar findings [18, 20], although one study found differences represented by pain score habituation in controls and potentiation in migraineurs [21]. Also, de Tommaso et al. [19] demonstrated pain score habituation in controls and only a habituation tendency in migraineurs, but they did compare the groups statistically.

Variation in applied methods may explain some of the discrepancy mentioned above (Table 6). For instance, three

Table 6 Studies on LEP-habituation in migraine

Author	Aim/ habituation measure		♀	♂	Age	Incl	Excl	Freq	Blinding	Laser	Intensity	Block	Stim	ISI	IBI	Comp	Sites	Main habituation results[a]
Valeriani 2003 (17)	Habituation/ % change	Mig:	14	10	33.7 ± 8.2	NR	NR	NR	NR/NR	CO_2	2.5 × STh	3	15–30[b]	8–12	5 m	N1 N2P2	Bilateral hands and face[c]	N1 hand: CO↘ Mig→
										10.6 μm								N1 face: CO → Mig→
		CO:	17	11	32.5 ± 6.4	NR	NR			2 mm								N2P2 hand: CO↘ > Mig↘
										10 ms								N2P2 face: CO↘ Mig→
de Tommaso 2005 (19)	Habituation/ ANOVA	Mig:	9	5	22–53	NR	NR	NR	NR/NR	CO_2	7.5 W	3	21	10	10s	N2P2	Rigth supraorbital	N2P2 face: CO↘ Mig→
										10.6 μm								
		CO:	7	3	21–50	NR	NR			2.5 mm								
										20 ms								
de Tommaso 2005 (21)	Interictal-ictal habituation/ ANOVA	Mig:	14	0	18–40	NR	NR	9.4 ± 4.6	NR/Yes	CO_2	7.5 W	3	20	10	10s	N2P2	Bilateral hands and supraorbital	N2P2 hand: CO↘ > Mig→
										10.6 μm								
		CO:	10	0	22–36	NR	NR			2.5 mm								N2P2 face: CO↘ > Mig→
										20 ms								
de Tommaso 2009 (18)	Pre-menstrual habituation/ Ratio	Mig:	9	0	26 ± 6.8	Outp	11	4 ± 2.94	NR/Yes	CO_2	7.5 W	3	20	10–15	5 m	N2P2	Right hand and supraorbital	N2P2 hand: CO > Mig
										10.6 μm								
		CO:	10	0	26.8 ± 5.3	Hosp staff	15			2 mm								N2P2 face: CO > Mig
										25 ms								
Di Clemente 2013 (20)	Intervention[d] / % change	Mig:	9	4	38.5 ± 12.0	NR	9	5.8 ± 2.2	NR/Yes	Nd:YAP	2.5 × STh	3	15	10	5 m	N1 N2P2	Right hand and supraorbital	N1 hand: CO > Mig
										NR								N1 face: CO > Mig
		CO:	10	5	30.9 ± 5.7	NR	0			NR								N2P2 hand: CO = Mig
										NR								N2P2 face: CO = Mig
Vecchio 2016 (22)	Intervention[e]/ % change	Mig:	23	9	35.5 ± 10	NR	1	6 ± 2.5	NR/Yes	CO_2	PTh + 1 W	3	7	10	10s	N2P2	Right hand and supraorbital	N2P2 hand: CO > Mig
										10.6 μm								
		CO:	12	4	36.0 ± 11	NR	0			2 mm								N2P2 face: CO > Mig
										25 ms								
Uglem 2017	Habituation by phase/ Multilevel mixed mod.	Mig:	41	8	40 ± 10	Adv	Yes[f]	4[g]	Yes/Yes	Nd:YAP	3–5.5 J	2	21	6–10	10s	N1 N2P2	Right hand	N1 hand: CO → =Mig→
										1.34 μm								
		CO:	25	5	38 ± 11	Adv				8 mm								N2P2 hand: CO↘ = Mig↘
										6 ms								

♀: number of females. ♂: number of males. Age is presented in mean ± SD or range. Incl: inclution/method of recruitment. Excl: number of exclusions. Freq: migraine attack frequency in mean ± SD days/monts. Blinding: blinding of investigators during examination/blinding of investigators during LEP-analysis. Laser: Type of laser, wavelength, beam diameter and stimulus duration. Block: number of blocks. Stim: number of stimuli per block. ISI: interstimuli interval in seconds. IBI: interblock interval. Comp: analyzed LEP-components. Mig: migraine. CO: control. NR: not reported. Outp: outpatients. Hosp staff: hospital staff. Adv: recruited by advertisement. STh: sensory threshold. PTh: pain threshold. ↘: habituation present. →: no significant habituation. >: increased habituation in the control group compared to the migraineur group. =: no significant difference in habituation between the groups

[a]Only results regarding habituation of N1 and/or N2P2-amplitudes are shown. The studies differ in how they analyzed habituation as some reported habituation in each group separately (results indicated by ↘ or →), some reported comparisons between groups (results indicated by > or =), and some reported both. Valeriani 2003 (17) reported both results for N2P2 hand, but not for the other amplitudes.

[b]Three blocks with 15 stimuli at each side of the face and three blocks with 30 stimuli at each hand.

[c]Data were collected from three centers that stimulated two different face regions. The perioral region was stimulated in all migraineurs and 17 of the control subjects, while the supraorbital region was stimulated in 13 controls. The reported number of controls from each center does not add up to the reported total of 28 controls.

[d]The study examined the effect of topiramate on LEPs.

[e]The study investigated the effect of transcranial direct current stimulation of the left primary motor cortex and left dorsolateral prefrontal cortex on LEPs.

[f]Exclutions and dropouts are presented in Additional file 1: Table S1.

[g]Frequency was recorded in blocks. The three blocks 1–3, 4–7 and 8–14 days/month contained 14, 30 and 5 migraineurs, respectively.

of the previous studies recorded LEPs from three blocks with a five-minute break in between while we recorded two blocks without delay. Therefore, the less pronounced habituation shown by those studies may represent late effects only present after about ten minutes of stimulation. A similar late effect has been shown in radiculopathy patients where the habituation of N2P2 was normal in the first three blocks of 25 stimuli (inter-stimuli interval 8–12 s, no break between blocks), but deficient in the fourth [25].

Strengths and limitations

The major strengths of this study are its relatively large size with a longitudinal design and rigorous blinding both during data collection and analysis. The level of arousal, attention, and distraction may affect LEPs [60, 61]. Therefore, within-study consistency of the laser stimulation procedure is important. Especially when comparing groups, blinding of the investigators performing the stimulations becomes a necessity. Unfortunately, none of the previous migraine LEP-studies reported blinding of the investigators during stimulation, although the majority analyzed the LEPs blind to diagnosis (Table 6).

The solid-state laser used in this study differs from the CO_2-lasers employed in previous studies in that it produces a laser beam with shorter wavelength with deeper skin penetration that activates nociceptors more directly. This increases the amplitude of N1 and N2 and shortens the latency of N2P2, but the distribution of brain generators remains equal [80]. We do not believe that these differences, or the subtle differences in target-intensity, can explain the discrepancy between previous and present results.

The longitudinal design ensured a substantial number of interictal and preictal measurements and an acceptable number of ictal measurements. The postictal estimates are the least reliable due to the lowest number of measurements in that phase [77], although the number is comparable to previous migraine LEP-studies [21, 23, 24]. Only first-session responses were included in the migraineur versus control analyses because the investigator could not be blinded to diagnosis for the subsequent sessions, and to avoid possible long-term habituation/sensitization effects in later exams. Nevertheless, the number of interictal responses in this study was equal to [17, 22] or considerably larger than in the previous studies whose findings we attempted to reproduce [18–21].

We always stimulated the right hand regardless of the side the migraineur predominantly experienced headache. We found no habituation differences of LEPs obtained ipsilateral and contralateral to a migraine headache in accordance with previous findings [17]. Hence, it is seemingly not necessary to adjust the stimulated side according to headache laterality. We did not collect information on clinical allodynia, which could be of importance as an explanatory variable. We recruited both migraineurs and controls from the general population, and this design may enhance the generalizability of our results to the standard migraine population [81]. Having a first-degree relative that suffers from migraine may influence the habituation in controls [82]. However, we found habituation in both groups, not lack of habituation, which would be the expected finding if migraine-related genes biased our control group. Also, only four of the controls in our study had a positive family history of migraine, and excluding them from the analyses did not change the conclusions (results not reported).

The use of symptomatic treatment may have influenced the results as both triptans and non-steroidal anti-inflammatory drugs may reduce the amplitudes during the ictal phase [83]. It is unlikely that the medication influenced other phases than the ictal phase due to short half-life. Lack of facial stimulation can also be considered a limitation. However, hand and face LEP habituation seems to agree quite well in previous studies (Table 6), and this is to be expected as LEP reflects activation of a large part of the bilateral cortical pain network, and our aim was to study the generalized effects. Also, other modalities like pain thresholds have shown abnormalities in hands (and face) [84–86], suggesting an eventual thalamocortical dysfunction in migraine, in line with the development of cutaneous allodynia demonstrated by Burstein et al. [87]. Nevertheless, the present results are valid only for the more global pain function in migraine. It is necessary to do a similar study with face stimulation to conclude about lateralized second order trigeminal medullar afferent sensitization can be detected by LEP-abnormalities.

Previous studies have calculated habituation differently (Table 6). The method we chose included all available data and estimated the amplitude-change without prior calculation/manipulation of the dependent variable. Also, the approach did not use listwise deletion of cases with missing values, as would be the case with ANOVA. We were thus able to compare all four phases in one model. We also included the N1-responses where the signal to noise ratio was too low, as interval censored variables instead of discarding them, to avoid exclusion bias [65].

Conclusion

Both imaging and neurophysiological studies have shown phasic alterations in migraineurs. However, we only found evidence of a subtle alteration of habituation of cerebral responses to painful laser stimulation in the ictal phase. We found comparable LEP-amplitudes and habituation to dorsal hand stimulation in migraineurs in the interictal phase and headache-free controls. Thus, in contrast to some previous studies, we conclude that cerebral responses to painful laser stimulation are normal interictally in migraineurs. LEPs seem to be stable throughout the migraine cycle, but we could not exclude small changes and recommend further studies on phase-related changes in pain-physiology.

Abbreviations

CI: Confidence interval; LEP: Laser-evoked potentials; NRS: Numerical rating scale; VEP: Visual evoked potentials

Acknowledgements

We thank all migraineurs and controls for their participation in the study, and Erling Tronvik, Lars Jacob Stovner, Knut Hagen, Mattias Linde, Lena Hoem Nordhaug, Jo Willy Gråwe and Morten Engstrøm for invaluable assistance.

Funding

This study received funding from NTNU, Norwegian University of Science and Technology.

Authors' contributions

MU wrote the first draft. PMO, TS, and MU did major revisions. All authors contributed to the final revision. All authors contributed to the planning of the study, supervised by TS. MS and GBG were responsible for inclusion, coordination, and follow-up of participants. Examinations, data processing, and statistics were done by MU, supervised by PMO and TS. All authors read and approved the final manuscript.

Competing interests

The authors declare that they have no competing interests.

Author details

[1]Department of Neuromedicine and Movement Science, NTNU, Norwegian University of Science and Technology, Trondheim, Norway. [2]Department of Neurology and Clinical Neurophysiology, St. Olavs Hospital, Trondheim, Norway. [3]Norwegian Advisory Unit on Headaches, St. Olavs Hospital, Trondheim, Norway. [4]NTNU, Faculty of Medicine and Health Sciences, P.B. 8905, N-7491 Trondheim, Norway.

References

1. Maniyar FH, Sprenger T, Monteith T, Schankin CJ, Goadsby PJ (2015) The premonitory phase of migraine–what can we learn from it? Headache 55:609–620
2. Bose P, Goadsby PJ (2016) The migraine postdrome. Curr Opin Neurol 29:299–301
3. Schulte LH, May A (2016) The migraine generator revisited: continuous scanning of the migraine cycle over 30 days and three spontaneous attacks. Brain 139:1987–1993
4. Sand T, Zhitniy N, White LR, Stovner LJ (2008) Brainstem auditory-evoked potential habituation and intensity-dependence related to serotonin metabolism in migraine: a longitudinal study. Clin Neurophysiol 119:1190–1200
5. Sand T, Zhitniy N, White LR, Stovner LJ (2008) Visual evoked potential latency, amplitude and habituation in migraine: a longitudinal study. Clin Neurophysiol 119:1020–1027
6. Uglem M, Omland PM, Nilsen KB, Tronvik E, Stovner LJ, Hagen K, Linde M, Sand T (2016) Does pain sensitivity change by migraine phase? A blinded longitudinal study. Cephalalgia. doi:10.1177/0333102416679955333102416679955
7. Harriott AM, Schwedt TJ (2014) Migraine is associated with altered processing of sensory stimuli. Curr Pain Headache Rep 18:458
8. Schulte LH, May A (2016) Functional Neuroimaging in Migraine: Chances and Challenges. Headache 56:1474–1481
9. de Tommaso M, Ambrosini A, Brighina F, Coppola G, Perrotta A, Pierelli F, Sandrini G, Valeriani M, Marinazzo D, Stramaglia S, Schoenen J (2014) Altered processing of sensory stimuli in patients with migraine. Nat Rev Neurol 10:144–155
10. Cruccu G, Sommer C, Anand P, Attal N, Baron R, Garcia-Larrea L, Haanpaa M, Jensen TS, Serra J, Treede RD (2010) EFNS guidelines on neuropathic pain assessment: revised 2009. Eur J Neurol 17:1010–1018
11. Garcia-Larrea L, Frot M, Valeriani M (2003) Brain generators of laser-evoked potentials: from dipoles to functional significance. Neurophysiol Clin 33:279–292
12. Treede RD, Lorenz J, Baumgartner U (2003) Clinical usefulness of laser-evoked potentials. Neurophysiol Clin 33:303–314
13. Bromm B, Treede RD (1984) Nerve fibre discharges, cerebral potentials and sensations induced by CO2 laser stimulation. Hum Neurobiol 3:33–40
14. Carmon A, Mor J, Goldberg J (1976) Evoked cerebral responses to noxious thermal stimuli in humans. Exp Brain Res 25:103–107
15. Iannetti GD, Zambreanu L, Cruccu G, Tracey I (2005) Operculoinsular cortex encodes pain intensity at the earliest stages of cortical processing as indicated by amplitude of laser-evoked potentials in humans. Neuroscience 131:199–208
16. Valentini E, Hu L, Chakrabarti B, Hu Y, Aglioti SM, Iannetti GD (2012) The primary somatosensory cortex largely contributes to the early part of the cortical response elicited by nociceptive stimuli. NeuroImage 59:1571–1581
17. Valeriani M, de Tommaso M, Restuccia D, Le Pera D, Guido M, Iannetti GD, Libro G, Truini A, Di Trapani G, Puca F, Tonali P, Cruccu G (2003) Reduced habituation to experimental pain in migraine patients: a CO(2) laser evoked potential study. Pain 105:57–64
18. de Tommaso M, Valeriani M, Sardaro M, Serpino C, Fruscolo OD, Vecchio E, Cerbo R, Livrea P (2009) Pain perception and laser evoked potentials during menstrual cycle in migraine. J Headache Pain 10:423–429
19. de Tommaso M, Libro G, Guido M, Losito L, Lamberti P, Livrea P (2005) Habituation of single CO2 laser-evoked responses during interictal phase of migraine. J Headache Pain 6:195–198
20. Di Clemente L, Puledda F, Biasiotta A, Vigano A, Vicenzini E, Truini A, Cruccu G, Di Piero V (2013) Topiramate modulates habituation in migraine: evidences from nociceptive responses elicited by laser evoked potentials. J Headache Pain 14:25
21. de Tommaso M, Lo Sito L, Di Fruscolo O, Sardaro M, Pia Prudenzano M, Lamberti P, Livrea P (2005) Lack of habituation of nociceptive evoked responses and pain sensitivity during migraine attack. Clin Neurophysiol 116:1254–1264
22. Vecchio E, Ricci K, Montemurno A, Delussi M, Invitto S, de Tommaso M (2016) Effects of left primary motor and dorsolateral prefrontal cortex transcranial direct current stimulation on laser-evoked potentials in migraine patients and normal subjects. Neurosci Lett 626:149–157
23. de Tommaso M, Guido M, Libro G, Losito L, Sciruicchio V, Monetti C, Puca F (2002) Abnormal brain processing of cutaneous pain in migraine patients during the attack. Neurosci Lett 333:29–32
24. de Tommaso M, Guido M, Libro G, Losito L, Difruscolo O, Puca F, Specchio LM, Carella A (2004) Topographic and dipolar analysis of laser-evoked potentials during migraine attack. Headache 44:947–960
25. Hullemann P, von der Brelie C, Manthey G, Dusterhoft J, Helmers AK, Synowitz M, Baron R (2017) Reduced laser-evoked potential habituation detects abnormal central pain processing in painful radiculopathy patients. Eur J Pain 21:918–926
26. de Tommaso M, Federici A, Santostasi R, Calabrese R, Vecchio E, Lapadula G, Iannone F, Lamberti P, Livrea P (2011) Laser-evoked potentials habituation in fibromyalgia. J Pain 12:116–124
27. Valeriani M, Sestito A, Le Pera D, De Armas L, Infusino F, Maiese T, Sgueglia GA, Tonali PA, Crea F, Restuccia D, Lanza GA (2005) Abnormal cortical pain processing in patients with cardiac syndrome X. Eur Heart J 26:975–982
28. Ioannidis JP (2014) How to make more published research true. PLoS Med 11:e1001747
29. Di Clemente L, Coppola G, Magis D, Fumal A, De Pasqua V, Schoenen J (2005) Nociceptive blink reflex and visual evoked potential habituations are correlated in migraine. Headache 45:1388–1393
30. Stankewitz A, Schulz E, May A (2013) Neuronal correlates of impaired habituation in response to repeated trigemino-nociceptive but not to olfactory input in migraineurs: an fMRI study. Cephalalgia 33:256–265
31. Katsarava Z, Giffin N, Diener HC, Kaube H (2003) Abnormal habituation of 'nociceptive' blink reflex in migraine–evidence for increased excitability of trigeminal nociception. Cephalalgia 23:814–819
32. Omland PM, Uglem M, Hagen K, Linde M, Tronvik E, Sand T (2016) Visual evoked potentials in migraine: Is the "neurophysiological hallmark" concept still valid? Clin Neurophysiol 127:810–816

33. Coppola G, Di Lorenzo C, Schoenen J, Pierelli F (2013) Habituation and sensitization in primary headaches. J Headache Pain 14:65
34. De Marinis M, Pujia A, Natale L, D'Arcangelo E, Accornero N (2003) Decreased habituation of the R2 component of the blink reflex in migraine patients. Clin Neurophysiol 114:889–893
35. Sand T, Vingen JV (2000) Visual, long-latency auditory and brainstem auditory evoked potentials in migraine: relation to pattern size, stimulus intensity, sound and light discomfort thresholds and pre-attack state. Cephalalgia 20:804–820
36. Chen WT, Wang SJ, Fuh JL, Lin CP, Ko YC, Lin YY (2009) Peri-ictal normalization of visual cortex excitability in migraine: an MEG study. Cephalalgia 29:1202–1211
37. Judit A, Sandor PS, Schoenen J (2000) Habituation of visual and intensity dependence of auditory evoked cortical potentials tends to normalize just before and during the migraine attack. Cephalalgia 20:714–719
38. Coppola G, Curra A, Di Lorenzo C, Parisi V, Gorini M, Sava SL, Schoenen J, Pierelli F (2010) Abnormal cortical responses to somatosensory stimulation in medication-overuse headache. BMC Neurol 10:126
39. Coppola G, Iacovelli E, Bracaglia M, Serrao M, Di Lorenzo C, Pierelli F (2013) Electrophysiological correlates of episodic migraine chronification: evidence for thalamic involvement. J Headache Pain 14:76
40. Kalita J, Bhoi SK, Misra UK (2014) Is lack of habituation of evoked potential a biological marker of migraine? Clin J Pain 30:724–729
41. Chen WT, Wang SJ, Fuh JL, Lin CP, Ko YC, Lin YY (2011) Persistent ictal-like visual cortical excitability in chronic migraine. Pain 152:254–258
42. Kropp P, Gerber WD (2005) Slow cortical potentials in migraine. Predictive value and possible novel therapeutic strategies to prevent an attack. Funct Neurol 20:193–197
43. Siniatchkin M, Averkina N, Andrasik F, Stephani U, Gerber WD (2006) Neurophysiological reactivity before a migraine attack. Neurosci Lett 400:121–124
44. Kropp P, Gerber WD (1995) Contingent negative variation during migraine attack and interval: evidence for normalization of slow cortical potentials during the attack. Cephalalgia 15:123–128 discussion 178-129
45. Evers S, Quibeldey F, Grotemeyer KH, Suhr B, Husstedt IW (1999) Dynamic changes of cognitive habituation and serotonin metabolism during the migraine interval. Cephalalgia 19:485–491
46. St. Olavs Hospital, Trondheim University Hospital. www.stolav.no/en. Accessed 25 March 2017
47. NTNU, Norwegian University of Science and Technology. www.ntnu.edu. Accessed 25 March 2017
48. Headache Classification Subcommittee of the International Headache Society (2004) The International Classification of Headache Disorders: 2nd edition. Cephalalgia 24 Suppl 1:9–160
49. Odegard SS, Omland PM, Nilsen KB, Stjern M, Gravdahl GB, Sand T (2015) The effect of sleep restriction on laser evoked potentials, thermal sensory and pain thresholds and suprathreshold pain in healthy subjects. Clin Neurophysiol 126:1979–1987
50. Iannetti GD, Leandri M, Truini A, Zambreanu L, Cruccu G, Tracey I (2004) Adelta nociceptor response to laser stimuli: selective effect of stimulus duration on skin temperature, brain potentials and pain perception. Clin Neurophysiol 115:2629–2637
51. Isak B, Tankisi H, Johnsen B, Pugdahl K, Finnerup NB, Fuglsang-Frederiksen A (2016) Laser and somatosensory evoked potentials in amyotrophic lateral sclerosis. Clin Neurophysiol 127:3322–3328
52. Di Stefano G, Celletti C, Baron R, Castori M, Di Franco M, La Cesa S, Leone C, Pepe A, Cruccu G, Truini A, Camerota F (2016) Central sensitization as the mechanism underlying pain in joint hypermobility syndrome/Ehlers-Danlos syndrome, hypermobility type. Eur J Pain 20:1319–1325
53. Cruccu G, Aminoff MJ, Curio G, Guerit JM, Kakigi R, Mauguiere F, Rossini PM, Treede RD, Garcia-Larrea L (2008) Recommendations for the clinical use of somatosensory-evoked potentials. Clin Neurophysiol 119:1705–1719
54. Garcia-Larrea L, Peyron R, Laurent B, Mauguiere F (1997) Association and dissociation between laser-evoked potentials and pain perception. Neuroreport 8:3785–3789
55. Lefaucheur JP, Debray S, Jarry G (2001) Laser evoked potentials using the Nd:YAG laser. Muscle Nerve 24:496–501
56. Treede RD, Meyer RA, Raja SN, Campbell JN (1995) Evidence for two different heat transduction mechanisms in nociceptive primary afferents innervating monkey skin. J Physiol 483(Pt 3):747–758
57. Truini A, Galeotti F, Romaniello A, Virtuoso M, Iannetti GD, Cruccu G (2005) Laser-evoked potentials: normative values. Clin Neurophysiol 116:821–826
58. de Tommaso M, Ricci K, Montemurno A, Vecchio E (2017) Age-related changes in laser-evoked potentials following trigeminal and hand stimulation in healthy subjects. Eur J Pain 21:1087–1097
59. Bromm B, Lorenz J (1998) Neurophysiological evaluation of pain. Electroencephalogr Clin Neurophysiol 107:227–253
60. Beydoun A, Morrow TJ, Shen JF, Casey KL (1993) Variability of laser-evoked potentials: attention, arousal and lateralized differences. Electroencephalogr Clin Neurophysiol 88:173–181
61. Lorenz J, Garcia-Larrea L (2003) Contribution of attentional and cognitive factors to laser evoked brain potentials. Neurophysiol Clin 33:293–301
62. Sand T, Zhitniy N, Nilsen KB, Helde G, Hagen K, Stovner LJ (2008) Thermal pain thresholds are decreased in the migraine preattack phase. Eur J Neurol 15:1199–1205
63. Kunde V, Treede RD (1993) Topography of middle-latency somatosensory evoked potentials following painful laser stimuli and non-painful electrical stimuli. Electroencephalogr Clin Neurophysiol 88:280–289
64. StataCorp (2013) intreg - interval regression. In: Stata 13 base reference manual, Stata Press. College Station, TX
65. Smithson M, Merkle EC (2013) Censoring and Truncation. In: Generalized Linear Models for Categorical and Continuous Limited Dependent Variables. CRC Press, Boca Raton, FL
66. Rabe-Hesketh S, Skrondal A (2012) Multilevel and longitudinal modeling using Stata : Vol. 1 : Continuous responses. Stata Press, College Station, Tex
67. Cohen J (1988) Statistical power analysis for the behavioral sciences. Laurence Erlbaum, Hillsdale, N. J
68. Coppola G, Ambrosini A, Di Clemente L, Magis D, Fumal A, Gerard P, Pierelli F, Schoenen J (2007) Interictal abnormalities of gamma band activity in visual evoked responses in migraine: an indication of thalamocortical dysrhythmia? Cephalalgia 27:1360–1367
69. Hodkinson DJ, Wilcox SL, Veggeberg R, Noseda R, Burstein R, Borsook D, Becerra L (2016) Increased Amplitude of Thalamocortical Low-Frequency Oscillations in Patients with Migraine. J Neurosci 36:8026–8036
70. De Ridder D, Vanneste S, Langguth B, Llinas R (2015) Thalamocortical Dysrhythmia: A Theoretical Update in Tinnitus. Front Neurol 6:124
71. Fuggetta G, Noh NA (2013) A neurophysiological insight into the potential link between transcranial magnetic stimulation, thalamocortical dysrhythmia and neuropsychiatric disorders. Exp Neurol 245:87–95
72. Schulman JJ, Cancro R, Lowe S, Lu F, Walton KD, Llinas RR (2011) Imaging of thalamocortical dysrhythmia in neuropsychiatry. Front Hum Neurosci 5:69
73. Jones EG (2010) Thalamocortical dysrhythmia and chronic pain. Pain 150:4–5
74. Schmidt S, Naranjo JR, Brenneisen C, Gundlach J, Schultz C, Kaube H, Hinterberger T, Jeanmonod D (2012) Pain ratings, psychological functioning and quantitative EEG in a controlled study of chronic back pain patients. PLoS One 7:e31138
75. Zambito-Marsala S, Erro R, Bacchin R, Fornasier A, Fabris F, Lo Cascio C, Ferracci F, Morgante F, Tinazzi M (2017) Abnormal nociceptive processing occurs centrally and not peripherally in pain-free Parkinson disease patients: A study with laser-evoked potentials. Parkinsonism Relat Disord 34:43–48
76. Schuh-Hofer S, Baumgartner U, Treede RD (2015) Effect of sleep deprivation on the electrophysiological signature of habituation to noxious laser stimuli. Eur J Pain 19:1197–1209
77. Button KS, Ioannidis JP, Mokrysz C, Nosek BA, Flint J, Robinson ES, Munafo MR (2013) Power failure: why small sample size undermines the reliability of neuroscience. Nat Rev Neurosci 14:365–376
78. Magis D, Vigano A, Sava S, d'Elia TS, Schoenen J, Coppola G (2013) Pearls and pitfalls: electrophysiology for primary headaches. Cephalalgia 33:526–539
79. Brighina F, Palermo A, Fierro B (2009) Cortical inhibition and habituation to evoked potentials: relevance for pathophysiology of migraine. J Headache Pain 10:77–84
80. Perchet C, Godinho F, Mazza S, Frot M, Legrain V, Magnin M, Garcia-Larrea L (2008) Evoked potentials to nociceptive stimuli delivered by CO2 or Nd:YAP lasers. Clin Neurophysiol 119:2615–2622

81. Rauschel V, Ruscheweyh R, Krafczyk S, Straube A (2016) Test-retest reliability of visual-evoked potential habituation. Cephalalgia 36:831–839
82. Lisicki M, Ruiz-Romagnoli E, D'Ostilio K, Piedrabuena R, Giobellina R, Schoenen J, Magis D (2016) Familial history of migraine influences habituation of visual evoked potentials. Cephalalgia. doi:10.1177/0333102416673207
83. de Tommaso M, Losito L, Libro G, Guido M, Di Fruscolo O, Sardaro M, Sciruicchio V, Lamberti P, Livrea P (2005) Effects of symptomatic treatments on cutaneous hyperalgesia and laser evoked potentials during migraine attack. Cephalalgia 25:359–368
84. Schwedt TJ, Krauss MJ, Frey K, Gereau RWt (2011) Episodic and chronic migraineurs are hypersensitive to thermal stimuli between migraine attacks. Cephalalgia 31:6–12
85. Schwedt TJ, Zuniga L, Chong CD (2015) Low heat pain thresholds in migraineurs between attacks. Cephalalgia 35:593–599
86. Engstrom M, Hagen K, Bjork MH, Stovner LJ, Gravdahl GB, Stjern M, Sand T (2013) Sleep quality, arousal and pain thresholds in migraineurs: a blinded controlled polysomnographic study. J Headache Pain 14:12
87. Burstein R, Cutrer MF, Yarnitsky D (2000) The development of cutaneous allodynia during a migraine attack clinical evidence for the sequential recruitment of spinal and supraspinal nociceptive neurons in migraine. Brain 123(Pt 8):1703–1709
88. Headache Classification Committee of the International Headache Society (2013) The International Classification of Headache Disorders, 3rd edition (beta version). Cephalalgia 33:629–808

19

Altered muscle activity during rest and during mental or physical activity is not a trait symptom of migraine - a neck muscle EMG study

Kerstin Luedtke[1,2†], Jan Mehnert[1†] and Arne May[1*]

Abstract

Background: Migraineurs have a high prevalence of neck pain prior to or during headache attacks. Whether neck pain is a symptom of migraine or an indicator for a constant neck muscle dysfunction potentially triggering migraine attacks is a topic of scientific debate. The presence of myofascial trigger points in neck muscles including the trapezius muscle, points towards muscle alterations associated with migraine. We measured electromyography (EMG) of the neck muscles in a large cohort to identify whether neck pain and neckmuscle tension reported by migraine patients can be attributed to increased neck muscle activation during rest, mental stress or physical activity.

Methods: Surface EMG responses of the trapezius muscle were recorded during a paradigm including rest periods, mental stress and physical activity of 102 participants (31 chronic migraine, 43 episodic migraine, 28 healthy participants).

Results: All groups showed increased trapezius activity during mental stress and physical activity compared to rest. There was no statistically significant difference between migraine patients and healthy controls for any of the 3 conditions except for the initial mental stress situation ($F(2,56.022) = 8.302$, $p = 0.001$), where controls increased tension by only 4.75%, episodic migraineurs by 17.39% and chronic migraineurs by 28.61%. Both migraine groups returned to resting EMG levels within the same timeframe as healthy controls.

Conclusions: Neck pain associated with migraine can therefore not be attributed to increased trapezius activity during rest, mental stress and physical activity or prolonged muscle activity and should not be seen as a constantly underlying trigger but rather as an accompanying symptom of migraine.

Keywords: Migraine, Trigger, Neck pain, Muscle tension, EMG, Stress

Background

The high prevalence of neck pain in patients with migraine [1–3] perpetuates an ongoing debate about the contribution of neck muscles to headache provocation and the frequency of attacks. While some authors claim that neck pain is simply a symptom of the migraine attack [2], others postulate that dysfunctions in neck muscles may trigger migraine attacks and thereby contribute to the transition from episodic to chronic migraine [4].

The latter hypothesis is based on publications that identified a higher prevalence of active and latent trigger points in neck muscles of patients with migraine compared to headache-free control populations [4–6]. This point of view is further supported by a study with a local anaesthetic (Ropivacaine) injection into these trigger points, which effectively reduced migraine frequency in approximately 60% of the participants in a non-controlled design including 52 chronic migraine patients [7] and another one which suggested beneficial effects of local therapy of active myofascial trigger points [8].

* Correspondence: a.may@uke.de
Kerstin Luedtke and Jan Mehnert contributed equally to this work.
†Equal contributors
[1]Department of Systems Neuroscience, University Medical Center Eppendorf, Martinistraße 52, 20246 Hamburg, Germany
Full list of author information is available at the end of the article

Other publications focusing on muscle tension in headache populations used surface electromyography (EMG) recordings either during rest or during physical or mental tasks. While higher levels of muscle tension, especially as a response to stressful mental tasks [9, 10], or to painful stimulation [11], are consistently found in patients with chronic tension-type headache (TTH), the evidence in migraine is conflicting: Sandrini et al. (1994) did not find altered EMG recordings from the frontalis muscle during mental arithmetic in migraine patients [10]. This was later confirmed by Leistad et al. (2006) who only found differences in trapezius muscle responses to 60-min periods of cognitive stress in patients with TTH but not in patients with migraine or in healthy controls [12]. Goudswaard and colleagues [13] reported that migraine patients consistently showed higher proportional EMG levels of the corrugator muscle during periods of experimental and real-life stress but patients who developed headaches during stress had lower levels of muscle tension than participants without headaches. The authors concluded that increased EMG activity during stress seems not to be the cause but rather a response to head pain [13]. A similar observation was reported by Pritchard and colleagues [14], who found that the occipital muscle output during an experimental stressor was significantly lower in the migraine group and higher in the tension-type group during the headache phase [14].

Opposing results were reported by van Boxtel et al. (1983) who recorded significantly higher EMG levels in the migraine and mixed headache groups when expressing the resting EMG levels as a percentage of the EMG level during maximal contraction [15]. In girls with "migraine-type" headache, a higher EMG/force ratio between the EMG of the left agonist sternocleidomastoid (SCM) muscle and the corresponding maximal neck flexion ($p = 0.030$) was observed [16]. Furthermore, during a physical task, a higher co-activation of the superficial extensor muscles (trapezius) was recorded in chronic migraineurs compared to healthy controls [17].

Interestingly, Leistad and colleagues (2006) reported a delayed recovery of migraine patients and controls from a painful stimulus as well as a delayed return of trapezius EMG activity to baseline, which was only significant in tension-type headaches but also more prolonged in migraine compared to healthy controls [12].

Neck muscle relaxation techniques including EMG biofeedback are frequently used as non-pharmacological additions to reduce the frequency of migraine attacks and are consequently recommended by national and international guidelines [18–20]. In a review, all relaxation methods including EMG, achieved an average reduction in migraine frequency of 35–45% [21], although blood-volume-pulse feedback yielded higher effect sizes than peripheral skin temperature feedback and electromyography feedback [22]. However, in a clinical trial, EMG biofeedback training had no additional effect over education [23].

The inconsistency of the existing evidence and two important additional questions triggered the design of the current study: question 1 is, whether activities of remote body parts, e.g. the lower limb will result in a higher activation of neck muscles in migraine patients, and question 2 is, whether neck muscle tension is prolonged after any type of stress or physical activity.

Therefore, the purpose of this study was to evaluate the level of muscle tension during voluntary relaxation and during mental and physical tasks as well as the ability to relax after periods of mental and physical stress in patients with migraine and headache-free control participants. The question was, whether migraine patients exhibit a constantly raised muscle tone or, if not, whether migraineurs are more susceptible to increased neck muscle tension under stress (mental of physical) which theoretically could also suggest that muscle tension is a trigger to induce migraine attacks.

- Hypothesis 1: The mean EMG response for both, physical and mental stress differs between healthy controls and patients.
- Hypothesis 2: Migraineurs' neck muscles need more time to recover from mental and physical tasks.

Methods

Subjects

There were no adequate previous publications to base a sample size calculation on. The difference between migraine patients and controls was anticipated to be rather large considering that neck pain is such a dominant symptom in migraineurs. A sample size of 102 was sufficient to detect an effect size (Cohen's d) of 0.4 with 95% power and an alpha level of 0.05 [24]. All consecutive patients attending a headache outpatient clinic in Germany that were diagnosed with migraine (with or without aura) according to the criteria published by the international headache society [25], by a neurologist specialized in the assessment and treatment of headache patients, were invited to participate. They received an information leaflet stating the inclusion/exclusion criteria and the data collection procedure in detail. Of those, who responded to this invitation, none had to be excluded.

Control participants were recruited using a university platform, social media and personal contacts, that had a maximum of 3 headache attacks per year that did not fulfil the criteria of migraine or any other primary headache type except sporadic episodic tension-type headache. For all groups, the following exclusion criteria were applied: not younger than 18 years, not suffering from a neurological, psychiatric or pain condition (other than migraine) as well as rheumatoid arthritis or diagnosed neck pathology (such as whiplash associated disorder or disc disease). Migraine patients were excluded if they took pain medication on more than 10 days in the past month or suffered from any relevant additional headache type.

After providing written informed consent, all patients were asked to fill out questionnaires regarding their quality of life reduced by headache (MIDAS [26], or neck dysfunctions (NDI [27], and the Patient Health Questionnaire (PHQ [28]). Furthermore, we assessed whether they had headache at the day of the examination, when the last and the next headache attack was, how many years of headache they had in their history, the number of days per month suffering from headache as well as the dominant headache side.

Experimental design

The experiment consisted of 7 experimental conditions alternated with relaxation periods, resulting in a total of 15 blocks. Three blocks were mentally stressful: participants had to count backwards from 100 in steps of 9 (from 80 in steps of 7 and from 60 in steps of 4, respectively for 3rd and 6th block) as fast as possible, while the other 4 conditions included physical lower limb activity: either pressing 1 foot down on a body weight scale and holding a minimum of 27 kg or resisted knee extension of one leg for 30 s. Tests were performed with each leg separately. At the start and end of the experiment further 2 min relaxation blocks were added. An overview of the experimental timeline can be found in Table 1.

Table 1 Experimental design

Block	Condition	Approx. duration [sec]
1	rest	120
2	counting backwards in steps of 9	45
3	Rest	60
4	counting backwards in steps of 7	45
5	Rest	60
6	counting backwards in steps of 4	35
7	rest	60
8	scale right leg	30
9	rest	60
10	scale left leg	30
11	rest	60
12	knee extension right	30
13	rest	60
14	knee extension left	30
15	rest	120

EMG data acquisition and pre-processing

During the experiment, electromyography was measured with two channels located at both sides of the neck over the upper trapezius muscle with a distance between electrodes of 20 cms. Surface EMG was recorded using a Schuhfried Biofeedback x-pert 2000 system (Dr. Schuhfried Medizintechnik GmbH, Wien, Austria) with a sampling frequency of 500 Hz in the frequency band of 100 to 200 Hz to measure muscle activity and a measuring range of 60 µV (resolution: 0.048 µV). A digital notch filter attenuated power line noise at 50 Hz. This system provides voltages for a moving temporal integral (250 ms) of absolute summed action potentials.

For further processing by self-written routines using the software Matlab (Mathworks, Version R2014a), data was down-sampled to 10 Hz and high frequency noise was reduced by 3 iterations of outlier reduction, where in a moving window of 20 sampling points values exceeding 4 times the standard deviation were replaced by the windows' mean. Sharp transients and ECG artifacts were eliminated with a median moving-window filter (filter order 500, build-in medfilt1 function in Matlab). Afterwards, data was segmented into the epochs of the experimental conditions described above (Table 1).

Data analysis

The person analyzing all data was blinded to the diagnosis. Differences across groups regarding migraine disability (MIDAS), depression (PHQ) and neck disability (NDI) were calculated using the Mann-Whitney-U test as a non-parametric option for not normally distributed data [29]). To test hypothesis 1 we calculated the proportion (percentage) of the difference to the previous relaxation block's mean for each of the 7 experimental conditions of the EMG signal. We tested the main effect of mental or physical stimulation with independent, one-sample t-tests and used one-way-ANOVAs to assess significant differences between the three groups for each condition separately. Whether the presumption of homoscedasticity was fulfilled was tested using Levene's test. Whenever this test was significant, Welch's test was used. To correct for multiple testing, Bonferroni correction was applied. Any significant difference was further tested for a relation to the side of headache. We therefore used point-biserial correlation as a special case of the Pearson's correlation to identify a correlation between the dominant headache side and the tested side of the neck. Subjects with bilateral headache were analyzed in both groups of dominant headache sides. As expected when including chronic migraine patients, a significant number of participating patients reported headache during the examination we further ran a two-sample t-test for all 7 blocks and 2 EMG channels to investigate the influence of acute headache on neck muscles tension. To further investigate an influence of the preictal phase we run two-sample t-tests between patients with headache in a 24 h (48 h, 72 h, respectively) period before the examination against patients which were headache free for the minimum of 4 days.

To test hypothesis 2 we calculated the time until the mean value within the relaxation block was reached after a mental or physical task and calculated a one-way-ANOVA between the three groups for each condition separately. All statistical analyses were performed using either Matlab (MathWorks, Version 2014a) or SPSS (IBM) Version 24.

Results

Clinical data

A total of 102 volunteers participated in the study between June 2016 and May 2107. Twenty eight were headache-free control participants (21 females; mean age 43.3 years (Standard deviation (SD) 12.2), min: 23 years, max: 70 years). Forty three subjects suffered from episodic migraine (38 females; mean age 39.12 years (SD 12.2), min: 18 years, max: 60 years), i.e. had headache on fewer than 14 days per month (mean 7.3 days, SD 3.6), and 31 patients were diagnosed with chronic migraine (30 females; mean age 39.3 years (SD 13.8), min: 20 years, max: 68 years) with 15 or more days of headache per month (mean: 21.7 days, SD: 5.6). Age was not significantly different between the three groups ($p > 0.3$, $F(2,98) = 1.065$, One-Way-ANOVA).

MIDAS, NDI and PHQ scores were significantly different between patient groups ($p = 0.02$, $p = 0.01$, and $p = 0.048$, respectively) with chronic patients suffering more (see Table 2).

Thirteen of the episodic patients (31.7%, 2 values missing) and 20 of the chronic patients (64.5%, 2 values missing) reported headache during the examination. Furthermore, 24 episodic (58.5%) and 24 (82.8%) chronic patients had headache within the 48 h before the examination and 21 (56.8%) episodic and 23 (85.2%) chronic patients had headache within 48 h after the examination.

EMG

All groups showed increased bilateral trapezius muscle activity during mental as well as physical stress (for all tasks $p < 0.05$). There was no difference across groups for the mean EMG increase (relative to the previous relaxation block) during any of the tasks apart from the first mental stress task which showed significantly higher EMG activity on the right side during counting backwards in steps of 9 (Fig. 1). Levene's test for homoscedasticity was significant, therefore Welch's Test was used ($F(2,56.022) = 8.302$, $p = 0.001$). The mean EMG amplitude change was 4.75% (SD 10.29%) for the healthy subjects, 17.39% (SD 25.34%) in the episodic migraine group, and 28.61% (SD 40.12%) in the chronic migraine group in the electrode covering the right neck muscle. The difference between the two migraine groups was not statistically significant in the Bonferroni corrected post-hoc testing ($p = 0.28$) and neither the difference between healthy controls and episodic migraineurs (p = 0,20), Nevertheless, the comparison between healthy controls and chronic migraineurs yielded Bonferroni corrected significance (Bonferroni, $p = 0.005$). There was no significant (point-biserial) correlation between the dominant headache side and the recorded side of the neck. Furthermore, we could not find any significant differences between patients with and without acute headache during the examination ($p > 0.05$ in all two-sampled t-test) as well as between preictal patients (in a 24 h, 48 h as well as 72 h period) and patients which were free of headache since at least 4 days.

Table 2 Clinical characteristics of participants

	Control (*n*=28)	Episodic migraine (*n*=43)	Chronic migraine (*n*=31)
Age [mean (SD)/range]	43.3 (12.2)/23-70	39.12 (12.2)/18-60	39.3 (13.8)/20-68
Gender [female / male]	21 / 7	38 / 5	30 / 1
Duration of disease (years) [mean (SD)]		17.3 (10.7)	15.0 (15.3)
Intensity (0-10) [mean (SD)]		6.5 (1.6)	6.9 (1.7)
Frequency (days per month) [mean (SD)]		7 (4)	22 (5)
MIDAS [mean (SD)]		35.8 (31.4)	68.5 (61.6)
NDI [mean (SD)]	3.0 (3.1)	12.0 (6.1)	16.6 (6.1)
PHQ [mean (SD)]	3.7 (3.9)	6.9 (3.8)	8.7 (4.4)
Days since last headache [mean (SD)]		4 (6)	2 (3)
Days until next headache [mean (SD)]		5 (8)	1 (2)

MIDAS migraine disability assessment test, *NDI* neck disability index, *PHQ* patient health questionnaire, *SD* standard deviation

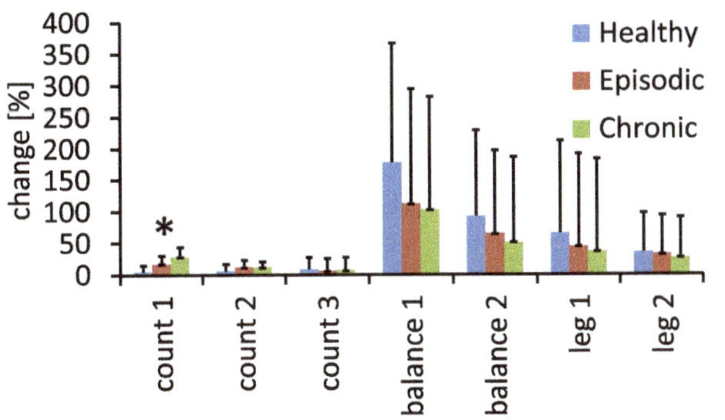

Fig. 1 EMG changes relative to rest blocks in the electrode over the right neck muscle for the three individual groups and each experimental condition. The errorbars represent standard deviations. The asterisk marks a significant group difference ($p < 0.05$)

The second hypothesis, that the time required to relax after a stressful task differs between migraine patients and healthy controls, had to be rejected, because there was no significant difference across groups for any of the relaxing periods as tested by a one-way ANOVA (Fig. 2).

Discussion

The migraine population did not differ from healthy participants regarding EMG-recorded muscle tension of the upper trapezius during mental and physical tasks, except for the first task (counting backwards from 100 in steps of 9). Furthermore, the results did not indicate a delayed recovery of trapezius EMG activity from mental or physical tasks, as previously reported for tension-type headache [12]. This unanticipated result suggests that altered muscle activity during rest or during mental or physical activity is not a trait symptom of migraine, in contrast to tension-type headache [9, 30–32]. Hence, the frequently observed neck pain before or during the migraine attack [1–3] is more likely a symptom of the migraine attack and less likely an indicator for a neck muscle pathology that subsequently triggers an attack. Headache status on the day of testing did not significantly influence the results, therefore neck pain or perceived muscle tension does not seem to be quantifiable with surface EMG data.

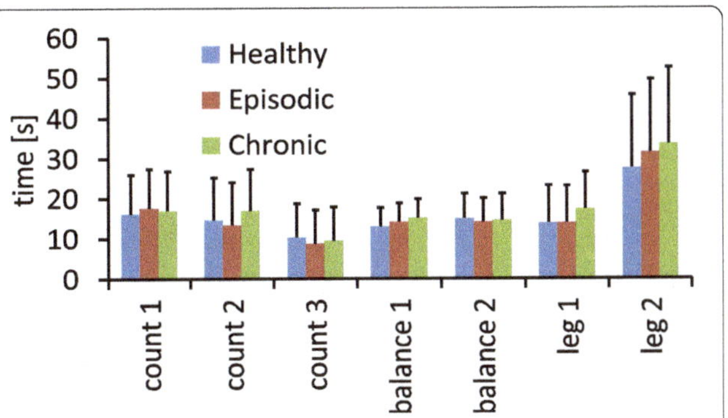

Fig. 2 Duration until the average relaxation value within the resting blocks was reached in the electrode over the right neck muscle for the three individual groups and each experimental condition. The errorbars represent standard deviations

It further suggests, that the migraine reducing effect of neck muscle EMG-biofeedback is probably not attributed to a reduction in muscle tension but to a general relaxation effect, further supported by Nestoriuc and Martin (2007) who reported that blood-volume-pulse feedback yielded higher effect sizes than peripheral skin temperature feedback or EMG feedback [22]. Our results are in line with the results from Leistad et al. (2006) who used a slightly different paradigm (60 min of cognitive stress preceding 30 min of relaxation) but reported no difference regarding EMG recordings from the neck muscles between migraine patients and controls [12]. Furthermore, Sandrini and colleagues also applied EMG measurements as a diagnostic tool and reported significantly altered muscle activity in patients with tension-type headache but not in patients with migraine [10]. The higher EMG levels reported by van Boxtel and colleagues refer to the temporalis muscle and not to muscles in the neck [15].

Significantly increased trapezius muscle tension in chronic migraine patients compared to controls during a physical task was reported by Florencio et al. (2016). Participants were required to perform a test aiming to measure deep cervical flexor activity. During this task chronic migraine patients showed significantly more co-activation of the extensor muscles than controls and episodic migraine patients. The authors explain their findings with pain-induced alterations of motor patterns [17]. While this might be a motor strategy for localized tasks such as upper cervical flexion, our findings reveal that altered motor patterns are not generalizable to activities of the lower limb, indicating that there is no tendency towards increased neck muscle tension in situations that do not require neck muscle strength.

One of the limitations of this study was that only one muscle was tested, hence not allowing to compare neck muscle tension with tension in e.g. the jaw muscles. Furthermore, EMG recordings were standardized using voluntary relaxation rather than contraction. And surface EMG recordings are not as precise as needle EMG recordings, which, however, would not have been feasible in our trial. An additional limitation is that headache assessment was based on history and not on headache diaries. However, patients were recruited at a specialised headache clinic. Most of the participants had used diaries for several month prior to participation, hence headache frequency was established based not only on recollection.

Our results from this study neither indicate higher levels of neck muscle tension nor increased durations of tension after stressful incidents in patients with frequent episodic or chronic migraine compared to headache-free controls. Perceived neck muscle tension during the premonitory phase or accompanying migraine headache is therefore more likely a subjective perception not quantifiable by EMG and should be regarded as a symptom of the attack and not as a trapezius muscle dysfunction triggering an attack. This conclusion was based on the evaluation of the trapezius muscle; whether it can be generalized to all neck muscles remains to be investigated by future studies.

Abbreviations

EMG: Electromyography; NDI: Neck disability index; PHQ: Patient health questionnaire; SCM: Sternocleidomastoid; SD: Standard deviation; TTH: Tension type headache

Acknowledgements

The authors thank Ines Garcia-May for helping with data acquisition.

Funding

This work was supported by the 7th Framework EU-project EuroHeadPain (#602633) and by the German Research Foundation, SFB936/A5 to A.M. The funding sources did not influence study conduction in any way.

Authors' contributions

KL: Data acquisition and analysis. Drafting and writing of the manuscript, JM: Data analysis, drafting and writing of the manuscript, AM: Study concept and design, drafting and writing of the manuscript, study supervision. All authors read and approved the final manuscript.

Competing interests

All authors have seen and agreed to the content. All authors declare that they have no competing interests.

Author details

[1]Department of Systems Neuroscience, University Medical Center Eppendorf, Martinistraße 52, 20246 Hamburg, Germany. [2]Department of Academic Physiotherapy, University of Luebeck, Luebeck, Germany.

References

1. Ashina S, Bendtsen L, Lyngberg AC et al (2015) Prevalence of neck pain in migraine and tension-type headache: a population study. Cephalalgia 35: 211–219. https://doi.org/10.1177/0333102414535110
2. Lampl C, Rudolph M, Deligianni CI, Mitsikostas DD (2015) Neck pain in episodic migraine: premonitory symptom or part of the attack? J Headache Pain 16:566. https://doi.org/10.1186/s10194-015-0566-9
3. Calhoun AH, Ford S, Millen C et al (2010) The prevalence of neck pain in migraine. Headache 50:1273–1277. https://doi.org/10.1111/j.1526-4610.2009.01608.x
4. Fernández-de-Las-Peñas C, Cuadrado ML, Pareja JA (2006) Myofascial trigger points, neck mobility and forward head posture in unilateral migraine. Cephalalgia 26:1061–1070. https://doi.org/10.1111/j.1468-2982.2006.01162.x
5. Calandre EP, Hidalgo J, García-Leiva JM, Rico-Villademoros F (2006) Trigger point evaluation in migraine patients: an indication of peripheral sensitization linked to migraine predisposition? Eur J Neurol 13:244–249. https://doi.org/10.1111/j.1468-1331.2006.01181.x
6. Ferracini GN, Chaves TC, Dach F et al (2016) Relationship between active trigger points and head/neck posture in patients with migraine. Am J Phys Med Rehabil 95:831–839. https://doi.org/10.1097/PHM.0000000000000510
7. García-Leiva JM, Hidalgo J, Rico-Villademoros F et al (2007) Effectiveness of ropivacaine trigger points inactivation in the prophylactic management of patients with severe migraine. Pain Med 8:65–70. https://doi.org/10.1111/j.1526-4637.2007.00251.x
8. Giamberardino MA, Tafuri E, Savini A et al (2007) Contribution of myofascial trigger points to migraine symptoms. J Pain 8:869–878. https://doi.org/10.1016/j.jpain.2007.06.002
9. Bansevicius D, Westgaard RH, Sjaastad OM (1999) Tension-type headache: pain, fatigue, tension, and EMG responses to mental activation. Headache 39:417–425
10. Sandrini G, Antonaci F, Pucci E et al (1994) Comparative study with EMG, pressure algometry and manual palpation in tension-type headache and migraine. Cephalalgia 14:451–457 discussion 394–395
11. Göbel H, Weigle L, Kropp P, Soyka D (1992) Pain sensitivity and pain reactivity of pericranial muscles in migraine and tension-type headache. Cephalalgia 12:142–151
12. Leistad RB, Sand T, Westgaard RH et al (2006) Stress-induced pain and muscle activity in patients with migraine and tension-type headache. Cephalalgia 26:64–73. https://doi.org/10.1111/j.1468-2982.2005.00997.x
13. Goudswaard P, Passchier J, Orlebeke JF (1988) EMG in common migraine: changes in absolute and proportional EMG levels during real-life stress. Cephalalgia 8:163–174
14. Pritchard DW (1989) EMG cranial muscle levels in headache sufferers before and during headache. Headache 29:103–108
15. van Boxtel A, Goudswaard P, Janssen K (1983) Absolute and proportional resting EMG levels in muscle contraction and migraine headache patients. Headache: J Head Face Pain 23:215–222. https://doi.org/10.1111/j.1526-4610.1983.hed2305215.x
16. Oksanen A, Pöyhönen T, Ylinen JJ et al (2008) Force production and EMG activity of neck muscles in adolescent headache. Disabil Rehabil 30:231–239. https://doi.org/10.1080/09638280701265430
17. Florencio LL, Oliveira AS, Lemos TW et al (2016) Patients with chronic, but not episodic, migraine display altered activity of their neck extensor muscles. J Electromyogr Kinesiol 30:66–72. https://doi.org/10.1016/j.jelekin.2016.06.003
18. Pryse-Phillips W, Dodick DW, Edmeads JG et al (1998) Guidelines for the nonpharmacologic management of migraine in clinical practice. CMAJ 159:47–54
19. Straube A et al (2007) Therapie primärer chronischer Kopfschmerzen: Chronische Migräne, chronischer Koppfschmerz vom Spannungstyp und andere chronische tägliche Kopfschmerzen. Nervenheilkunde 26(03):186–199 Deutsche Migräne-und Kopfschmerzgesellschaft
20. Duncan CW, Watson DPB, Stein A (2008) Diagnosis and management of headache in adults: summary of SIGN guideline. BMJ 337:a2329. https://doi.org/10.1136/bmj.a2329
21. Fritsche G, Kröner-Herwig B, Kropp P et al (2013) Psychological therapy of migraine: systematic review. Schmerz 27:263–274. https://doi.org/10.1007/s00482-013-1319-9
22. Nestoriuc Y, Martin A (2007) Efficacy of biofeedback for migraine: a meta-analysis. Pain 128:111–127. https://doi.org/10.1016/j.pain.2006.09.007
23. Mullally WJ, Hall K, Goldstein R (2009) Efficacy of biofeedback in the treatment of migraine and tension type headaches. Pain Physician 12:1005–1011
24. Faul F, Erdfelder E, Lang A-G, Buchner A (2007) G*power 3: a flexible statistical power analysis program for the social, behavioral, and biomedical sciences. Behav Res Methods 39:175–191
25. Headache Classification Committee of the International Headache Society (IHS) (2013) The international classification of headache disorders, 3rd edition (beta version). Cephalalgia 33:629–808. https://doi.org/10.1177/0333102413485658
26. Stewart WF, Lipton RB, Kolodner K et al (1999) Reliability of the migraine disability assessment score in a population-based sample of headache sufferers. Cephalalgia 19:107–114 discussion 74
27. Vernon H, Mior S (1991) The neck disability index: a study of reliability and validity. J Manip Physiol Ther 14:409–415
28. Spitzer RL, Kroenke K, Williams JB (1999) Validation and utility of a self-report version of PRIME-MD: the PHQ primary care study. Primary care evaluation of mental disorders. Patient health questionnaire. JAMA 282: 1737–1744

29. Mann HB, Whitney DR (1947) On a test of whether one of two random variables is stochastically larger than the other. Ann Math Stat 18:50–60. https://doi.org/10.1214/aoms/1177730491
30. Sohn J-H, Choi H-C, Jun A-Y (2013) Differential patterns of muscle modification in women with episodic and chronic tension-type headache revealed using surface electromyographic analysis. J Electromyogr Kinesiol 23:110–117. https://doi.org/10.1016/j.jelekin.2012.08.001
31. Fernández-de-las-Peñas C, Falla D, Arendt-Nielsen L, Farina D (2008) Cervical muscle co-activation in isometric contractions is enhanced in chronic tension-type headache patients. Cephalalgia 28:744–751. https://doi.org/10.1111/j.1468-2982.2008.01584.x
32. Schoenen J, Gerard P, De Pasqua V, Juprelle M (1991) EMG activity in pericranial muscles during postural variation and mental activity in healthy volunteers and patients with chronic tension type headache. Headache 31: 321–324

20

Characterization of the trigeminovascular actions of several adenosine A_{2A} receptor antagonists in an in vivo rat model of migraine

Kristian A. Haanes[1†], Alejandro Labastida-Ramírez[1†], Kayi Y. Chan[1], René de Vries[1], Brian Shook[2], Paul Jackson[2], Jimmy Zhang[2], Christopher M. Flores[2], Alexander H. J. Danser[1], Carlos M. Villalón[3] and Antoinette MaassenVanDenBrink[1*]

Abstract

Background: Migraine is considered a neurovascular disorder, but its pathophysiological mechanisms are not yet fully understood. Adenosine has been shown to increase in plasma during migraine attacks and to induce vasodilation in several blood vessels; however, it remains unknown whether adenosine can interact with the trigeminovascular system. Moreover, caffeine, a non-selective adenosine receptor antagonist, is included in many over the counter anti-headache/migraine treatments.

Methods: This study used the rat closed cranial window method to investigate in vivo the effects of the adenosine A_{2A} receptor antagonists with varying selectivity over A_1 receptors; JNJ-39928122, JNJ-40529749, JNJ-41942914, JNJ-40064440 or JNJ-41501798 (0.3–10 mg/kg) on the vasodilation of the middle meningeal artery produced by either CGS21680 (an adenosine A_{2A} receptor agonist) or endogenous CGRP (released by periarterial electrical stimulation).

Results: Regarding the dural meningeal vasodilation produced neurogenically or pharmacologically, all JNJ antagonists: (i) did not affect neurogenic vasodilation but (ii) blocked the vasodilation produced by CGS21680, with a blocking potency directly related to their additional affinity for the adenosine A_1 receptor.

Conclusions: These results suggest that vascular adenosine A_{2A} (and, to a certain extent, also A_1) receptors mediate the CGS21680-induced meningeal vasodilation. These receptors do not appear to modulate prejunctionally the sensory release of CGRP. Prevention of meningeal arterial dilation might be predictive for anti-migraine drugs, and since none of these JNJ antagonists modified per se blood pressure, selective A_{2A} receptor antagonism may offer a novel approach to antimigraine therapy which remains to be investigated in clinical trials.

Keywords: Adenosine receptor, CGS21680, Dural vasodilation, Rat, vasodepressor response

Background

Migraine is a neurovascular disorder associated with activation of the trigeminovascular system and release of calcitonin gene-related peptide (CGRP) from trigeminal sensory perivascular nerves, which results in cranial vasodilation and stimulation of sensory nerve transmission [1]. In line with these neurovascular mechanisms: (i) plasma levels of CGRP, which increase during migraine, are normalized by triptans in parallel with amelioration of headache [2]; and (ii) CGRP receptor antagonists [1] and antibodies against CGRP or its receptor [3] are

* Correspondence: a.vanharen-maassenvandenbrink@erasmusmc.nl
Kristian A. Haanes and Alejandro Labastida-Ramírez contributed equally to this work.
†Equal contributors
[1]Division of Vascular Medicine and Pharmacology, Department of Internal Medicine, Erasmus MC, Rotterdam, Dr Molewaterplein 50, 3015, GE, Rotterdam, The Netherlands
Full list of author information is available at the end of the article

effective in migraine treatment. Although there seem to be some full-responders, the average reduction in migraine days compared to placebo is only in the excess of 1 day per month when administering any CGRP antibody [4]. This limited efficacy resulting from inhibiting CGRP effects suggests that the pathogenesis of migraine could involve additional mechanisms.

Interestingly, adenosine (released centrally and peripherally as a breakdown product of ATP) is another neuromodulator that seems to play a role in migraine pathophysiology [5]. Indeed: (i) adenosine plasma levels have been reported to be increased during migraine attacks [6]; (ii) exogenous adenosine may trigger migraine attacks [7]; (iii) dipyridamole, an adenosine uptake inhibitor, may increase the frequency of migraine attacks [8]; and (iv) an adenosine gene haplotype has been associated with migraine with aura [9]. Accordingly, adenosine receptor antagonists may have potential therapeutic usefulness in the treatment of migraine; while caffeine, a non-selective adenosine receptor antagonist [5], is already present in several over-the-counter anti-headache/migraine medications [10].

The conjunction of structural, transductional and operational criteria has shown that adenosine can activate four subtypes of G-protein-coupled receptors [11, 12], namely adenosine: (i) A_1 and A_3 receptors (coupled to G_i proteins), which mediate vascular smooth muscle constriction; and (ii) A_{2A} and A_{2B} receptors (coupled to G_s proteins), which mediate direct and endothelium-dependent vasodilation [13, 14]. Moreover, the A_1 receptor can also mediate endothelium-dependent vasodilation [15, 16].

Within this framework, it has been shown ex vivo that adenosine and CGS21680, a stable A_{2A} receptor agonist (with about 10–100-fold selectivity for A_{2A} receptors over A_1 and A_3 receptors and poor affinity for A_{2B} receptors [17]), dilate middle meningeal and cerebral arteries respectively, a response blocked by A_{2A} receptor antagonists [13, 18].

The above findings, coupled to the demonstration that the trigeminal ganglion expresses A_{2A} receptors [19] and the ability of this receptor to facilitate CGRP release in the hippocampus [20], beg the questions of whether adenosine A_{2A} receptors can induce meningeal vasodilation in vivo, and also whether they could be involved in neurogenic vasodilation either per se or as modulators of CGRP release in the trigeminovascular system.

Hence, this study used the rat closed cranial window method, a model predictive of antimigraine action [21], to investigate the effects of five novel adenosine A_{2A} receptor antagonists (Fig. 1) on the vasodilation of the middle meningeal artery produced by either CGS21680 or endogenous CGRP (released by periarterial electrical stimulation). These antagonists (JNJ-41942914, JNJ-39928122, JNJ-40529749, JNJ-40064440 and JNJ-41501798) were developed as described by Shook et al. [22] and display a varying degree of selectivity for A_{2A} over A_1 receptors (Table 1).

Methods

Intravital microscopy experiments

Animals

Fifty seven normotensive male Sprague-Dawley rats (300–400 g), purchased from Harlan (Horst, The Netherlands),

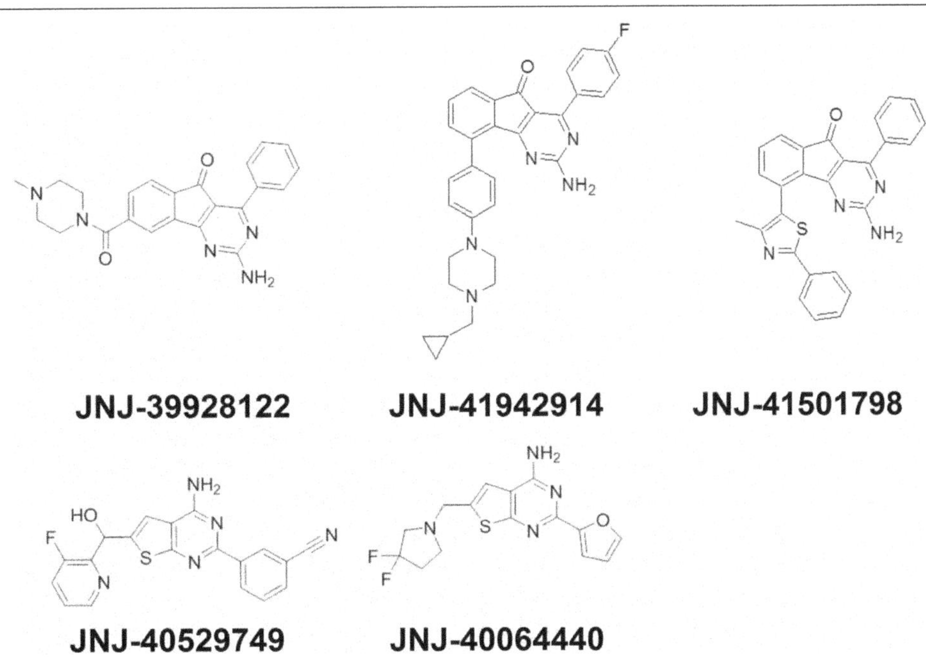

Fig. 1 Molecular structures of the JNJ antagonists from Janssen Research & Development

Table 1 Affinity constants indicated as IC_{50} in nM (and the corresponding pIC_{50}) for the compounds used in the present study

Compound	A_{2A}	A_1	Fold selectivity Selectivity A_{2A} vs. A_1
CGS21680[33]	22 nM (7.6)	3100 nM (5.5)	141
Caffeine[28]	8100 nM (5.1)	20,000 nM (4.7)	2.5
JNJ-39928122[a]	7.9 nM [λ] (8.1)	55.1 nM [λ] (7.3)	7
JNJ-40529749[a]	4.9 nM (8.3)	89.1 nM (7.1)	18
JNJ-41942914[a]	8.3 nM (8.1)	1093 nM (6.0)	132
JNJ-40064440[a]	8.2 nM (8.1)	1240 nM (5.9)	151
JNJ-41501798[a]	11.5 nM (7.9)	7997 nM (5.1)	695

The JNJ antagonists were developed by Johnson & Johnson Pharmaceutical Research & Development, L.L.C
Hutchison et al. 1989 [33]; Fredholm et al. 1999 [28]; [a], Paul Jackson (Janssen Research & Development, personal communication); [λ], Indicates K_i values

were maintained at a 12/12-h light-dark cycle (with light beginning at 7 a.m.) and housed at a constant temperature (22 ± 2°C) and humidity (50%), with food and water ad libitum. Only male rats were used to avoid crosstalk between CGRP and hormonal fluctuations during the female oestrus cycle [23]. The animals were anaesthetized with an intraperitoneal (i.p.) injection of sodium pentobarbital (60 mg/kg, followed by 18 mg/kg i.v. per hour when necessary). The adequacy of anaesthesia was judged by a negative tail flick test and the absence of ocular reflexes, amongst others. All experimental protocols of this study were approved by our Institutional Ethics Committee [Erasmus MC; permission protocol number EMC 1931 (118–09-04)], in accordance with the NIH guide for the Care and Use of Laboratory Animals in U.S.A. and the ARRIVE guidelines for reporting experiments in animals [24]. All rats were randomly assigned into the different experimental protocols (see experimental protocol section).

General methods

After anesthesia, the trachea was cannulated and connected to a pressure ventilator (small animal ventilator SAR-830 series, CWE Inc., Ardmore, PA, U.S.A.). End-tidal pCO_2 was monitored (Capstar-100 CWE Inc., PA, U.S.A.) and kept between 35 and 48 mmHg. The left femoral vein and artery were cannulated for intravenous (i.v.) administration of drugs and continuous monitoring of blood pressure, respectively. Two or three samples of blood (at the beginning and at the end of the experiment) were withdrawn via the femoral artery to monitor blood gases and other parameters, which were kept between normal values (pH: 7.35–7.48; pCO_2: 35–48 mmHg; pO_2: 100–120 mmHg). The body temperature of each rat was monitored via a rectal thermometer and maintained throughout the experiment (36.5 °C–37.5 °C) by a homeothermic blanket system for rodents (Harvard Instruments, Edenbridge, Kent, U.K.). The rats were placed in a stereotaxic frame and the parietal bone overlying a segment of the dural meningeal artery was carefully drilled thin, applying cold saline (4 °C) until the artery was visible. Since skull drilling induces vasodilation, we allowed the animal to recover for 1 h before the experimental protocol. The drilled area was covered with mineral oil to prevent drying and to facilitate visualization of the meningeal artery. The artery was captured with an intravital microscope (model MZ 16; Leica microsystem Ltd., Heerbrugg, Switzerland) using a cyan blue filter on a cold source of light. A zoom lens (80–450 × magnification) and a camera was used to display images with the blood vessel diameter (30–40 μm at baseline) being continuously monitored and measured with a video dimension analyser (Living Systems Instrumentation Inc., Burlington, VT, U.S.A.). In rats where periarterial electrical stimulation was used to evoke dural vasodilation, a bipolar stimulating electrode (NE 200X, Clark Electromedical, Edenbridge, Kent, U.K.) was placed on the surface of the cranial window approximately within 200 μm from the vessel of interest. The cranial window surface was stimulated at 5 Hz, 1 ms for 10 s (Stimulator model S88, Grass Instruments, West Warwick, RI, U.S.A.). For neurogenic dural vasodilation, we initially started with a current intensity (monitored on an oscilloscope, model 54601A, Hewlett Packard, Palo Alto, CA, U.S.A.) of 100 μA and increased with 50 μA steps until a maximal level of dilatation was achieved, usually at 200 μA. The resulting data were displayed and recorded using a WINDAQ data acquisition system (Version 2.54; DataQ Instruments Inc., Akron, OH, U.S.A.).

Experimental protocols

First, 6 animals were used to determine the effect of i.v. adenosine and caffeine on the middle meningeal artery diameter. The doses of adenosine (1 mg/kg) and caffeine (40 mg/kg) were based on previously published work [15, 25]. Further, 51 animals were divided into two groups which received, respectively, periarterial electrical stimulation (150–250 μA; $n = 27$) and the adenosine A_2 receptor agonist CGS21680 (10 μg/kg, i.v., $n = 24$; the optimal dose as determined in 7 pilot experiments, data not shown). Dural vasodilator responses remained unchanged after repeated treatment for 4 times (data not shown) and in the presence of the vehicle captisol, which was used for dissolving most of the antagonists. Thirty min were allowed between each of these treatments for recovery to the baseline diameter. Subsequently, each of these groups was subdivided into five subgroups ($n = 3$–6 each) which were given (after 30 min) i.v. bolus injections of, respectively, the adenosine A_{2A} receptor antagonists JNJ-41942914 (0.3, 1, and 3 mg/kg), JNJ-39928122, JNJ-40529749, JNJ-40064440 and JNJ-41501798 (all 1, 3 and up to 10 mg/kg). Based on their binding affinities (see Table 1), only doses up until significant blockade, were tested for the CGS21580 response. Each antagonist dose was administered 5 min before periarterial electrical stimulation or CGS21680, except for caffeine (15 min) as previously reported [25]. The duration of each experiment was approximately 2.5 h after stabilization.

Data presentation and statistical evaluation

All data are presented as mean ± SEM. The peak increases in dural meningeal artery diameter are expressed as percent change from baseline. Changes in mean arterial blood pressure (MAP) were expressed as absolute values (mm Hg). The difference between the variables within one group was compared by using a one-way repeated measures analysis of variance followed by Dunnet's test. Dunnet's test does not give individual *P*-values, hence statistical significance was accepted at $P < 0.05$. When there was only one dose applied (for caffeine), two-tailed paired Student's T-test was used.

Drugs

The compounds used in this study were: sodium pentobarbital (Nembutal; Ceva Sante Animale B.V., Maassluis, The Netherlands); caffeine, adenosine and CGS21680 hydrochloride hydrate (2-p-(2-Carboxyethyl)phenethylamino-5′-N-ethylcarboxamido adenosine hydrochloride hydrate) (Sigma Chemicals Co., Steinheim, Germany); JNJ-41942914, JNJ-39928122, JNJ-40064440, JNJ-40529749 and JNJ-41501798 (gift courtesy from Janssen Research & Development, L.L.C., Raritan, NJ, U.S.A.). Caffeine, adenosine, CGS21680 and JNJ-40064440 were dissolved in distilled water, whereas JNJ-39928122, JNJ-41942914, JNJ-40529749 and JNJ-41501798 were dissolved in captisol (sulfobutylether β-cyclodextrin; Ligand Pharmaceuticals, San Diego, U.S.A.). The suspensions of JNJ-40529749 and JNJ-41501798 were sonicated and filtrated. All solutions were further diluted in saline.

Results

General considerations

In order to facilitate the interpretation of the following results, the five JNJ antagonists (Table 1) were sub-divided, a priori, into 3 groups (indicated in different grey-tones): (i) JNJ-39928122 and JNJ-40529749 have ~ 10 fold selectivity for A_{2A} over A_1 receptors; (ii) JNJ-41942914 and JNJ-40064440 are ~ 100 fold selective for A_{2A} over A_1 receptors; and (iii) JNJ-41501798 is ~ 700 fold selective for A_{2A} over A_1 receptors. It is also worth mentioning that caffeine has ~ 2.5 fold selectivity for the rat and ~ 5 fold selectivity for the human A_{2A} vs. A_1 receptors [K_D values, [26]]; however, caffeine also inhibits A_{2B} receptor with similar affinity as for A_1, which is not the case for the JNJ antagonists.

Effects of i.v. adenosine and caffeine on dural diameter and MAP

We initially set out to determine the effect of adenosine on the dural diameter in vivo. Figure 2 shows that (i) 1 mg/kg adenosine caused a dural artery dilation of 50 ± 6% and a drop in blood pressure to 53 ± 4 mmHg; (ii) 40 mg/kg caffeine caused a non-significant dural artery dilation of 12 ± 5%, while blood pressure was increased significantly by 14 ± 3 mmHg; (iii) after a stabilizing period post-caffeine, the second dural artery dilation produced by adenosine was reduced to 25 ± 6% ($n = 6$, $p = 0.003$, which was accompanied by a significantly attenuated drop in blood pressure, to 69 ± 5 mmHg ($p = 0.004$).

Effect of the JNJ antagonists on the dural dilatation by periarterial electrical stimulation

In order to investigate whether the dural dilation induced by periarterial electrical stimulation could be in part dependent on adenosine release, either as direct activation of vascular adenosine receptors or prejunctional modulation

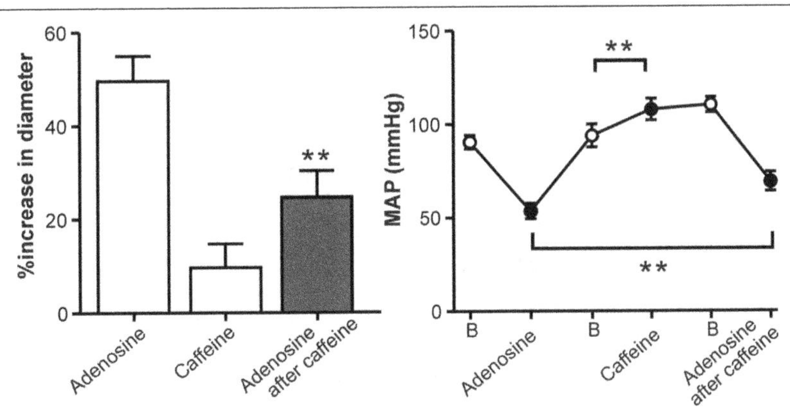

Fig. 2 The effect of caffeine on adenosine-induced dural vasodilation. Adenosine (1 mg/kg) was injected i.v. after a recovery period of 30 min. Then, caffeine (40 mg/kg) was injected slowly, and a second adenosine injection (1 mg/kg) was injected 15 min after the caffeine injection (adenosine after caffeine). Left panel illustrates increase in diameter and right panel changes in mean arterial blood pressure, in response to adenosine. Data are ± SEM, $n = 6$, ** $p < 0.01$ compared to the control. Open circles represent baseline measurements before injections, B=Baseline

of trigeminal CGRP release, the JNJ antagonists (given i.v.) were investigated in their capability to modify the dural vasodilation produced by electrical stimulation. As shown in Fig. 3 (left panels), neurogenic stimulation induced, overall, an immediate increase in dural artery diameter of 83 ± 7% ($n = 27$). Surprisingly, none of the JNJ antagonists affected this neurogenic vasodilation (left panels). Suggesting that neither A_1 nor A_{2A} receptors are involved.

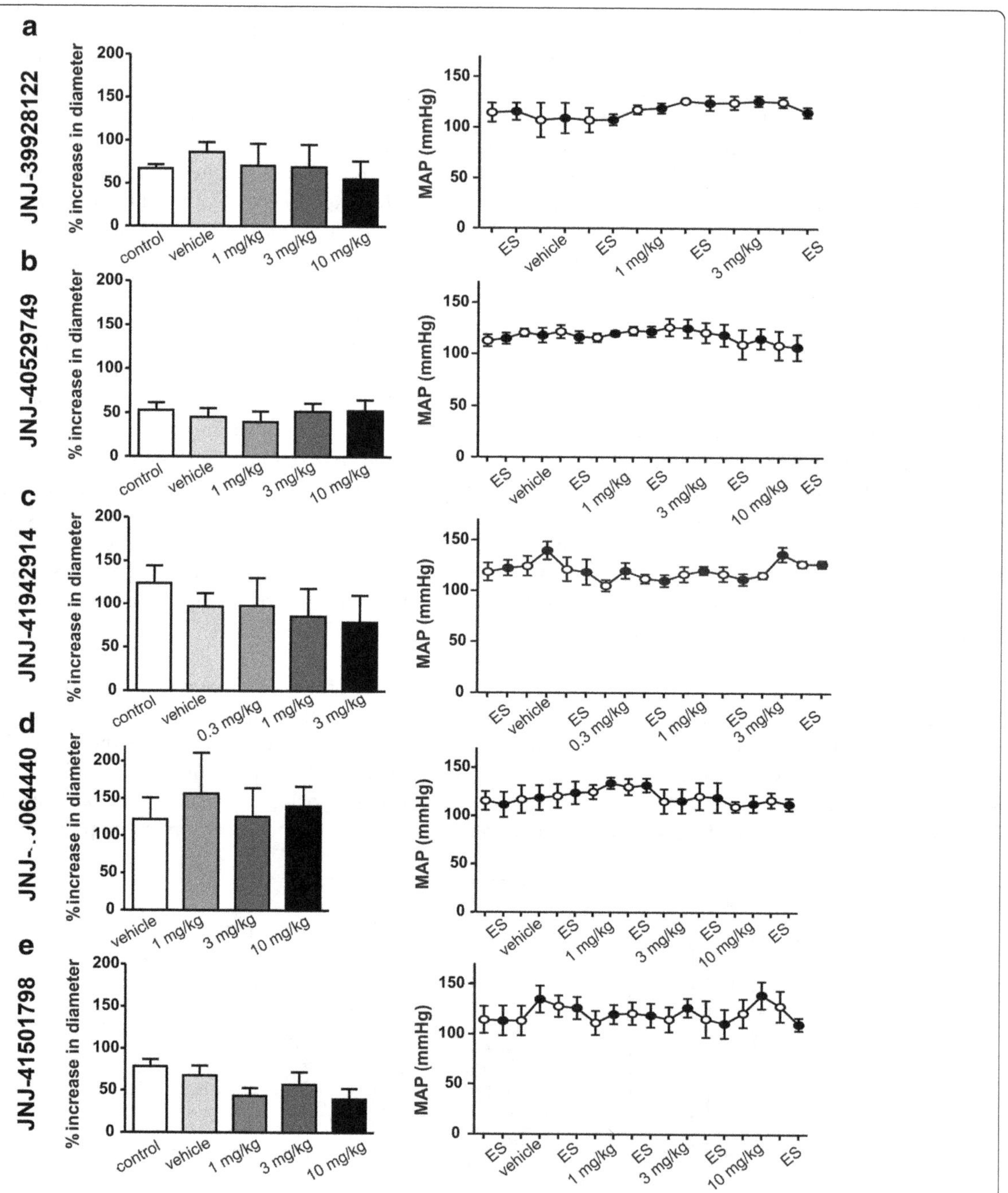

Fig. 3 Effect of A_{2A} antagonists on perivascular electrical stimulation of the dural artery. Perivascular electrical stimulation (150–250 μA) in the absence or presence of vehicle, or varying doses of JNJ-39928122 (A, $n = 4$), JNJ-40529749 (B, n = 4–5), JNJ-41942914 (C, n = 6), JNJ-40064440 (D, n = 4), or JNJ-41501798 (E, $n = 7$–8). Data are presented as percentage of increase in diameter, left panels) and changes in mean arterial blood pressure (mm Hg, right panels) induced by periarterial electrical stimulation (ES). Note that none of the treatments produced any significant changes ($p > 0.05$ compared to the vehicle). Open circles represent baseline measurements before injections/ES. JNJ-40064440 was dissolved in water, so vehicle measurements equal control

The effect of the JNJ antagonists on MAP before and during neurogenic dural stimulation

As shown in Fig. 3 (right panels), both periarterial electrical stimulation and the JNJ antagonists were devoid of any effect per se on MAP.

Effects of CGS21680 on dural artery diameter and MAP

Although adenosine A_{2A} or A_1 receptors did not appear to be important in the vasodilation observed after neurogenic dural stimulation, adenosine vasodilates dural arteries in vivo (Fig. 2), most likely via both A_{2A} and A_{2B} receptors as previously reported ex vivo [13]. Since our study set out to study specifically the role of the adenosine A_{2A} receptor, we continued our study using CGS21680, which is a more biologically stable, highly selective for A_{2A} over A_{2B} receptor agonist [17].

As shown in Fig. 4, CGS21680 (10 μg/kg before administration of JNJ antagonists; $n = 24$) mimicked adenosine in its capability to produce: (i) a marked dilation of the dural artery diameter (66 ± 9%; left panels); and (ii) a drop in blood pressure (53 ± 9 mmHg; right panels) and hence excluding the involvement of A_{2B} receptors.

The lower the selectivity (A_{2A} over A_1 receptors) the higher the potency of JNJ antagonists to block CGS21680-induced dural vasodilation

To further uncover the nature of the adenosine receptors in the dural vasculature, we explored the effect of the JNJ antagonist with varying selectivity (A_{2A} over A_1 receptors). Figure 4 (left panels) also shows that all JNJ antagonists significantly blocked the CGS21680-induced dural vasodilation with varying degrees of potency. Specifically, the vasodilation to CGS21680 was: (i) abolished by 1 mg/kg (− 1 ± 2%) of JNJ-39928122 (Fig. 4a); (ii) abolished at 1 mg/kg (− 2 ± 1%) of JNJ-40529749 (Fig. 4b); (iii) significantly attenuated (but not abolished) by 3 mg/kg (21 ± 11%) of JNJ-41942914 (Fig. 4c); (iv) significantly attenuated by 3 mg/kg (23 ± 15%) and abolished (1 ± 3%) by 10 mg/kg of JNJ-40064440 (Fig. 4d); and (v) dose-dependently blocked, and practically abolished by 10 mg/kg (5 ± 4%) of JNJ-41501798 (Fig. 4e). Clearly, the lower the selectivity of A_{2A} vs. A_1 (Table 1) the higher the potency of JNJ antagonists to block CGS21680-induced dural vasodilation.

Effect of JNJ antagonists on CGS21680-induced vasodepressor responses

Similarly, the vasodepressor responses to CGS21680 were blocked by the JNJ antagonists as follows: (i) very potently by the less selective antagonists JNJ-39928122 and JNJ-40529749; and (ii) less potently by the highest doses of the more selective antagonists JNJ-41942914, JNJ-40064440 and JNJ-41501798, which display from low to very low affinity for the A_1 receptor (Table 1).

Discussion

Comparison between in vivo and in vitro vascular responses to adenosine

The adenosine receptor antagonists SCH58261 (478-fold A_{2A} over A_1 selective [27]) and caffeine (non-selective $A_{1/2A/2B}$ [28]) have been shown to block the ex vivo adenosine-induced dilation of endothelium-denuded middle meningeal arteries [18]. In these experiments, not only did caffeine (50 μM) or SCH58261 (1 μM) prevent the dural dilation, but a vasoconstriction to adenosine was unmasked. Interestingly, this effect was not observed in vivo, which could be due to the fact that the artery used for the myograph (outer diameter ~ 100 μm) had a larger diameter than in this study (outer diameter ~ 35 μm) and that there potentially are less A_3 receptors expressed in smaller vessels, as we see no indirect involvement of A_3 (i.e. vasoconstriction) in the current experiments. These differences require further investigation, but it is known that receptor expression changes along different vascular beds [29].

General considerations

In addition to the implications discussed below, the present study shows that: (i) both adenosine and CGS21680 produced rat dural vasodilation in vivo; and (ii) for JNJ antagonists, the lower the selectivity (A_{2A} over A_1 receptors) the higher the potency to block the dural vasodilation and vasodepressor responses induced by CGS21680 (implying that blockade of A_1 receptors is also necessary to completely block the dural vasodilation in vivo). The latter finding is most likely due to endothelial A_1 receptors, as the main difference between the in vivo (present study) and the ex vivo studies [18] is the absence of endothelium. Indeed, Honey et al. [21] have shown the presence of adenosine A_1 receptors mediating vasodilation in the rat middle meningeal artery in vivo.

The potential role of A_{2A} and A_1 receptors in the dural vasodilation as prejunctional modulators of neurogenic dural vasodilation or produced by CGS21680

The simplest interpretation of the fact that the JNJ antagonists had no effect on neurogenic dural vasodilation (Fig. 3), which involves CGRP release [1], implies that: (i) adenosine is not released by periarterial electrical stimulation; (ii) A_{2A} receptors do not constitute a positive feedback mechanism for CGRP release, as expected from its transductional properties (positive coupling to G_s proteins; [11]); or (iii) cAMP increase, induced by CGRP, is so high that this could have masked the small increase in cAMP levels mediated by A_{2A} receptors [26]. Interestingly, adenosine A_1 receptors [coupled to G_i

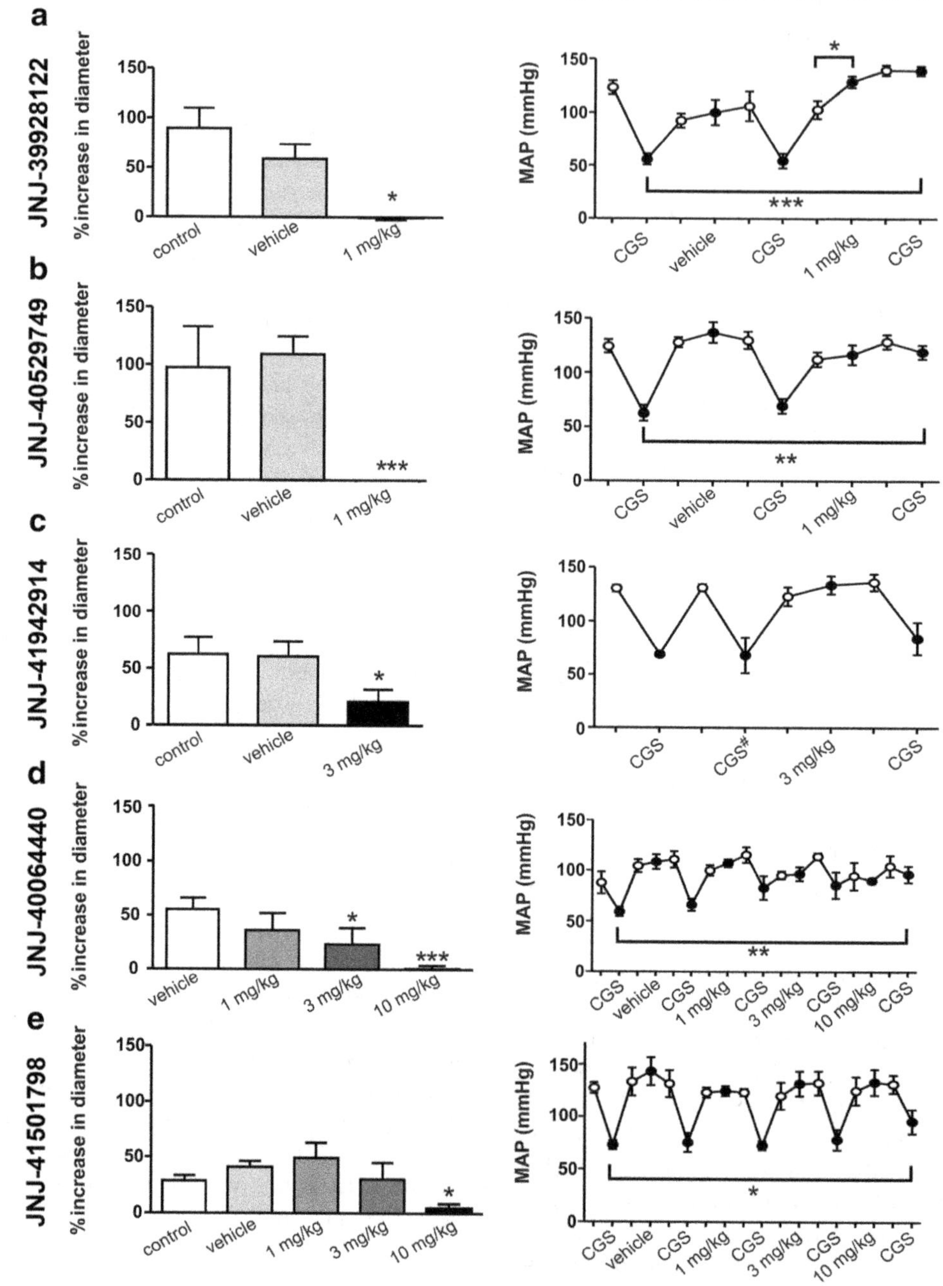

Fig. 4 Effect of i.v. CGS21680 on the dural diameter. CGS21680 (10 μg/kg) was injected followed by an injection of vehicle and varying doses of JNJ-39928122 (**a**), $n = 5$, Dunnet critical value: 1014), JNJ-40529749 (**b**), $n = 3$–5, Dunnet critical value: 3791) JNJ-41942914 (**c**), $n = 4$, Dunnet critical value: 6008), JNJ-40064440 (**d**), $n = 3$–4, Dunnet critical value: 8446), or JNJ-41501798 (**e**), $n = 5$–6, Dunnet critical value: 5848). Data are presented as percentage of increase in diameter (left panels) and changes in mean arterial blood pressure (mm Hg, right panels) induced by CGS21680 (left lower panels). CGS, 10 μg/kg CGS21680 i.v.; * $p < 0.05$, ** $p < 0.01$, *** $p < 0.001$ compared to the vehicle. #CGS in presence of vehicle. Open circles represent baseline measurements before injections. JNJ-40064440 was dissolved in water, so vehicle measurements equal control

proteins; [11]] can produce a prejunctional inhibition of the neurogenic dural vasodilation in rats [21]. However, the weakly selective JNJ antagonists (JNJ-39928122 and JNJ-40529749), which would be theoretically expected to block (at least in part) this mechanism, did not increase neurogenic dural vasodilation (Fig. 3).

Several lines of evidence have previously shown in other systems that: (i) the vasodilation produced by adenosine and related agonists is mainly mediated by vascular and endothelial A_{2A} receptors [13, 14] as well as by endothelial A_1 receptors [16]; and (ii) the trigeminovascular system expresses A_{2A} receptors [19]. In keeping with these findings, our results further demonstrate that the JNJ antagonists blocked CGS21680-induced dural vasodilation (Fig. 4), with a different profile of blockade (dependent on A_{2A} vs. A_1 selectivity; see below). This reinforces the involvement of adenosine A_{2A} and, probably to a lesser extent, of A_1 receptors. In addition, based on the poor affinity of CGS21680 for the A_{2B} receptors [17] and similar responses to adenosine, our data did not show any strong involvement of the A_{2B} receptors.

Systemic effects of JNJ antagonists on A_{2A} and A_1 receptors

Caffeine is a non-selective adenosine A_1, A_{2A} and A_{2B} receptor antagonist that does not affect A_3 receptors at the doses used [28]. Accordingly, caffeine produced a slight increase in blood pressure (Fig. 2), as previously reported [25]. Interestingly, the fact that none of the JNJ antagonists increased blood pressure (Fig. 4, right panel), even at doses that blocked the dural vasodilation to CGS21680 (Fig. 4, left panel) suggests that there is no strong "adenosine vascular tone". In addition, it is worth emphasizing that A_{2B} receptors are involved in the blood pressure effects of adenosine [30], which would explain the minor difference between caffeine and the JNJ antagonists in our study.

It is well established that A_{2A} receptor agonists lower blood pressure [12, 31]. The A_1 receptor agonists GR79236 and N6-cyclopentyladenosine (CPA), although less studied, also decrease blood pressure with higher potency than CGS21680, and both cause direct production of endothelial NO [15, 16, 31]. Hence, the vasodepressor response to adenosine in A_1 −/− mice is reduced [32]. In the present study, the less selective (JNJ-39928122 and JNJ-40529749) A_{2A} vs. A_1 antagonists potently blocked the decrease in blood pressure, whereas the more selective (JNJ-40064440 and JNJ-41501798) A_{2A} antagonists were less potent, and only effective at 10 mg/kg. These high doses of JNJ-4006440 and JNJ-41501798 also induced inihibition of A_1 receptors. Blockade of the adenosine A_{2A} and A_1 receptors prevents systemic vasodilation in response to adenosine, and therefore the block in blood pressure.

In vivo effects of CGS21680

In binding affinity studies, CGS21680 is 141-fold selective for A_{2A} over A_1 receptors [33]. However, our study raises the concern whether CGS21680 is a specific A_{2A} receptor agonist in vivo in rats, as it appears that higher blocking affinities for the A_1 receptor causes a more potent blockade of the vasodepressor and dural vasodilator responses. For the human adenosine receptors, the selectivity for A_{2A} over A_1 receptors is minimal [34].

The most obvious explanation for the apparent discrepancy between the binding affinity selectively and the in vivo effects, is the location of adenosine receptors, as A_1 receptors are on the endothelium, whereas the A_{2A} receptors are mainly located on vascular smooth muscle [12]; hence the endothelium will be directly exposed to an apparently higher concentration. In addition, there are opposing findings on the selectivity of CGS21680. For example CGS21680 binds with high affinity (around 1 nM) to A_1 receptors in the hippocampus of A_{2A}−/− mice [35], in contrast, in the same mice CGS21680 had no effect on blood pressure [36].

Comparing our findings with previous studies in rats, the vasodepressor response to CGS21680 (10 μg/kg) was completely blocked by 3 mg/kg of the A_{2A} receptor antagonists ZM241385 [319-fold A_{2A} over A_1; [15, 27]] or CGS15943 [9-fold A_{2A} over A_1; [37]]. Clearly, ZM241385 has a higher A_{2A} over A_1 selectivity, but its K_i for A_1 receptors is 255 nM. Since these binding data are similar to those of our less selective compounds, A_{2A} and also A_1 receptors would be blocked in these studies.

Possible clinical implications

On the basis of the above lines of evidence, the antimigraine potential of selective adenosine A_{2A} receptor antagonists would be of particular relevance in those patients whose adenosine plasma levels are markedly increased during a migraine attack. Although our findings indicate that adenosine is not released by perivascular electrical stimulation, inhibition of dural vasodilation is a shared mechanism of current (ergots and triptans) and prospective (CGRP (receptor) antagonists and antibodies) antimigraine drugs [1, 38]. Whether this (antimigraine) mechanism alone is sufficient to attenuate the trigeminal nociceptive transmission associated with migraine headache, remains to be determined. Additionally, other studies have shown that: (i) activation of A_{2A} receptors facilitates the action of CGRP and VIP in the rat hippocampus [20]; (ii) A_{2A} receptor knockout mice are hypoalgesic [36]; and (iii) A_{2A} receptors are expressed in the rat trigeminovascular system [19] as well as in the rat trigeminal ganglion, together with A_1, A_{2B} and A_3 receptors [18]. Furthermore, intra-articular administration of adenosine and N6-cyclohexyladenosine (CHA, an adenosine A_1 receptor agonist), but not CGS21680, significantly increased ketorolac antinociception [39]. These findings, taken together: (i) argue in favor of selective blockade of adenosine A_2 receptors as a potential antimigraine strategy; and (ii) imply that blockade of A_1 receptors would be a disadvantage in antimigraine treatment. Obviously, further clinical studies should evaluate the JNJ antagonist(s) with the optimal oral bioavailability based on their pharmacokinetic properties.

Conclusions

In conclusion, all the JNJ antagonists were capable of blocking CGS21680-induced dural vasodilation without affecting neurogenic dural vasodilation (suggesting no modulation of trigeminal CGRP release). This blockade was more potent when showing lower A_{2A} over A_1 selectivity, and that both these receptors are involved in the dural artery vasodilation. On this basis, and considering that the JNJ antagonist were devoid of any effect per se on blood pressure, selective A_{2A} receptor antagonism may offer a novel approach to antimigraine therapy that remains to be determined in clinical trials.

Abbreviations
CGRP : Calcitonin gene-related peptide; i.p. : Intraperitoneal; i.v. : Intravenous

Acknowledgments
Dr. Antoinette MaassenVanDenBrink was supported by the Netherlands Organisation for Scientific Research (Vidi grant 917.113.349), whereas Prof. Carlos M. Villalón and Alejandro Labastida-Ramírez were supported by Consejo Nacional de Ciencia y Tecnología (CONACyT; Grant No. 219707 to CMV and fellowship No. 410778 to ALR; Mexico City). Dr. Kristian A. Haanes was supported by a postdoctoral fellowship from the International Headache Society.

Funding
This study was supported by a grant from Janssen Research & Development.

Authors' contributions
Participated in research design: KAH, ALR, KYC, CMV, AMVDB. Conducted Experiments: KAH, ALR, KYC, RDV. Contributed reagents or analytical tools: BS, PJ, JZ, AHJD, AMVDB. Performed data analysis: KAH, ALR, KYC, CMV, AMVDB. Wrote or contributed to the writing of the manuscript: KAH, ALR, KYC, BS, PJ, JZ, CMF, AHJD, CMV, AMVDB. All authors read and approved the final manuscript.

Competing interests
The authors have nothing to disclose. Jannsen was not involved in the experimental design or the interpretation of the results.

Author details
[1]Division of Vascular Medicine and Pharmacology, Department of Internal Medicine, Erasmus MC, Rotterdam, Dr Molewaterplein 50, 3015, GE, Rotterdam, The Netherlands. [2]Janssen Research & Development, L.L.C, Welsh and McKean Roads, Spring House, PA 19477, USA. [3]Departamento de Farmacobiología, Cinvestav-Coapa, Czda. de los Tenorios 235, Col. Granjas-Coapa, Deleg. Tlalpan, C.P, 14330 Ciudad de México, Mexico.

References
1. Edvinsson L, Villalón CM, MaassenVanDenBrink A (2012) Basic mechanims of migraine and its acute treatment. Pharmacol Ther 136:319–333
2. Goadsby PJ, Edvinsson L (1993) The trigeminovascular system and migraine: studies characterizing cerebrovascular and neuropeptide changes seen in humans and cats. Ann Neurol 33:48–56
3. Mitsikostas DD, Reuter U (2017) Calcitonin gene-related peptide monoclonal antibodies for migraine prevention: comparisons across randomized controlled studies. Curr Opin Neurol 30:272–280
4. Deen M, Correnti E, Kamm K, Kelderman T, Papetti L, Rubio-Beltrán E et al (2017) Blocking CGRP in migraine patients - a review of pros and cons. J Headache Pain 18:96
5. Shapiro RE (2007) Caffeine and headaches. Neurol Sci 28(Suppl 2):S179–S183
6. Guieu R, Devaux C, Henry H, Bechis G, Pouget J, Mallet D et al (1998) Adenosine and migraine. Can J Neurol Sci 25:55–58
7. Brown SG, Waterer GW (1995) Migraine precipitated by adenosine. Med J Aust 162(389):391
8. Hawkes CH (1978) Dipyridamole in migraine. Lancet 2:153
9. Hohoff C, Marziniak M, Lesch KP, Deckert J, Sommer C, Mossner R (2007) An adenosine A2A receptor gene haplotype is associated with migraine with aura. Cephalalgia 27:177–181
10. Derry CJ, Derry S, Moore RA (2014) Caffeine as an analgesic adjuvant for acute pain in adults. Cochrane Database Syst Rev 12:CD009281
11. Burnstock G (2007) Purine and pyrimidine receptors. Cell Mol Life Sci 64: 1471–1483
12. Burnstock G, Ralevic V (2014) Purinergic signaling and blood vessels in health and disease. Pharmacol Rev 66:102–192
13. Ngai AC, Coyne EF, Meno JR, West GA, Winn HR (2001) Receptor subtypes mediating adenosine-induced dilation of cerebral arterioles. Am J Physiol Heart Circ Physiol 280:H2329–H2335
14. Shin HK, Park SN, Hong KW (2000) Implication of adenosine A2A receptors in hypotension-induced vasodilation and cerebral blood flow autoregulation in rat pial arteries. Life Sci 67:1435–1445
15. Kirkup AJ, Eastwood C, Grundy D, Chessell IP, Humphrey PP (1998) Characterization of adenosine receptors evoking excitation of mesenteric afferents in the rat. Br J Pharmacol 125:1352–1360
16. Ray CJ, Marshall JM (2006) The cellular mechanisms by which adenosine evokes release of nitric oxide from rat aortic endothelium. J Physiol 570:85–96
17. Liang BT, Urso M, Zambraski E, Jacobson KA. Adenosine A3 receptors in muscle protection. A3 Adenosine Receptors from Cell Biology to Pharmacology and Therapeutics. Dordrecht: Springer; 2010. p. 257–280
18. Haanes KA, Edvinsson L (2014) Expression and characterization of purinergic receptors in rat middle meningeal artery-potential role in migraine. PLoS One 9:e108782
19. Lu W, Li B, Chen J, Su Y, Dong X, Su X et al (2016) Expression of calcitonin gene-related peptide, adenosine A2a receptor and adenosine A1 receptor in experiment rat migraine models. Biomed Rep 4:379–383
20. Sebastiao AM, Macedo MP, Ribeiro JA (2000) Tonic activation of a(2A) adenosine receptors unmasks, and of a(1) receptors prevents, a facilitatory action of calcitonin gene-related peptide in the rat hippocampus. Br J Pharmacol 129:374–380
21. Honey AC, Bland-Ward PA, Connor HE, Feniuk W, Humphrey PP (2002) Study of an adenosine A1 receptor agonist on trigeminally evoked dural blood vessel dilation in the anaesthetized rat. Cephalalgia 22:260–264
22. Shook BC, Rassnick S, Hall D, Rupert KC, Heintzelman GR, Hansen K et al (2010) Methylene amine substituted arylindenopyrimidines as potent adenosine a(2A)/a(1) antagonists. Bioorg Med Chem Lett 20:2864–2867
23. Labastida-Ramírez A, Rubio-Beltrán E, Villalón CM, MaassenVanDenBrink A (2017) Gender aspects of CGRP in migraine. Cephalalgia 333102417739584. https://doi.org/10.1177/0333102417739584
24. McGrath J, Drummond G, McLachlan E, Kilkenny C, Wainwright C (2010) Guidelines for reporting experiments involving animals: the ARRIVE guidelines. Br J Pharmacol 160:1573–1576
25. Meno JR, Nguyen TS, Jensen EM, Alexander West G, Groysman L, Kung DK et al (2005) Effect of caffeine on cerebral blood flow response to somatosensory stimulation. J Cereb Blood Flow Metab 25:775–784
26. Arslan G, Kull B, Fredholm BB (1999) Signaling via A2A adenosine receptor in four PC12 cell clones. Naunyn Schmiedeberg's Arch Pharmacol 359:28–32
27. Ongini E, Dionisotti S, Gessi S, Irenius E, Fredholm BB (1999) Comparison of CGS 15943, ZM 241385 and SCH 58261 as antagonists at human adenosine receptors. Naunyn Schmiedeberg's Arch Pharmacol 359:7–10
28. Fredholm BB, Battig K, Holmen J, Nehlig A, Zvartau EE (1999) Actions of caffeine in the brain with special reference to factors that contribute to its widespread use. Pharmacol Rev 51:83–133
29. Haanes KA, Spray S, Syberg S, Jorgensen NR, Robaye B, Boeynaems JM et al (2016) New insights on pyrimidine signalling within the arterial vasculature - different roles for P2Y2 and P2Y6 receptors in large and small coronary arteries of the mouse. J Mol Cell Cardiol 93:1–11
30. Teng B, Fil D, Tilley SL, Ledent C, Krahn T, Mustafa SJ (2013) Functional and RNA expression profile of adenosine receptor subtypes in mouse mesenteric arteries. J Cardiovasc Pharmacol 61:70–76
31. Schindler CW, Karcz-Kubicha M, Thorndike EB, Muller CE, Tella SR, Ferre S et al (2005) Role of central and peripheral adenosine receptors in the cardiovascular responses to intraperitoneal injections of adenosine A1 and A2A subtype receptor agonists. Br J Pharmacol 144:642–650

32. Koeppen M, Eckle T, Eltzschig HK (2009) Selective deletion of the A1 adenosine receptor abolishes heart-rate slowing effects of intravascular adenosine in vivo. PLoS One 4:e6784
33. Hutchison AJ, Webb RL, Oei HH, Ghai GR, Zimmerman MB, Williams M (1989) CGS 21680C, an A2 selective adenosine receptor agonist with preferential hypotensive activity. J Pharmacol Exp Ther 251:47–55
34. de Lera Ruiz M, Lim YH, Zheng J (2014) Adenosine A2A receptor as a drug discovery target. J Med Chem 57:3623–3650
35. Halldner L, Lopes LV, Dare E, Lindstrom K, Johansson B, Ledent C et al (2004) Binding of adenosine receptor ligands to brain of adenosine receptor knock-out mice: evidence that CGS 21680 binds to A1 receptors in hippocampus. Naunyn Schmiedeberg's Arch Pharmacol 370:270–278
36. Ledent C, Vaugeois JM, Schiffmann SN, Pedrazzini T, El Yacoubi M, Vanderhaeghen JJ et al (1997) Aggressiveness, hypoalgesia and high blood pressure in mice lacking the adenosine A2a receptor. Nature 388:674–678
37. Patel M, Sheehan MJ, Strong P (1994) Failure of CGS15943A to block the hypotensive action of agonists acting at the adenosine A3 receptor. Br J Pharmacol 113:741–748
38. Rivera-Mancilla E, Aviles-Rosas VH, Manrique-Maldonado G, Altamirano-Espinoza AH, Villanueva-Castillo B, MaassenVanDenBrink A et al (2017) The role of alpha1- and alpha2-adrenoceptor subtypes in the vasopressor responses induced by dihydroergotamine in ritanserin-pretreated pithed rats. J Headache Pain 18:104
39. Aguirre-Banuelos P, Castaneda-Hernandez G, Lopez-Munoz FJ, Granados-Soto V (1999) Effect of coadministration of caffeine and either adenosine agonists or cyclic nucleotides on ketorolac analgesia. Eur J Pharmacol 377: 175–182

21

Survival outcome and mortality rate in patients with migraine

Tomor Harnod[1,2], Cheng-Li Lin[3,4] and Chia-Hung Kao[5,6,7*]

Abstract

Background: Whether the patients with migraine have an elevated mortality risk in Taiwan is unclear.

Methods: We analyzed a subset of the National Health Insurance Research Database of Taiwan and enrolled patients (≥20 years old) who received a diagnosis of migraine between 2000 and 2012. The migraine cohort was further divided into the ones ever with status migrainosus (SM) and non-status migraine (NM) subcohort and compared with a 1:4 age-, sex-, comorbidity-, and index date-matched comparison cohort. We calculated the adjusted hazard ratios (aHRs) and 95% confidence intervals (CIs) for subsequent mortality risk after adjustment for age, sex, and comorbidities.

Results: Compared with the comparison cohort, the corresponding aHRs for mortality were 0.81 (95% CI = 0.76–0.87), 0.89 (95% CI = 0.80–0.98), and 0.78 (95% CI = 0.72–0.84) in the total migraine, SM, and NM cohorts, respectively. SM, male sex, comorbid alcohol-related illness, depression, and mental disorders were identified as risk factors for subsequent mortality. Comorbid alcohol-related illness significantly increased the mortality risk in patients with migraine.

Conclusion: Taiwanese patients with migraine require comprehensive and universal medical care. These patients would benefit from controlling their migraines and reducing the subsequent mortality.

Keywords: Cohort study, Migraine, Mortality, National Health Insurance

Background

Migraine is a major disabling disease worldwide. Numerous epidemiological studies conducted in developed Western countries have found that migraines affect approximately 20% of the general population [1, 2]. An international study in developing Asian countries showed that migraine accounts for 66.6% (range: 50.9%–85.8%) of all headache services at neurological clinics [3]. Globally, migraine is approximately 2 times more prevalent in women than in men, particularly in young and middle-aged women during menstruation [2, 4, 5]. Migraine not only affects the central nervous system and disrupts daily life but also increases life-threatening comorbid psychological and cardiovascular diseases in patients [6, 7]. The prevalence for migraine has been investigated a lot for the past 50 years and described the burden of migraine on individuals and communities worldwide [5, 8]. Researchers have proposed that patients with migraine have a higher risk of mortality due to a high vulnerability to other fatal diseases. Although numerous studies have examined the markers for the long-term outcomes of migraine, the actual mortality risk in patients with migraine has remained unclear so far [5, 8, 9]. Therefore, further investigation is required to understand the correlated mortality in patients with migraine to elucidate future treatment strategies for migraine.

Treatment-resistant migraine or status migrainosus (SM) poses a unique and difficult challenge to headache specialists. Patients with such a condition may experience considerably more disability than patients with a classic, non-status migraine (NM) and thus may require specific pharmacological treatment or adopt psychological strategies to reduce the burden of the disease [10]. There might be different mortality risks in these 2

* Correspondence: d10040@mail.cmuh.org.tw; dr.kaochiahung@gmail.com
[5]Graduate Institute of Biomedical Sciences and School of Medicine, College of Medicine, China Medical University, No. 2, Yuh-Der Road, Taichung 404, Taiwan
[6]Department of Nuclear Medicine and PET Center, China Medical University Hospital, Taichung, Taiwan
Full list of author information is available at the end of the article

groups of patients compared with the general population. We used a nationwide, population-based database to investigate the subsequent mortality rates in patients ever with SM and NM. The findings of this study might constructively inform the development and implementation of effective treatment strategies to reduce the migraine burden in Taiwan.

Methods

Data source

This population-based cohort study used the Longitudinal Health Insurance Database (LHID) provided by the National Health Research Institutes in Taiwan. Since March 1995, the Taiwanese government has managed a National Health Insurance (NHI) program that provides comprehensive universal health insurance to approximately 99.9% of the Taiwan population (more than 23 million individuals) [11, 12]. The details of the LHID and NHI program have been well documented [13, 14]. In this study, diagnoses were coded according to the International Classification of Diseases, Ninth Revision, Clinical Modification (ICD-9-CM). This study was approved by the Ethics Review Board of China Medical University in Taiwan (CMUH-104-REC2–115).

Participants

The migraine cohort was composed of patients with newly diagnosed SM (ICD-9-CM code 346.9, and without code 346.90 or 346.91) or NM (ICD-9-CM code 346.x except 346.9) from January 1, 2000 to December 31, 2012. The date of the diagnosis was defined as the index date. The comparison cohort comprised patients without a migraine diagnosis in the LHID. For each identified patient with migraine, 4 non-migraine participants from the LHID were randomly selected for the comparison cohort and were frequency matched with age (each 5-year span); sex; and comorbidities of depression (ICD-9-CM 296.2, 296.3, 296.82, 300.4, and 311), mental disorders (ICD-9-CM 290–319), insomnia (ICD-9-CM 307.4 and 780.5), alcohol-related illness (ICD-9-CM 291, 303, 305.00, 305.01, 305.02, 305.03, 571.0, 571.1, 571.3, 790.3, and V11.3), and anxiety (ICD-9-CM 300.00); and index date (year). Patients aged < 20 years or with incomplete demographic information were excluded (Fig. 1). The participants were followed until death, withdrawal from the NHI, or the end of 2013, whichever occurred first.

Statistical analysis

The distributions of demographic characteristics, including age, sex, and comorbidities, were compared between the migraine and non-migraine cohorts. The differences were examined using the chi-square and t tests for categorical and continuous variables, respectively. We calculated the incidence density rates of subsequent mortality for the total migraine, SM, NM, and comparison cohorts. Univariable and multivariable Cox proportional hazard regression analyses were used to assess the risk of mortality associated with migraine compared with the comparison cohort. Hazard ratios (HRs) and 95% confidence intervals (CIs) were estimated in the Cox models. In a multivariable model, we adjusted for age, sex, and comorbidities of depression, mental disorders, insomnia, alcohol-related illness, and anxiety, all of

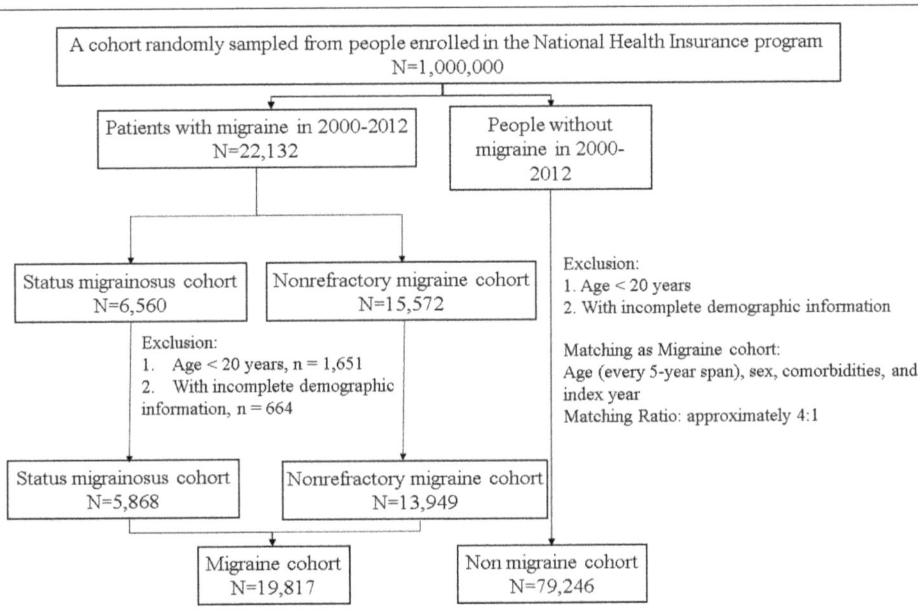

Fig. 1 The flowchart of participant selection in the study cohorts

which had a significant difference in the univariable model. A multivariable regression analysis was used to estimate the average number of hospital days per year for all-cause admissions and frequency of migraine-related medical visits annually, and those associated with the risk factors in patients with migraine were determined using a stepwise selection method. We used SAS (version 9.4, Statistical Analysis System Institute Inc., Cary, NC, USA) for the data analyses. A two-tailed P value of < 0.05 was considered indicative of statistical significance.

Results

In total, 19,817 patients with migraine were selected (70.4% NM and 29.6% ever with SM). In both migraine and comparison cohorts, the mean age was 46 years (standard deviation [SD] = 15), proportion of women was 73.3%, and insomnia was the major comorbidity, followed by mental disorders and anxiety (Table 1).

The overall incidence density rates of mortality were 9.74, 7.95, 9.02, and 7.49 per 1000 person-years in the comparison, total migraine, SM, and NM cohorts, respectively (Table 2). Compared with the comparison cohort, the corresponding adjusted HRs (aHRs; 95% CIs) of the mortality were 0.81 (0.76–0.87), 0.89 (0.80–0.98), and 0.78 (0.72–0.84) for the total migraine, SM, and NM cohorts, respectively. Patients aged 50–64 years (aHR = 2.57, 95% CI = 2.40–2.75) and ≥ 65 years (aHR = 10.5, 95% CI = 9.84–11.1) had a higher risk of mortality when compared with those aged 20–49 years. In the multivariable model, the mortality risk was higher in men (aHR = 1.78, 95% CI = 1.70–1.87) and in patients with comorbid depression (aHR = 1.33, 95% CI = 1.24–1.43), mental disorders (aHR = 1.19, 95% CI = 1.12–1.27), and alcohol-related illness (aHR = 2.18, 95% CI = 1.98–2.40). Furthermore, the NM cohort had a significantly lower mortality risk (aHR = 0.89, 95% CI = 0.79–0.99) than did the SM cohort (Table 2).

Table 3 shows that the mortality risk, stratified by sex, age, and comorbidities; it was significantly lower in the total migraine and NM cohorts than in the comparison cohort. The aHRs of mortality were 0.68–0.86 and 0.64–0.84 in the total migraine and NM cohorts, respectively. In the total migraine cohort, patients with comorbidities demonstrated higher mortality rate than did those without. In patients with SM, the relative risk of mortality was lower in those aged 20–49 years (aHR = 0.79, 95% CI = 0.64–0.98) and in those without comorbidities (aHR = 0.73, 95% CI = 0.57–0.94; Table 3).

Table 4 shows the stepwise regression analysis for evaluating the factors associated with the average all-cause hospital days annually among the patients with migraine. Compared with the comparison cohort, the average hospitalization duration was 0.66 days longer for the patients ever with SM. Furthermore, alcohol-related illness, male sex, depression, mental disorders, and age increased the hospitalization duration by 4.10, 1.98, 1.08, 0.81, and 0.11 days in the patients with migraine (Table 4). Table 5 shows the stepwise regression analysis used to evaluate the factors associated with the frequency of

Table 1 Distribution of age, sex, and comorbidities between the migraine and comparison cohorts

	Migraine						Comparison		p-value[b]
	Total N = 19,817		Status migrainosus N = 5868		Non-status migraine N = 13,949		N = 79,246		
	n	%	n	%	n	%	n	%	
Age, year									0.99
20–49	12,641	63.8	3685	62.8	8956	64.2	50,552	63.8	
50–64	4683	23.6	1388	23.7	3295	23.6	18,732	23.6	
65+	2493	12.6	795	13.6	1698	12.2	9962	12.6	
Mean (SD)[a]	45.9	14.9	46.3	15.3	45.7	14.8	45.8	15.2	0.37
Sex									0.99
Female	14,533	73.3	4199	71.6	10,334	74.1	5819	73.3	
Male	5284	26.7	1669	28.4	3615	25.9	21,127	26.7	
Comorbidity									
Depression	2536	12.8	663	11.3	1873	13.4	10,129	12.8	0.95
Mental disorders	10,928	55.1	3033	51.7	7895	56.6	43,690	55.1	0.97
Insomnia	13,414	67.7	3774	64.3	9640	69.1	53,645	67.7	0.99
Alcohol-related illness	746	3.76	199	3.39	547	3.92	2964	3.74	0.87
Anxiety	7316	36.9	2045	34.9	5271	37.8	29,248	36.9	0.98

Chi-square test; [a]t test
[b]Total migraine vs. comparison

Table 2 Incidence and hazard ratios of mortality and associated risk factors

	HR (95% CI)					
	Event no	Person-years	Rate	Crude	Adjusted[a]	Adjusted[a]
Migraine						
None	5567	582,126	9.74	1.00	1.00	
Total	1167	146,776	7.95	0.82(0.77, 0.87)***	0.81(0.76, 0.87)***	
Status migrainosus	401	44,471	9.02	0.92(0.83, 1.02)	0.89(0.80, 0.98)*	1.00
Non-status migraine	766	102,304	7.49	0.77(0.72, 0.83)***	0.78(0.72, 0.84)***	0.89(0.79, 0.99)*
Age, year						
20–49	1753	475,258	3.69	1.00	1.00	1.00
50–64	1667	171,118	9.74	2.65(2.48, 2.84)***	2.57(2.40, 2.75)***	3.05(2.58, 3.61)***
65+	3414	82,525	41.4	11.4(10.8, 12.1)***	10.5(9.84, 11.1)***	12.4(10.6, 14.4)***
Sex						
Female	3693	538,264	6.86	1.00	1.00	1.00
Male	3141	190,637	16.5	2.41(2.29, 2.52)***	1.78(1.70, 1.87)***	1.96(1.74, 2.21)***
Comorbidity						
Depression						
No	5771	643,710	8.97	1.00	1.00	1.00
Yes	1063	85,192	12.5	1.41(1.32, 1.50)***	1.33(1.24, 1.43)***	1.27(1.07, 1.52)**
Mental disorders						
No	2279	320,327	7.11	1.00	1.00	1.00
Yes	4555	408,575	11.2	1.56(1.49, 1.64)***	1.19(1.12, 1.27)***	1.19(1.02, 1.39)*
Insomnia						
No	1985	263,064	7.55	1.00	1.00	1.00
Yes	4849	465,838	10.4	1.41(1.34, 1.48)***	0.95(0.89, 1.00)	1.05(0.92, 1.21)
Alcohol-related illness						
No	6367	708,326	8.99	1.00	1.00	1.00
Yes	467	20,575	22.7	2.61(2.37, 2.86)***	2.18(1.98, 2.40)***	1.95(1.53, 2.49)***
Anxiety						
No	3970	463,834	8.56	1.00	1.00	1.00
Yes	2864	265,067	10.8	1.27(1.21, 1.33)***	0.81(0.76, 0.87)***	0.79(0.67, 0.92)**

Rate per 1000 person-years

[a]: multivariable analysis of age, sex, and comorbidities of depression, mental disorders, insomnia, alcohol-related illness, and anxiety

*$P < 0.05$, ** $P < 0.01$, ***$P < 0.001$

medical visits annually in the patients with migraine. We found that only age was a mild positive predictor (0.04 higher frequency of medical visits) in patients with migraine (Table 5).

Discussion

In this study, Taiwanese patients with migraine demonstrated a lower all-cause subsequent mortality rate. Overall, 9.74 and 7.95 mortality events per 1000 person-years occurred in the comparison and total migraine cohorts. In the patients with NM, the protective effects against mortality might have been due to the frequent medical care and physical examinations, particularly for the female patients. Women usually tend to use more medical services and spend more on health care than men do, with regard to primary care, physical therapy, and other medical support [15, 16]. However, the life expectancy for women generally being higher than that for men and the higher mortality risk among men can be confounding factors [17]. In the SM cohort, fewer protective effects were observed and those were noted only in patients aged < 50 years; even the frequency of medical visits increased with age in these patients.

We observed some common trends between the increase of average all-cause hospitalization duration annually and higher mortality risk in the cohorts. In addition to the risk factors of age and the condition of SM, alcohol-related illness, male sex, depression, and mental disorders were major risk factors for all-cause hospitalization and mortality in patients with migraine.

Table 3 Incidence and hazard ratios of mortality stratified by age, sex, and comorbidity for patients with migraine comparing with those without migraine

	Comparison N = 79,246		Migraine								
			Total N = 19,817			Status migrainosus N = 5868			Non-status migraine N = 13,949		
	Event no	Rate	Event no	Rate	HR[a] (95% CI)	Event no	Rate	HR[a] (95% CI)	Event no	Rate	HR[a] (95% CI)
Age, year											
20–49	1495	3.94	258	2.70	0.68(0.60, 0.78)***	91	3.13	0.79(0.64,0.98)*	167	2.51	0.64(0.54, 0.75)***
50–64	1373	10.0	294	8.54	0.85(0.75, 0.96)**	86	8.53	0.85(0.68, 1.06)	208	8.55	0.85(0.73, 0.98)*
65+	2799	42.6	615	36.7	0.86(0.79, 0.94)***	224	42.0	0.97(0.85, 1.11)	391	34.2	0.81(0.73, 0.90)***
Sex											
Female	3090	7.19	603	5.57	0.78(0.71, 0.85)***	205	6.39	0.88(0.77, 1.02)	398	5.22	0.73(0.66, 0.81)***
Male	2577	16.9	564	14.7	0.86(0.78, 0.94)**	196	15.8	0.89(0.77, 1.03)	368	14.1	0.84(0.75, 0.94)**
Comorbidity											
None	986	7.56	172	5.20	0.69(0.59, 0.81)***	68	5.52	0.73(0.57, 0.94)*	104	5.02	0.66(0.54, 0.81)***
With any one	4681	10.4	995	8.75	0.84(0.79, 0.90)***	333	10.4	1.00(0.89, 1.11)	662	8.12	0.78(0.72, 0.85)***

Rate per 1000 person-years
[a]: multivariable analysis including age, sex, and comorbidities of depression, mental disorders, insomnia, alcohol-related illness, and anxiety
*$P < 0.05$, **$P < 0.01$, ***$P < 0.001$

Among the comorbidities, alcohol-related illness was the strongest risk factor for hospital admission and mortality in patients with migraine. In general, a small amount of alcohol may not trigger migraine. Several recent studies could not conclusively show whether alcohol triggers migraines [18–20]. Differences in cultural and ethnic values and practices affect alcohol consumption, which increases complexity in studying the relationship between alcohol drinking and migraine. In this study, we considered alcohol-related illness a major comorbidity and risk factor; it should be due to that the patients with this comorbidity had already experienced toxic effects from alcohol consumption along with their migraine. Migraine alters peoples' neuroendocrinal, neurophysiological, and neuropsychological conditions [5–8], and increases the risk of cardiovascular diseases. In addition to cardiovascular risk, this study reveals that alcohol-related illness is another risk factor to cause premature mortality in Taiwanese patients with migraine.

Table 4 Stepwise regression analysis for average hospital days per year (all-cause admission) among patients with migraine

Variable	Parameter Estimate	Standard Error	95% CI
Intercept	−3.71	0.30	(−4.30, − 3.12)***
Status migrainosus	0.66	0.20	(0.27, 1.05)***
Age	0.11	0.01	(0.09, 0.12)***
Sex (male vs. female)	1.98	0.21	(1.57, 2.39)***
Alcohol-related illness	4.10	0.49	(3.15, 5.06)***
Mental disorders	0.81	0.20	(0.41, 1.21)***
Depression	1.08	0.29	(0.51, 1.65)***

***$P < 0.001$

To our knowledge, this is the first study to show the long-term mortality rates in patients with migraine: patients with SM and NM demonstrated diverse survival outcomes. After the NHI was implemented in Taiwan, the annual mortality rate in general population significantly decreased by 5.83% from 1996 to 1999 [21]. In this study, we only analyzed the mortality risks in patients with migraine who died after being treated at inpatient facilities, excluding mortality cases outside a hospital. The NHI program has been over 20 years which is a universally compulsive insurance covering more than 99% of Taiwan's population and it is operated by the government in Taiwan. NHI guarantees the residents of Taiwan equal access of medical service regardless of socioeconomic status, background, and critical problems existing or not [12, 22]. The Taiwan's universal healthcare system showed very few disparities in accessing inpatient service and ultimate outcomes between different hospitals and areas in Taiwan [23, 24], and the proportion of migraineurs died outside a hospital should be very rare. However, the detail underlying mechanisms need to be studied in the future to explain why Taiwanese patients with migraine have a lower mortality risk depicted in this study. Furthermore, patients ever with SM, of the male sex, and with alcohol-related illness, depression, or mental disorders have fewer protective

Table 5 Stepwise regression analysis for frequency of migraine-related visits per year among patients with migraine

Variable	Parameter Estimate	Standard Error	95% CI
Intercept	−0.49	0.91	(−2.29, 1.30)
Age	0.04	0.02	(0.002, 0.08)*

*$P < 0.05$

effects from premature mortality, and could be said to have a malignant course of migraine. We hope that our findings highlight a future strategy for providing proper medical care to patients with migraine.

Because of our study design, which included a nationwide, population-based sample with little risk of recall and selection bias, our findings should be considered convincing in Taiwan and other developing Asian countries with a heritage similar to that of Taiwan. However, this study has several limitations. First, we could not directly contact our patients because their identities were anonymized in the LHID. Therefore, the study design did not include details regarding the migraines, such as duration and frequency, psychological burden, and whether or how the migraines were treated with medication. Whether any migraine medications and other comorbid disorders influence the mortality rate is unknown. Second, any mortality cases occurring outside a hospital were out of the scope of our study. We intentionally designed our study in those died after being treated at inpatient facilities to achieve results with high validity, despite the slight possibility of introducing underestimation bias into the results. Third, we have to admit there was a possible bias that missed or underdiagnosed SM and NM. However, the NHIRD covers a highly representative sample of Taiwan's general population because the reimbursement policy is universal and operated by a single-buyer, the government in Taiwan. All insurance claims should be scrutinized by medical reimbursement specialists and peer review according to the standard diagnosed criteria in the study. If these doctors or hospitals make wrong diagnoses or coding, they will be punished with a lot of penalties. Therefore, the diagnoses of SM and NM in this study were highly reliable and our results indicate that the sample size was sufficient to statistically demonstrate the mortality risk in patients with migraine in Taiwan.

Conclusions

This study revealed that Taiwanese patients with migraine benefit from comprehensive and universal health care for not only controlling their migraines but also reducing subsequent mortality risk. Our findings provide vital information for clinicians and for assisting global efforts for understanding and treating migraine.

Abbreviations

aHR: Adjusted hazard ratio; CI: Confidence interval; ICD-9-CM: International Classification of Diseases, Ninth Revision, Clinical Modification; NHIRD: National Health Insurance Research Database

Acknowledgements

This work was supported by grants from the Ministry of Health and Welfare, Taiwan (MOHW107-TDU-B-212-123004), China Medical University Hospital (DMR-107-192); Academia Sinica Stroke Biosignature Project (BM10701010021); MOST Clinical Trial Consortium for Stroke (MOST 106-2321-B-039-005-); Tseng-Lien Lin Foundation, Taichung, Taiwan; and Katsuzo and Kiyo Aoshima Memorial Funds, Japan. The funders had no role in study design, data collection and analysis, decision to publish, or preparation of the manuscript. No additional external funding received for this study.

Authors' contributions

All authors have contributed significantly, and that all authors are in agreement with the content of the manuscript: Conception/Design: TH, C-HK; Provision of study materials: C-HK; Collection and/or assembly of data: All authors; Data analysis and interpretation: All authors; Manuscript writing: All authors; Final approval of manuscript: All authors.

Competing interests

The authors declare that they have no competing interests.

Author details

[1]Department of Neurosurgery, Hualien Tzu Chi General Hospital, Buddhist Tzu Chi Medical Foundation, Hualien, Taiwan. [2]College of Medicine, Tzu Chi University, Hualien, Taiwan. [3]Management Office for Health Data, China Medical University Hospital, Taichung, Taiwan. [4]College of Medicine, China Medical University, Taichung, Taiwan. [5]Graduate Institute of Biomedical Sciences and School of Medicine, College of Medicine, China Medical University, No. 2, Yuh-Der Road, Taichung 404, Taiwan. [6]Department of Nuclear Medicine and PET Center, China Medical University Hospital, Taichung, Taiwan. [7]Department of Bioinformatics and Medical Engineering, Asia University, Taichung, Taiwan.

References

1. Streel S, Donneau AF, Hoge A, Albert A, Schoenen J, Guillaume M (2015) One-year prevalence of migraine using a validated extended French version of the ID migraine™: a Belgian population-based study. Rev Neurol (Paris) 171:707–714
2. Stovner LJ, Zwart JA, Hagen K, Terwindt GM, Pascual J (2006) Epidemiology of headache in Europe. Eur J Neurol 13:333–345
3. Wang SJ, Chung CS, Chankrachang S, Ravishankar K, Merican JS, Salazar G, Siow C, Cheung RT, Phanthumchinda K, Sakai F (2008) Migraine disability awareness campaign in Asia: migraine assessment for prophylaxis. Headache 48:1356–1365
4. Wang SJ, Fuh JL, Young YH, Lu SR, Shia BC (2000) Prevalence of migraine in Taipei, Taiwan: a population-based survey. Cephalalgia 20:566–572
5. Lipton RB, Stewart WF, Diamond S, Diamond ML, Reed M (2001) Prevalence and burden of migraine in the United States: data from the American migraine study II. Headache 41:646–657
6. Rambarat CA, Elgendy IY, Johnson BD, Reis SE, Thompson DV, Sharaf BL, Bittner V, Sopko G, Bairey Merz CN, Pepine CJ, Ahmed B (2017) Migraine headache and long-term cardiovascular outcomes: an extended follow-up of the women's ischemia syndrome evaluation. Am J Med 130:738–743
7. Nović A, Kõlves K, O'Dwyer S, De Leo D (2016) Migraine and suicidal behaviors: a systematic literature review. Clin J Pain 32:351–364
8. Leonardi M (2015) Burden of migraine: what should we say more? Neurol Sci 36(Suppl 1):1–3
9. Granella F, Cavallini A, Sandrini G, Manzoni GC, Nappi G (1998) Long-term outcome of migraine. Cephalalgia 18:30–33
10. Colombo B, Dalla Libera D, Dalla Costa G, Comi G (2013) Refractory migraine: the role of the physician in assessment and treatment of a problematic disease. Neurol Sci 34(Suppl 1):109–112
11. Database NHIR. Taiwan. http://nhird.nhri.org.tw/en/index.html (cited in 2017)
12. Ministry of Health and Welfare (2017). Taiwan health and welfare report. available at: http://www.mohw.gov.tw
13. Lin FY, Yang YC, Lin CL, Lee LJ (2018) Increased risk of overactive bladder in patients with idiopathic Parkinson's disease: insight from a nationwide population-based cohort study. PLoS One 13:e0193783. https://doi.org/10.1371/journal.pone.0193783 eCollection 2018
14. Lin SY, Lin CL, Lin CC, Wang IK, Hsu WH, Kao CH (2018) Risk of acute coronary syndrome and peripheral arterial disease in chronic liver disease

and cirrhosis: a nationwide population-based study. Atherosclerosis 270: 154–159. https://doi.org/10.1016/j.atherosclerosis.2018.01.047

15. Kaur S, Stechuchak KM, Coffman CJ, Allen KD, Bastian LA (2007) Gender differences in health care utilization among veterans with chronic pain. J Gen Intern Med 22:228–233
16. Owens GM (2008) Gender differences in health care expenditures, resource utilization, and quality of care. J Manag Care Pharm 14(Supp I):2–6
17. Kochanek KD, Murphy SL, Xu J, Arias E (2015) Mortality in the United States, 2014. NCHS Data Brief 229:1–8
18. Dueland AN (2015) Headache and alcohol. Headache 55:1045–1049
19. Panconesi A, Franchini M, Bartolozzi ML, Mugnai S, Guidi L (2013) Alcoholic drinks as triggers in primary headaches. Pain Med 14:1254–1259
20. Krymchantowski AV, da Cunha Jevoux C (2014) Wine and headache. Headache 54:967–975
21. Lee YC, Huang YT, Tsai YW, Huang SM, Kuo KN, McKee M, Nolte E (2010) The impact of universal National Health Insurance on population health: the experience of Taiwan. BMC Health Serv Res 10:225
22. Lee YH, Ang TFA, Chiang TC, Kaplan WA (2018) Growing concerns and controversies to Taiwan National Health Insurance- what are the lessons from mainland China, South Korea and Singapore? Int J Health Plann Manag 33:e357–e366. https://doi.org/10.1002/hpm.2387
23. Huang N, Yip W, Chang HJ, Chou YJ (2006) Trends in rural and urban differentials in incidence rates for ruptured appendicitis under the National Health Insurance in Taiwan. Public Health 120:1055–1063
24. Shu CC, Lin JW, Lin YF, Hsu NC, Ko WJ (2011) Evaluating the performance of a hospitalist system in Taiwan: a pioneer study for nationwide health insurance in Asia. J Hosp Med 6:378–382

22

Fremanezumab blocks CGRP induced dilatation in human cerebral, middle meningeal and abdominal arteries

Lena Ohlsson[1,4*], Erik Kronvall[2,4], Jennifer Stratton[3,4] and Lars Edvinsson[1,4]

Abstract

Background: Fremanezumab (TEV-48125) is a fully humanized anti-calcitonin gene-related peptide (CGRP) monoclonal antibody (mAb) that has shown positive results in the prevention of episodic migraine and chronic migraine. Previous preclinical studies have revealed CGRP antagonistic effects on intracranial arteries (ICA). The aim of the study was to evaluate the in vitro antagonistic effects of fremanezumab on human arteries.

Methods: Arteries were removed in conjunction with neurosurgery (cerebral, CA, and middle meningeal artery, MMA, $n = 7$) or reconstructive abdominal surgery (abdominal artery, AA, $n = 6$). Ring segments of the vessels were mounted in a sensitive myograph, the functional responses of vasoactive intestinal peptide (VIP), substance P and CGRP in increasing concentrations (10^{-10}–10^{-7} M) were studied using pre-contraction with 30 mM potassium chloride (KCl). The concentrations of fremanezumab or isotype control antibody (66.7 nM, 0.33 μM, 0.67 μM) were given 30 min prior to CGRP administration.

Results: All included arteries responded with a strong stable contraction to the application of 30 mM KCl. During this pre-contraction, CGRP caused a concentration-dependent relaxation which differed slightly in maximum effect (I_{max}) between the types of arteries (ICA = 100%; AA 80%). Fremanezumab (66.7 nM) showed a shift in the IC_{50} value of CGRP, but no significant change in I_{max}. At higher doses there was also a reduction of I_{max}. For AA, the I_{max} decreased from 71% at 66.7 nM, to 4.5% with 0.33 μM of fremanezumab. Isotype control antibody did not modify the responses. There was no effect on concentration-dependent relaxation with VIP with 66.7 nM of fremanezumab or isotype control.

Conclusion: CGRP relaxes pre-contracted human arteries by 80–100%, but with different IC_{50}; the potency range was ICA < AA. The antagonistic effect and potency of fremanezumab was similar, suggesting that there are vasodilatory CGRP receptors present in all studied arteries and that the antibody may have effect in all studied vessels.

Keywords: CGRP, CGRP receptor antagonist, Antibody, Fremanezumab, Human vessels

Background

Calcitonin gene-related peptide alpha (αCGRP) is a 37-amino acid neuropeptide belonging to the calcitonin family of peptides. It is abundant in the circulation. CGRP is widely distributed throughout the central, peripheral and enteric nervous systems [1] and has strong vasodilatory properties, especially in the peripheral microvasculature [2] and in the cerebral circulation [3]. CGRP increases cAMP in human, feline and rodent vascular smooth muscle cells (VSMC) [4, 5] and is also active in endothelium-denuded cerebral arteries as well as in meningeal arteries [6]. The vasomotor actions of αCGRP are implied in a variety of both physiological and pathological processes, including migraine and other primary headaches as well as cerebral vasospasm after subarachnoid hemorrhage [7].

Monoclonal antibodies against CGRP or its receptor are currently being evaluated for the prevention of episodic migraine and chronic migraine; all available

* Correspondence: Lena.Ohlsson@med.lu.se
[1]Department of Clinical Sciences, Division of Experimental Vascular Research, Lund University, BMC A13, Sölvegatan 17, SE-223 62 Lund, Sweden
[4]Department of Internal Medicine and Neurosurgery, University Hospital, Lund, Sweden
Full list of author information is available at the end of the article

clinical trials have shown positive results [8–11]. However, as with all new medications, care has to be taken in order to evaluate possible risks of adverse events such as stroke, hypertension, and myocardial infarction; one way is to study human vessels [12].

Fremanezumab is a fully humanized monoclonal antibody that potently and selectively binds to both isoforms (α and β) of CGRP and thereby prevents CGRP from binding to the CGRP receptor. Therapeutic monoclonal antibodies to CGRP such as fremanezumab have been developed because of the very high target specificity, long pharmacokinetic half-lives, and markedly low potential for hepatic toxicity [8, 13] and in phase 2 and 3 clinical studies, fremanezumab was shown to be an effective and safe migraine treatment [8, 14, 15]. Recently, Edvinsson et al. explained the long time it has taken from finding CGRP to the new medications like gepants (small molecules) and the monoclonal antibodies against CGRP or against the CGRP receptor. Human cranial arteries have been a method to understand how CGRP blocking agents modify the vascular responses to CGRP [16].

The present study was designed to evaluate the in vitro vascular effects of fremanezumab (TEV-48125, formerly LBR-101) on isolated human cerebral, middle meningeal and abdominal arteries.

Methods

Human meningeal ($n = 4$) and cerebral cortical ($n = 3$) arteries were removed during neurosurgical operations for intracranial tumors (4 male and 3 female). Human subcutaneous arteries ($n = 6$, female) were obtained from reconstructive abdominal surgery. The study was approved by the human ethics committee of Lund (LU818–01) and written informed consent was given by all vessel donors.

After removal, the vessels were immediately immersed in 4 °C cold cell culture medium (DMEM containing essential nutrients and antibiotics) (Gipco, ThermoFisher Scientific, Waltham, MA USA 02451). The vessels were carefully dissected and transferred to cold sodium buffer solution (NaCl 119 mM, $NaHCO_3$ 15 mM, KCl 4.6 mM, $CaCl_2$ 1.5 mM, NaH_2PO_4 1.2 mM, MgCl 1.2 mM and glucose 5.6 mM), pH 7.4, and stored in refrigerator at 4°Covernight.

Substances

CGRP, vasoactive intestinal peptide (VIP) and substance P were purchased from Bio-Techne (Abingdon, UK). Common substances for buffer preparation were purchased from Sigma-Aldrich (St Louis, MO, USA).

Myography

In order to evaluate the dilatory response to CGRP (10^{-10} – 10^{-7} M), VIP (10^{-10} – 10^{-7} M) and substance P (10^{-9} – 10^{-8} M), in human arteries a Mulvany-Halpern Wire Myograph (Danish Myo Technology A/S, Aarhus, Denmark) was used as has been previously described [17]. Vessel segments (1–2 mm) were placed in a tissue bath in 5 ml sodium buffer solution (NaCl 119 mM, $NaHCO_3$ 15 mM, KCl 4.6 mM, $CaCl_2$ 1.5 mM, NaH_2PO_4 1.2 mM, MgCl 1.2 mM and glucose 5.6 mM). The solution was kept at 37 °C and was continuously aerated with air with 5% CO_2 to maintain pH at 7.4. Depending on the thickness of the artery, the vessels were mounted either on pins 200 μm thick or on two 40 μm wires, which were inserted into the vessel lumen. The pins/wires were connected to a force transducer and a micrometer screw. Normalization was performed by successive manipulation of the micrometer screw until the vessel segments were stretched to 90% of the normal internal circumference, which is the diameter they would have if relaxed under a transmural pressure of 100 mmHg [18]. After 30 min of recovery, viability of the vessel segments were determined by replacing the sodium buffer with a 63.5 mM potassium buffer [19] (NaCl 119 mM, $NaHCO_3$ 15 mM, KCl 63.5 mM, $CaCl_2$, 1.5 mM, NaH_2PO_4, 1.2 mM, MgCl 1.2 mM, and glucose 5.6 mM); the contractile response was measured as 100% contraction by the respective vessel segment. After observing the contractile response to high potassium twice, tissue baths were washed in the above mentioned sodium buffer. Endothelial viability was then tested by pre-contract the vessels with 30 mM potassium-buffer, and after stabilization, successive concentrations of substance P 10^{-8} – 10^{-7} M were added, which, if the endothelium was viable, would induce a transient vasodilation. After this step, the potassium buffer was again washed out and replaced with the above mentioned sodium buffer. The vessels were pre-treated with either fremanezumab antibody or the isotype control antibody (KLH) for 20 min. To test the dilatory response to CGRP, the vessels were pre-contracted with 30 mM potassium-buffer for 10 min followed by dose response of antibody. The concentrations of the antibodies were 10, 50, and 100 μg/ml (66.7 nM, 0.33 μM, 0.67 μM, respectively) in the vessel baths, which was in the same range as used in the chronic migraine clinical study [8, 20]. Contraction forces were recorded through a PowerLab unit (ADInstruments, Chalgrove, UK).

Statistics

Relaxations are expressed as percentage of the pre-tension induced by 30 mM potassium buffer. All concentration-response curves were analyzed by iterative non-linear regression analysis using GraphPad Prism 7.02 (GraphPad Corp, San Diego, CA, USA). I_{max} is the maximal response developed to the agonist. IC_{50} is the concentration that produced half maximum dilatation. Results are given as mean +/− standard error of the mean (SEM) and n is the number of patients used in the respective group. Statistical analyses were performed with non-parametric Mann-Whitney (two groups) and Kruskal-Wallis followed by Dunn's multiple comparison test (three or four groups) non-parametric tests. Results were considered as significant if $p < 0.05$.

Results

Arteries from human subcutaneous and intracranial arteries were found to have functional endothelium as tested in artery segments pre-contracted by performing the experiments in a buffer containing 30 mM potassium. The addition of substance P resulted in a concentration-dependent relaxation of the artery segments. For subcutaneous arteries, 10^{-9} M substance P dilated pre-contracted arteries by 49.8% ± 22.7 and at 10^{-8} M by 66.2% ± 21.4 (mean ± SEM). The relaxant responses were at the same concentrations of substance P in meningeal and cortical arteries 17.3% ± 16.2 and 26.1% ± 20.6, respectively.

Following washout with standard buffer solution, the vessels relaxed to baseline and after equilibrium, again the 30 mM potassium buffer was added. In these arteries, CGRP resulted in relaxation by as much as 80–100% of the pre-contraction by increasing concentrations of CGRP (10^{-10} – 10^{-7} M) (Figs 1 and 2). We observed no difference in the responses to the endothelial function check at these two time-points.

At the lowest concentration of fremanezumab in the tissue bath (10 mg/L, 66.7 nM), the results showed that the I_{max} was the same as in the control, but the IC_{50} was increased (a shift to the right) for all three types of arteries. In addition, no effect was seen by fremanezumab per se (neither dilatation nor contraction).

At the higher dose of fremanezumab, a delayed dilatation of abdominal arteries was observed with concentrations > 1 nM CGRP. With 100 nM fremanezumab and control, the I_{max} was reduced and the IC_{50} increased (Table 1, Fig. 1). After pre-treatment with 50 or 100 µg/mL (0.33 or 0.67 µM) fremanezumab or isotype control, there was no dilatation

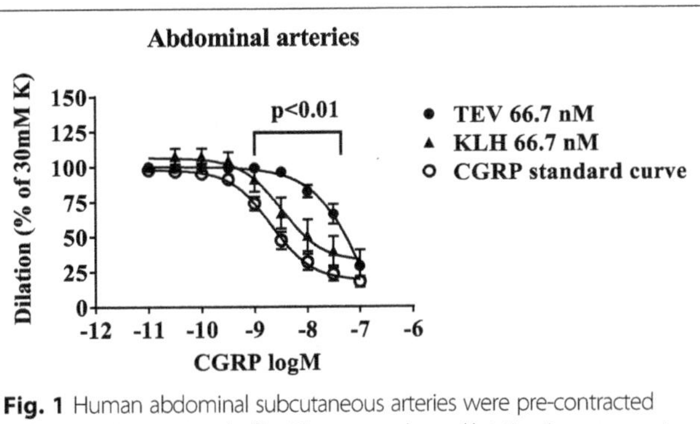

Fig. 1 Human abdominal subcutaneous arteries were pre-contracted with 30 mM potassium buffer. The curves show dilatation in response to increasing concentrations of αCGRP 10^{-11} to 10^{-7} M in the presence of 66.7 nM of the monoclonal antibody against CGRP (fremanezumab) or an isotype control (KLH). The data show mean ± SEM, n = 2–4 for each concentration. CGRP:calcitonin gene-related peptide; K:potassium; TEV:Teva

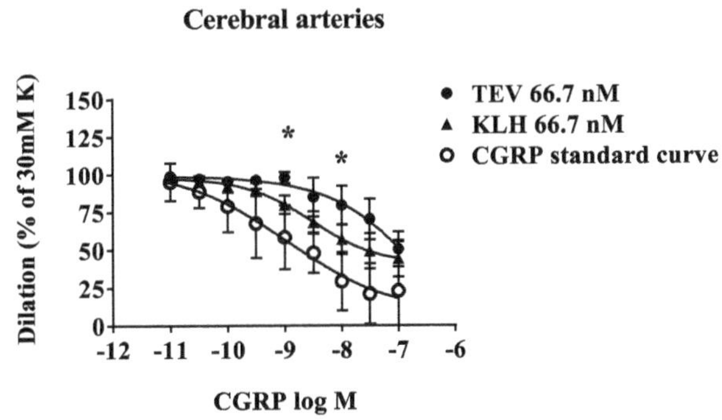

Fig. 2 Human intracranial arteries were pre-contracted with 30 mM potassium buffer. The curves show dilatation in response to increasing concentrations of αCGRP 10^{-11} to 10^{-7} M in the presence of 66.7 nM of the monoclonal antibody against CGRP (fremanezumab) or an isotype control (KLH). The data show mean ± SEM, n = 2–4 for each concentration. CGRP:calcitonin gene-related peptide; K:potassium; TEV:Teva

with any concentration of CGRP (tested up to 0.1 µM, data not shown). Due to the similar effect in this assay with the isotype control, the effect of these higher antibody concentrations on dilatation cannot be attributed to the sequestration of CGRP.

Cerebral and middle meningeal arteries responded in a similar manner with a significantly delayed dilatation in the presence of 10 µg/mL (66.7 nM) fremanezumab antibody (Fig. 2, Table 1). There was a shift in IC_{50} towards the right indicating change in I_{max}. Result also showed no relaxation by fremanezumab or the isotype antibody control per se in ICA (data not shown). Addition of 50 µg/mL (0.33 µM) fremanezumab or its isotype control inhibited the CGRP-induced dilatation completely. Therefore, no higher concentration was tested.

In abdominal and intracranial arteries, the study tested whether the antibodies had any effect on vasodilatation induced by VIP (Figs. 3 and 4). Neither fremanezumab nor the isotype control antibody had any effect on the VIP-induced dilatation of the cerebral arteries at the doses of 66.7 nM (Figs. 3 and 4) or 0.33 µM (data not shown).

Table 1 Relaxant responses to CGRP in the presence or absence of 66.7 nM fremanezumab or its isotype control

	Abdominal arteries		Intracranial arteries	
	I_{max} (%)	IC_{50} (nM)	I_{max} (%)	IC_{50} (nM)
CGRP control curve	82 ± 4	2.1 ± 0.1	78 ± 22	1.1 ± 0.5
+ fremanezumab 66.7 nM	71 ± 3	182 ± 1.0	49 ± 11	752 ± 9
+ isotype control 66.7 nM	71 ± 9	3.2 ± 0.2	55 ± 12	2.9 ± 0.4

CGRP: calcitonin gene-related peptide, IC_{50}: concentration of CGRP in nM that produced half the maximum dilatation, I_{max}: maximum dilatation induced by CGRP when the pre-contraction by 30 mM potassium buffer is set to 100%
Values are mean ± SEM

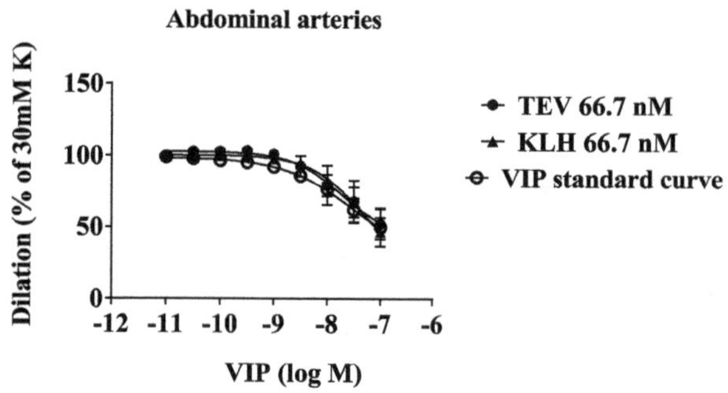

Fig. 3 Human abdominal subcutaneous arteries were pre-contracted with 30 mM potassium buffer. The curves show dilatation in response to increasing concentrations of VIP 10^{-11} to 10^{-7} M in the presence of 66.7 nM of the monoclonal antibody against CGRP (fremanezumab) or an isotype control (KLH). The data show mean ± SEM, $n = 2–4$ for each concentration. K:potassium; TEV:Teva; VIP:vasoactive intestinal peptide

Discussion

The present study shows that the monoclonal antibody against CGRP, fremanezumab, effectively and selectively blocks the vasomotor responses to CGRP in preparations of human intracranial and peripheral arteries.

Migraine is a highly prevalent disorder characterized by attacks of headache and associated symptoms such as nausea, photophobia, and phonophobia. Most individuals with migraine have episodic migraine, but some have a more severe form known as chronic migraine. The burden of episodic or chronic migraine on the person with migraine, their family, and society at large is substantial [21].

CGRP, a neuropeptide with two isoforms (αCGRP and βCGRP), is believed to be crucial to the pathophysiology of migraine and is therefore an attractive target in the development of migraine preventive strategies. CGRP seems to be involved in peripheral events in migraine (vasodilation, inflammation, and protein extravasation) and is abundantly distributed in the trigeminal ganglion and in the brain [21]. Inhibition of the CGRP pathway has demonstrated efficacy in the acute and preventive treatment of migraine [16, 22, 23]. The first suggestion to use a CGRP receptor antagonist for migraine therapy was made in 1985 [24], however, it has taken more than three decades to reach the clinic [16]. The subsequent testing of such a receptor antagonist or an antagonist antibody on cerebral [25] and middle meningeal arteries [26]. The likely site of action residing outside the blood-brain barrier (BBB) putatively on meningeal vessels or trigeminal ganglion [27, 28].

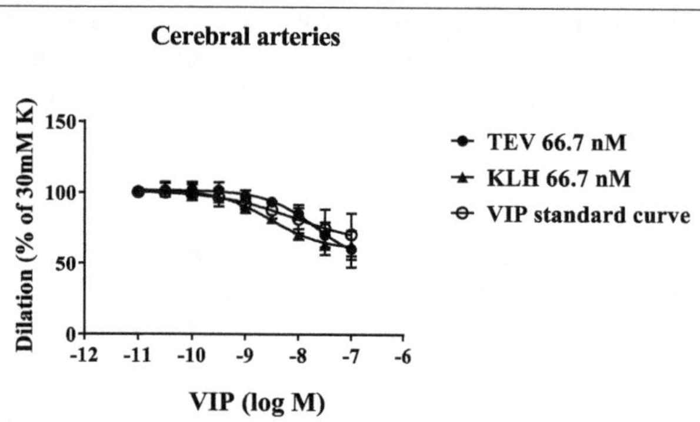

Fig. 4 Human intracranial arteries were pre-contracted with 30 mM potassium buffer. The curves show dilatation in response to increasing concentrations of VIP 10^{-11} to 10^{-7} M in the presence of 66.7 nM of the monoclonal antibody against CGRP (fremanezumab) or an isotype control (KLH). The data show mean ± SEM, $n = 2–4$ for each concentration. K:potassium; TEV:Teva; VIP:vasoactive intestinal peptide

This study was designed to study in some detail the antagonistic effects of fremanezumab, a fully humanized monoclonal antibody that targets CGRP, on the CGRP-mediated dilatation of human cerebral, meningeal, and abdominal arteries at clinically relevant concentrations. One clear effect was the lack of effect per se of the antibody, thus indicating no tonus by CGRP in these circulations [7]. We observed that the CGRP-induced relaxations in pre-contracted segments behave rather similarly in all three vascular regions and was in concert with previous work (with same IC_{50} and I_{max}) [29]. At the lowest concentration of fremanezumab (66.7 nM), CGRP-induced relaxation showed a parallel shift to the right with no change in maximum dilatation and no effect by the isotype control antibody solution. At higher concentrations of fremanezumab, the arterial response to CGRP was markedly reduced or even absent as a sign of strong antagonism. However, the isotype control also had equal effect on arterial relaxation but only at the highest concentration as well, suggesting that some of these data at the higher concentrations may be artefact and is not a contribution of CGRP sequestration. This is commonly seen with high antibody concentrations using in vitro assays and is one of the reasons that we use an isotype control antibody.

It is unknown if fremanezumab may have an effect on several of the receptors belonging to the calcitonin family receptors; future studies may be designed to evaluate also the effects of fremanezumab on the vascular responses to the other calcitonin family member peptides (adrenomedullin, intermedin, amylin and calcitonin). These peptides also activate CGRP receptors so essentially, we are only looking at one component of the receptor action in this in vitro system, which may not represent the normal milieu of peptides occurring in patients.

Previous studies using gepants [29] revealed a competitive antagonistic response with a shift of the concentration-response curve to the right, allowing the calculation of the dissociation constant. The behavior of fremanezumab thus differs from gepants, because the antibody acts as a "sink" in removing CGRP from the myography test system, a likely manner of interaction in patients. The specificity at the 66.7 nM concentration of fremanezumab was verified by unaltered relaxant responses to

VIP (a known peptide mediator of VIPR1 and VIPR2 receptors, but has no effect on CGRP receptors) and the contractile effects of 30 mM potassium buffer.

The antibody fremanezumab appears to have a direct functional effect on CGRP-induced relaxation in the tested human arteries with no change in maximum dilatation at the 66, 7 nM concentration. The fremanezumab/CGRP dissociation constant cannot be determined in this experiment due to its extremely high affinity for CGRP, and because the off rate is substantially longer than the time frame of each experiment.

Conclusion

The results of this study showed that the humanized monoclonal antibody fremanezumab can compete with CGRP to a similar extent in different human arteries. The long half-life of the interaction is relevant in a "chronic" situation or in prophylaxis because a patient will be exposed to the antibody for a longer period of time and will therefore, at some point, be at steady state with respect to the equilibrium constant of the antibody/antigen interaction. The antagonistic effect and potency of fremanezumab was similar in the different arteries studied, suggesting that there are vasodilatory CGRP receptors present in all studied arteries and that the antibody may have effect in all studied vessels.

Abbreviations

AA: Abdominal artery; BBB: Blood brain barrier; CA: Cerebral artery; CGRP: Calcitonin gene-related peptide; ICA: Intracranial artery; MMA: Middle meningeal artery; VIP: Vasoactive intestinal peptide; VSMC: Vascular smooth muscle cell

Acknowledgments

Prof. Lars Edvinsson was supported by Vetenskapsrådet Grant No. VR5958.

Funding

Prof. Lars Edvinsson was supported by Vetenskapsrådet Grant No. VR5958. The material for the study was funded by TEVA Pharmaceuticals Ltd.

Authors' contributions

Participated in research design: JS, LE, EH. Clinical surgery: EH. Conducted experiments: LO. Performed data analysis: LO, LE. Wrote or contributed to the writing of the manuscript: LE, JS, EH, LO. All authors read and approved the final manuscript.

Competing interests

The authors have nothing to disclose. JS is an employee of TEVA Pharmaceuticals Ltd., but was not involved in the interpretation of the results.

Author details

[1]Department of Clinical Sciences, Division of Experimental Vascular Research, Lund University, BMC A13, Sölvegatan 17, SE-223 62 Lund, Sweden. [2]Department of Clinical sciences, Neurosurgery, Skane University Hospital, Lund, Sweden. [3]Teva Biologics R&D, Redwood City, California, USA. [4]Department of Internal Medicine and Neurosurgery, University Hospital, Lund, Sweden.

References

1. Uddman R, Edvinsson L, Ekblad E, Hakanson R, Sundler F (1986) Calcitonin gene-related peptide (CGRP): perivascular distribution and vasodilatory effects. Regul Pept 15(1):1–23
2. Brain SD, Williams TJ, Tippins JR, Morris HR, MacIntyre I (1985) Calcitonin gene-related peptide is a potent vasodilator. Nature 313(5997):54–56
3. Uddman R, Edvinsson L, Ekman R, Kingman T, McCulloch J (1985) Innervation of the feline cerebral vasculature by nerve fibers containing calcitonin gene-related peptide: trigeminal origin and co-existence with substance P. Neurosci Lett 62(1):131–136
4. Crossman DC, Dashwood MR, Brain SD, McEwan J, Pearson JD (1990) Action of calcitonin gene-related peptide upon bovine vascular endothelial and smooth muscle cells grown in isolation and co-culture. Br J Pharmacol 99(1):71–76
5. Edvinsson L, Fredholm BB, Hamel E, Jansen I, Verrecchia C (1985) Perivascular peptides relax cerebral arteries concomitant with stimulation of cyclic adenosine monophosphate accumulation or release of an endothelium-derived relaxing factor in the cat. Neurosci Lett 58(2):213–217.
6. Edvinsson L, Mulder H, Goadsby PJ, Uddman R (1998) Calcitonin gene-related peptide and nitric oxide in the trigeminal ganglion: cerebral vasodilatation from trigeminal nerve stimulation involves mainly calcitonin gene-related peptide. J Auton Nerv Syst 70(1–2):15–22
7. Goadsby PJ, Holland PR, Martins-Oliveira M, Hoffmann J, Schankin C, Akerman S (2017) Pathophysiology of migraine: a disorder of sensory processing. Physiol Rev 97(2):553–622. https://doi.org/10.1152/physrev.00034.2015
8. Bigal ME, Edvinsson L, Rapoport AM, Lipton RB, Spierings EL, Diener HC et al (2015b) Safety, tolerability, and efficacy of TEV-48125 for preventive treatment of chronic migraine: a multicentre, randomised, double-blind, placebo-controlled, phase 2b study. Lancet Neurol 14(11):1091–1100. https://doi.org/10.1016/S1474-4422(15)00245-8
9. Dodick DW, Goadsby PJ, Spierings EL, Scherer JC, Sweeney SP, Grayzel DS (2014) Safety and efficacy of LY2951742, a monoclonal antibody to calcitonin gene-related peptide, for the prevention of migraine: a phase 2, randomised, double-blind, placebo-controlled study. Lancet Neurol 13(9): 885–892. https://doi.org/10.1016/S1474-4422(14)70128-0
10. Goadsby PJ, Sprenger T (2010) Current practice and future directions in the prevention and acute management of migraine. Lancet Neurol 9(3):285–298. https://doi.org/10.1016/S1474-4422(10)70005-3
11. Sun H, Dodick DW, Silberstein S, Goadsby PJ, Reuter U, Ashina M et al (2016) Safety and efficacy of AMG 334 for prevention of episodic migraine: a randomised, double-blind, placebo-controlled, phase 2 trial. Lancet Neurol 15(4):382–390. https://doi.org/10.1016/S1474-4422(16)00019-3
12. MaassenVanDenBrink A, Meijer J, Villalon CM, Ferrari MD (2016) Wiping out CGRP: potential cardiovascular risks. Trends Pharmacol Sci 37(9):779–788. https://doi.org/10.1016/j.tips.2016.06.002
13. Schuster NM, Rapoport AM (2016) New strategies for the treatment and prevention of primary headache disorders. Nat Rev Neurol 12(11):635–650. https://doi.org/10.1038/nrneurol.2016.143
14. Bigal ME, Dodick DW, Rapoport AM, Silberstein SD, Ma Y, Yang R et al (2015a) Safety, tolerability, and efficacy of TEV-48125 for preventive treatment of high-frequency episodic migraine: a multicentre, randomised, double-blind, placebo-controlled, phase 2b study. Lancet Neurol 14(11): 1081–1090. https://doi.org/10.1016/S1474-4422(15)00249-5
15. Silberstein SD, Dodick DW, Bigal ME, Yeung PP, Goadsby PJ, Blankenbiller T et al (2017) Fremanezumab for the preventive treatment of chronic migraine. N Engl J Med 377(22):2113–2122. https://doi.org/10.1056/NEJMoa1709038
16. Edvinsson L, Haanes KA, Warfvinge K, Krause DN (2018) CGRP as the target of new migraine therapies - successful translation from bench to clinic. Nat Rev Neurol 14(6):338–350. https://doi.org/10.1038/s41582-018-0003-1
17. Edvinsson L, Ekman R, Goadsby PJ (2010b) Measurement of vasoactive neuropeptides in biological materials: problems and pitfalls from 30 years of experience and novel future approaches. Cephalalgia 30(6):761–766
18. Mulvany MJ, Halpern W (1977) Contractile properties of small arterial resistance vessels in spontaneously hypertensive and normotensive rats. Circ Res 41(1):19–26
19. Hogestatt ED, Andersson KE, Edvinsson L (1983) Mechanical properties of rat cerebral arteries as studied by a sensitive device for recording of mechanical activity in isolated small blood vessels. Acta Physiol Scand 117(1):49–61. https://doi.org/10.1111/j.1748-1716.1983.tb07178.x

20. Cohen-Barak O, Weiss S, Rasamoelisolo M, Faulhaber N, Yeung PP, Loupe PS et al (2018) A phase 1 study to assess the pharmacokinetics, safety, and tolerability of fremanezumab doses (225 mg, 675 mg and 900 mg) in Japanese and Caucasian healthy subjects. Cephalalgia:333102418771376. https://doi.org/10.1177/0333102418771376
21. Warfvinge K, Edvinsson L (2017) Distribution of CGRP and CGRP receptor components in the rat brain. Cephalalgia:333102417728873. https://doi.org/10.1177/0333102417728873
22. Edvinsson L, Linde M (2010) New drugs in migraine treatment and prophylaxis: telcagepant and topiramate. Lancet 376(9741):645–655. https://doi.org/10.1016/S0140-6736(10)60323-6
23. Ho TW, Edvinsson L, Goadsby PJ (2010) CGRP and its receptors provide new insights into migraine pathophysiology. Nat Rev Neurol 6(10):573–582. https://doi.org/10.1038/nrneurol.2010.127
24. Edvinsson L (1985) Functional-role of perivascular peptides in the control of cerebral-circulation. Trends Neurosci 8(3):126–131. https://doi.org/10.1016/0166-2236(85)90050-5
25. Edvinsson L (2007) Novel migraine therapy with calcitonin gene-regulated peptide receptor antagonists. Expert Opin Ther Targets 11(9):1179–1188. https://doi.org/10.1517/14728222.11.9.1179
26. Juhl L, Edvinsson L, Olesen J, Jansen-Olesen I (2007) Effect of two novel CGRP-binding compounds in a closed cranial window rat model. Eur J Pharmacol 567(1–2):117–124. https://doi.org/10.1016/j.ejphar.2007.04.004
27. Eftekhari S, Salvatore CA, Johansson S, Chen TB, Zeng Z, Edvinsson L (2014) Localization of CGRP, CGRP receptor, PACAP and glutamate in trigeminal ganglion. Relation to the blood-brain barrier. Brain Res. https://doi.org/10.1016/j.brainres.2014.11.031
28. Lundblad C, Haanes KA, Grande G, Edvinsson L (2015) Experimental inflammation following dural application of complete Freund's adjuvant or inflammatory soup does not alter brain and trigeminal microvascular passage. J Headache Pain 16:91. https://doi.org/10.1186/s10194-015-0575-8
29. Edvinsson L, Chan KY, Eftekhari S, Nilsson E, de Vries R, Saveland H et al (2010a) Effect of the calcitonin gene-related peptide (CGRP) receptor antagonist telcagepant in human cranial arteries. Cephalalgia 30(10):1233–1240. https://doi.org/10.1177/0333102410362122

Multi-frequency analysis of brain connectivity networks in migraineurs: a magnetoencephalography study

Di Wu[1], Yuchen Zhou[1], Jing Xiang[2], Lu Tang[1], Hongxing Liu[1], Shuyang Huang[1], Ting Wu[3], Qiqi Chen[3] and Xiaoshan Wang[1*]

Abstract

Background: Although alterations in resting-state neural network have been previously reported in migraine using functional MRI, whether this atypical neural network is frequency dependent remains unknown. The aim of this study was to investigate the alterations of the functional connectivity of neural network and their frequency specificity in migraineurs as compared with healthy controls by using magnetoencephalography (MEG) and concepts from graph theory.

Methods: Twenty-three episodic migraine patients with and without aura, during the interictal period, and 23 age- and gender-matched healthy controls at resting state with eye-closed were studied with MEG. Functional connectivity of neural network from low (0.1–1 Hz) to high (80–250 Hz) frequency ranges was analyzed with topographic patterns and quantified with graph theory.

Results: The topographic patterns of neural network showed that the migraineurs had significantly increased functional connectivity in the slow wave (0.1–1 Hz) band in the frontal area as compared with controls. Compared with the migraineurs without aura (MwoA), the migraineurs with aura (MwA) had significantly increased functional connectivity in the theta (4–8 Hz) band in the occipital area. Graph theory analysis revealed that the migraineurs had significantly increased connection strength in the slow wave (0.1–1 Hz) band, increased path length in the theta (4–8 Hz) and ripple (80–250 Hz) bands, and increased clustering coefficient in the slow wave (0.1–1 Hz) and theta (4–8 Hz) bands. The clinical characteristics had no significant correlation with interictal MEG parameters.

Conclusions: Results indicate that functional connectivity of neural network in migraine is significantly impaired in both low- and high-frequency ranges. The alteration of neural network may imply that migraine is associated with functional brain reorganization.

Keywords: Migraine, Magnetoencephalography (MEG), Multi-frequency, Functional connectivity, Neural network, Graph theory

Background

Migraine is characterized by episodic headache attacks and is frequently accompanied by nausea, vomiting, yawning, photophobia, and phonophobia [1]. Our conceptualization of migraine has evolved from primarily a vascular disorder to a neurovascular disorder and currently to a brain disorder, primarily a disorder of neurons rather than a disorder of blood vessels [2, 3]. Numerous neuroimaging studies have used functional connectivity analysis to detect alterations in brain function in migraineurs and have revealed that neuroimaging alterations correlate with longer migraine duration and increased migraine frequency [4–8].

Functional connectivity has been considered an approach to describe how brain regions communicate information with each other [9]. During the resting state, correlated spontaneous fluctuations occur within spatially distinct and functionally related groups of

* Correspondence: lidou2005@126.com
[1]Department of Neurology, Nanjing Brain Hospital, Nanjing Medical University, 264 Guangzhou Road, Nanjing, Jiangsu 210029, China
Full list of author information is available at the end of the article

cortical and subcortical regions, consisting of the human brain's functional connectivity networks [10]. Functional connectivity measures the statistical interdependencies between two time series (brain signals), and different functional connectivity patterns reflect different models that brain regions work together [11]. The introduction of graph theory to neuroscience allows us to quantify different networks and further characterize the features of brain functional topology [12]. According to concepts from graph theory, the brain can be considered a mathematical network consisting of a set of nodes and links. Nodes in large-scale brain networks represent brain regions, and connections signify the communication among distinct brain regions (i.e., functional connectivity [13, 14]). Subsequently, graph theory has been extensively used to gain insight into how brain regions coordinate to support higher cognitive functions [15].

Electroencephalography (EEG) has been used in the study of functional connectivity or neural network in migraine [16–18]. By analysis of EEG signals in 0.5–30 Hz, de Tommaso and colleagues have found that migraineurs have increased connectivity between the bilateral temporal-parietal and the frontal regions around the midline as compared with healthy controls after laser stimulation [16]. It has been shown that neural network can reproduce the abnormality of the neurophysiological dysfunction in migraine [17]. An EEG study has demonstrated that MwA and MwoA are associated with different patterns of functional and effective connectivity in ongoing EEG under repetitive photic stimulation [18]. Functional magnetic resonance imaging (fMRI) study of migraine has also extended the focus from a single region or structure to a network of regions and structures and the interactions among them [19–21]. Tedeschi and colleagues have found that migraineurs exhibit an increased resting-state visual network connectivity, which may be related to the initiation and propagation of the migraine aura [19]. Mickleborough and colleagues have revealed that migraineurs lack suppression of unattended events and have heightened orienting to sudden onset stimuli in peripheral locations [20]. By using effective connectivity analysis of resting-state fMRI, Ting and colleagues have indicated that the dysfunctional ascending and descending pain network at the thalamic-level may play an important role in the study of migraine [21]. Though previous EEG and fMRI studies revealed the alteration of neural network in migraine, it remains unclear if the neural network impairment in migraine is frequency-dependent.

Magnetoencephalography (MEG), a relatively new clinical neuroimaging modality, is well suited for noninvasively detecting and localizing neuromagnetic signals [22]. MEG is considered to be superior to scalp EEG because the skull, skin, and other tissues can distort electric signals, whereas magnetic signals can pass through these tissues without significant distortion [23, 24]. Analysis of functional connectivity with MEG can investigate the functional organization of the brain based on temporal correlations in neuromagnetic signal fluctuations in different brain regions. Previous studies have used MEG with graph theory to reveal the features of the intrinsic functional network of the brain [25]. The changed features during the resting state may serve as a marker to reflect the progress of multiple diseases, such as Alzheimer's disease [12], Parkinson's disease [26], and Autism spectrum disorder [27]. Combining multi-frequency MEG analysis with graph theory, the neural network topology and its frequency specificity can be systematically demonstrated in both low- and high-frequency ranges.

The aim of this study was to investigate whether the functional connectivity neural networks are abnormal in migraineurs relative to healthy controls in low- and high-frequency ranges and whether the neural networks are different between the MwA and MwoA.

Methods

This study was approved by the Institutional Review Board at Nanjing Brain Hospital. All subjects signed a consent form after the experimental procedures were fully explained.

Subjects

The inclusion criteria for patients with migraine were based on the International Classification of Headache Disorders Second Edition (ICHD-II) [28, 29]. Exclusion criteria included the following: (1) existence of other neurological disease; and (2) use of prescription medications within a week prior to the study. Healthy controls were recruited to match subjects in the migraine group in terms of age and gender. Inclusion criteria included the following: (1) no history of any neurologic disorder; and (2) no first-degree relative with a history of any type of migraine. Exclusion criteria for all participants included the following: (1) presence of an implant (e.g., braces or pacemaker), which could produce visible magnetic noise in MEG data; (2) demonstration or expression of noticeable anxiety and/or inability to communicate readily with personnel operating the MEG equipment; (3) inability to keep still; and (4) pregnant patients or those with claustrophobic tendencies (for MRI scans).

Twenty-three patients with episodic migraine with or without aura (15 females; mean age: 30.04 years, standard deviation: 6.62 years, range: 20–40 years) were recruited from Nanjing Brain Hospital (Table 1). Ten (six

Table 1 Demographic and Clinical Characteristics of Migraineurs

Patients	Sex	Age (years)	Aura	History (years)	Attack Frequency	Duration (hours)	Pain Type	Pain Loacation	Pain Intensity	Onset to scan(days)
1	Female	27	No	10	2–3/month	24	Throbbing	Unilateral	5	5
2	Male	23	No	13	4/month	10	Constant	Unilateral	7	6
3	Female	36	No	12	1/month	20	Throbbing	Bilateral	7	4
4	Female	39	Yes	30	1/month	6	Pressure	Unilateral	6	15
5	Male	20	Yes	5	1–2/month	6	Pressure	Bilateral	7	7
6	Female	40	Yes	30	1–2/month	36	Throbbing	Unilateral	8	7
7	Female	34	No	12	2/month	4	Sharp	Unilateral	3	4
8	Female	40	Yes	16.5	1–2/month	48	Throbbing	Bilateral	7	5
9	Female	40	Yes	18	1–2/month	12	Pressure	Bilateral	7	10
10	Male	26	Yes	8	2/month	4	Throbbing	Unilateral	3	20
11	Female	26	No	3.5	3/month	72	Throbbing	Unilateral	8	5
12	Female	30	Yes	4.5	1–2/month	12	Pressure	Bilateral	6	4
13	Female	27	Yes	3.5	4/month	36	Constant	Unilateral	6	6
14	Female	32	No	2	1/month	48	Constant	Unilateral	5	7
15	Female	34	No	7	2/month	1	Pressure	Unilateral	6	7
16	Male	30	No	5.5	1/month	5	Pressure	Bilateral	3	4
17	Female	31	No	10	1–2/month	1.5	Stabbing	Unilateral	6	3
18	Male	24	No	7.5	1/month	12	Pressure	Unilateral	7	10
19	Male	20	No	4.5	3/month	12	Throbbing	Bilateral	5	6
20	Male	27	Yes	7	1/month	8	Pressure	Unilateral	7	5
21	Female	29	No	8	2–3/month	1	Squeezing	Unilateral	6	3
22	Female	35	No	10	1–2/month	2	Throbbing	Bilateral	7	4
23	Male	26	Yes	12	1/month	12	Throbbing	Unilateral	5	3

females; mean age: 31.50 years, standard deviation: 7.52 years, range: 20–40 years) of 23 patients with migraine had aura. Thirteen (nine females; mean age: 29.31 years, standard deviation: 5.02 years, range: 20–36 years) of 23 patients with migraine had no aura. All patients with migraine were right handed. Twenty-three age- and gender-matched, right-handed healthy controls (15 females; mean age: 29.83 years, standard deviation: 6.86 years, range: 20–40 years) were recruited. Patients had no migraine headache attack during MEG recording. All subjects were headache free at least 72 h (h) prior to the testing and 24 h after the scan.

MEG recording

MEG signals were recorded in a magnetically shielded room by using a whole-head CTF 275-Channel MEG system (VSM MedTech Systems, Inc., Coquitlam, BC, Canada) in the MEG Center at Nanjing Brain Hospital. Before data acquisition, every subject was asked to remove all metals from their body. Electromagnetic coils were attached to the nasion and to the left and right preauricular points of the subject. These three coils were subsequently activated at different frequencies to measure the head positions of the subject relative to the MEG sensors. MEG data were recorded at a sampling rate of 6000 Hz for 120 s. Subjects were placed in the supine position and instructed to keep their eyes closed during the recording, not to think of anything in particular, and not to fall asleep. After scanning, the subjects were asked if they remained awake during the whole procedure. The head positions were measured at the beginning and end of the scanning. If head movement during recording was beyond 5 mm, the dataset was indicated as "bad" and an additional dataset was recorded.

MRI scanning

Anatomical image data were recorded for all subjects by using a 1.5 T MRI scanner (Singa, GE, USA). Three fiducial points were placed at the same locations to facilitate co-registration of MEG and MRI data; these points were regarded as the positions of the three coils used in the MEG recordings before MRI scan. Subsequently, all anatomical landmarks digitized in the MEG study were identified during MRI scanning.

Data preprocessing

Similar to previous reports [30, 31], MEG waveforms were visually inspected for identifying magnetic noise and other artifacts. Any MEG data with noticeable magnetic noise or artifact (>6 pT) were excluded from the analyses. The MEG data were preprocessed by removing the direct current offset. The neural network at the sensor levels was analyzed by computing the coherence of MEG signals in multiple regions. A custom-designed program, MEG Processor, was used to compute and visualize functional networks at the sensor level [32, 33]. Neural activity (120 s) was filtered into seven frequency bands: slow wave (0.1–1 Hz), delta (1–4 Hz), theta (4–8 Hz), alpha (8–12 Hz), beta (12–30 Hz), gamma (30–80 Hz), and ripple (80–250 Hz). The distribution of the coherence for each possible pair of the 275 sensors was displayed in topographic patterns (network contourmaps, see Fig. 1). Red color indicated excitatory connection on contourmaps. An excitatory connection was a positive connection where the amplitude of signals in two connected sensors was positively correlated. Blue color indicated inhibitory connections on contourmaps. An inhibitory connection was a negative connection where the amplitude of signals in a sensor pair was negatively correlated. To compare migraineurs and controls, the same threshold value was used to exhibit contourmaps for all subjects.

Graph theory analysis [25] was performed to quantify the functional connectivity of networks at the sensor level. Neural networks were identified based on correlations among MEG signals from different brain regions. A total of 275 MEG sensors were considered a collection of nodes, whereas edges corresponded to functional connections between all pairs of these nodes. In this study, we focused on the network parameters of connection strength, path length, and clustering coefficient [13]. Average connection strength refers to the average functional connectivity between all possible connections of the entire MEG sensor array. The average path length refers to the average path length over each possible pair of nodes. This parameter is a measure of global integration of the network. The clustering coefficient of a node represents the ratio of all existing connections between the "neighbors" of a node (nodes that are one-step away) and the maximum possible number of edges between the neighbors. The average clustering coefficient of a network indicates the average clustering value over each node and represents a measure of the tendency of network elements to form local clusters.

Statistical analysis

Fisher's exact tests were used to analyze the odds ratio of functional connections in brain areas among the migraineurs and the controls. Analysis of variance analysis was applied to the power value difference between the migraineurs and the controls. Post-hoc comparison was conducted with two-tailed Student *t*-test for assessing the network parameters (strength, path length and clustering coefficient) between the migraine and control groups. The correlations between migraine clinical characteristics (age, headache history, attack frequency, duration, pain intensity and time from the last attack) and MEG parameters (topographic patterns of neural network and network parameters) were analyzed using Spearman correlation coefficients.

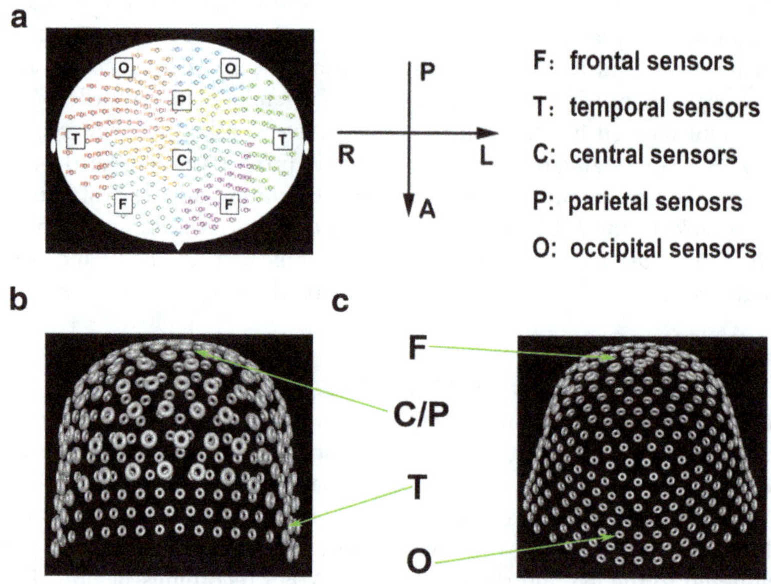

Fig. 1 Distribution map of MEG sensors. **a** 2D map of the distributionof all MEG sensors. **b** 3D front view of the distribution of all MEG sensors. **c** 3D bottom view of the distribution of all MEG sensors

A significance level of 0.05 (two-tailed) was accepted for each comparison. If multiple testing was considered, the significance level for each of these tests was reduced from 0.05 to 0.016 (three parameters, Bonferroni correction). Statistical analyses were performed using SPSS version 19.0 software package (IBM Inc.).

Results

Clinical characteristics

Of 23 patients with migraine, 15 (65 %) were females (eight were males, 35 %). Out of the 23 patients, 10 (43 %) had visual aura, 20 (87 %) presented moderate to severe headache, and 15 (65 %) manifested unilateral headache attacks (Table 1).

Topographic patterns of neural network

In the slow wave (0.1–1 Hz) band, a significant difference was observed in functional connectivity patterns in the frontal cortex between the migraineurs and the controls. Typical topographic distributions of functional connectivity patterns are shown in Fig. 2. The neural network revealed that both the migraine group and the controls had excitatory connections in the left and right temporal sensors, and the connections between the bilateral temporal sensors were inhibitory connections. However, most of the migraineurs (17 of 23) had excitatory connections in the frontal sensors, whereas the controls did not ($p = 0.001$, Fig. 3). This result indicated that the migraineurs had significantly increased functional connectivity in the frontal sensors than that of the controls. No significant difference was observed between the MwA and MwoA in this frequency band.

In the delta (1–4 Hz) band, no significant difference was observed in functional connectivity patterns between the migraineurs and the controls. The neural network showed that both the migraine group and the

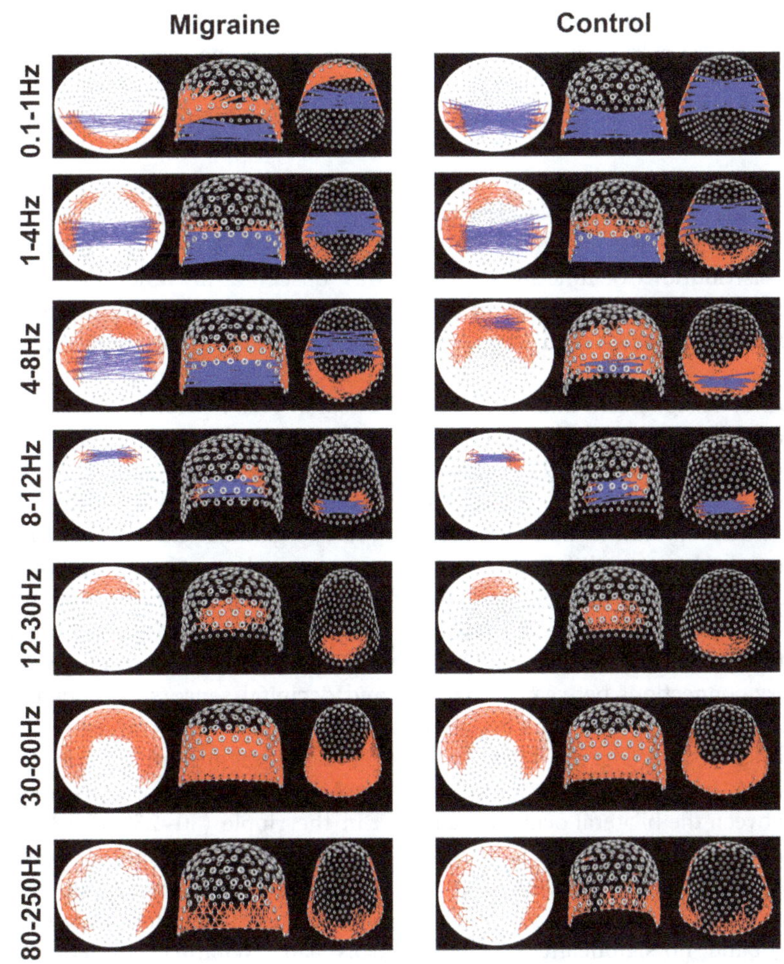

Fig. 2 Typical topographic distributions of functional connectivity patterns for seven frequency bands recorded from a migraineur and a control. The red color indicates excitatory connection and the blue color indicates inhibitory connections on contour maps. Compared with the controls, the migraineurs show significantly altered functional connectivity patterns in 0.1–1 Hz. Compared with the MwoA, the MwA shows significantly altered functional connectivity patterns in 4–8 Hz. The MwoA shows the same functional connectivity patterns as the controls in 4–8 Hz

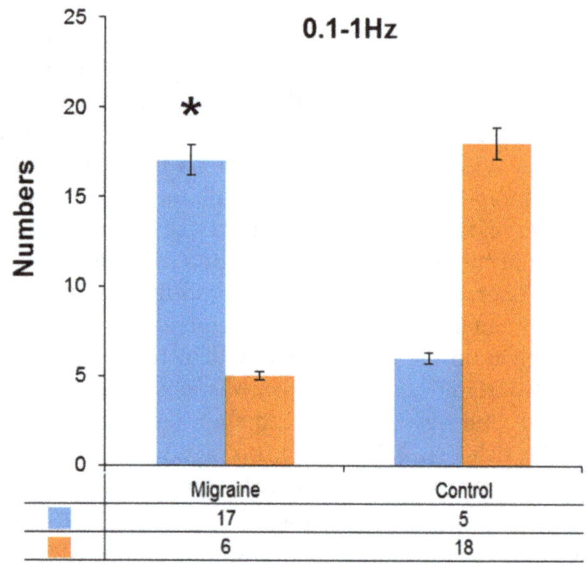

Fig. 3 Number of migraineurs and controls in different functional connectivity patterns in 0.1–1 Hz. Migraineurs have significantly higher odds of functional connectivity in the frontal area compared with controls. The blue bars indicate that excitatory connections are present in the frontal area. The orange bars indicate that no excitatory connections exist in the frontal area

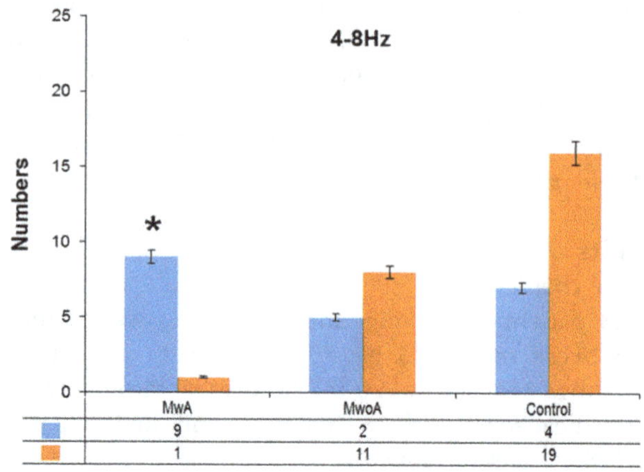

Fig. 4 Number of the MwA, MwoA, and controls in different functional connectivity patterns in 4–8 Hz. The MwoA and controls have significantly higher odds of inhibitory connections in the occipital area compared with the MwA. The blue bars indicate that no inhibitory connections exist in the occipital area, and the orange bars indicate that inhibitory connections exist in the occipital area

controls had excitatory connections in bilateral temporal and occipital sensors, and the connections between the bilateral temporal sensors were inhibitory connections. The typical topographic distributions of functional connectivity patterns are shown in Fig. 2. No significant difference was observed between the MwA and MwoA in this frequency band.

In the theta (4–8 Hz) band, no significant difference was observed between the MwoA and the controls. The neural network revealed that both the MwoA and the controls had excitatory connections in bilateral temporal and occipital sensors as well as inhibitory connections between the bilateral occipital sensors. However, differences were found between MwA and MwoA. The neural network revealed that the MwA had excitatory connections in bilateral temporal and occipital sensors. However, most MwA (9 of 10) had no inhibitory connections between bilateral occipital sensors and had inhibitory connections between bilateral temporal sensors ($p = 0.007$, Fig. 4). This result may indicate that the MwA had significantly increased functional connectivity between the bilateral occipital sensors than that of the MwoA and the controls. The typical topographic distributions of functional connectivity patterns are shown in Fig. 2.

In the alpha (8–12 Hz) band, no significant difference was observed in functional connectivity patterns between the migraineurs and the controls. The neural network revealed that both the migraineurs and the controls had excitatory connections in bilateral occipital sensors, and the connections between the bilateral occipital sensors were inhibitory connections. The typical topographic distributions of functional connectivity patterns are shown in Fig. 2. No significant difference was observed between the MwA and MwoA in this frequency band.

In the beta (12–30 Hz) band, no significant difference was observed in functional connectivity patterns between the migraineurs and the controls. The neural network revealed that both the migraineurs and the controls had excitatory connections in bilateral occipital sensors. The typical topographic distributions of functional connectivity patterns are shown in Fig. 2. No significant difference was observed between the MwA and MwoA in this frequency band.

In the gamma (30–80 Hz) band, no significant difference was observed in functional connectivity patterns between the migraineurs and the controls. The neural network revealed that both the migraineurs and the controls had excitatory connections in bilateral temporal and occipital sensors. The typical topographic distributions of functional connectivity patterns are shown in Fig. 2. No significant difference was observed between the MwA and MwoA in this frequency band.

In the ripple (80–250 Hz) band, no significant difference was observed in functional connectivity patterns between the migraineurs and the controls. The neural network revealed that both the migraineurs and the controls had excitatory connections in bilateral temporal and occipital sensors. The typical topographic distributions of functional connectivity patterns are shown in Fig. 2. No significant difference was observed between the MwA and MwoA in this frequency band.

Graph theory analysis

Strength

Group comparison revealed that the average connection strength of the functional connectivity network of the slow wave (0.1–1 Hz) band in migraineurs significantly increased compared with that of the controls ($p = 0.008$). No significant difference was observed between the migraineurs and controls in the other frequency bands. The average connection strength for migraineurs and controls in seven frequency bands are shown in Fig. 5.

Path

Group comparison revealed that the average path length of functional connectivity network in migraineurs significantly increased as compared with controls in the theta (4–8 Hz) ($p = 0.013$) and ripple (80–250 Hz) ($p = 0.002$) bands. No significant difference was observed between the migraineurs and controls in the other frequency bands. The average path length for migraineurs and controls in seven frequency bands are shown in Fig. 5.

Clustering coefficient

Group comparison revealed that the average clustering coefficient of functional connectivity network in migraineurs significantly increased compared with controls in the slow wave (0.1–1 Hz) ($p = 0.005$) and theta (4–8 Hz) bands ($p = 0.003$). No significant difference was observed between migraineurs and the controls in the other frequency bands. The average clustering coefficient for migraineurs and controls in seven frequency bands are shown in Fig. 5.

Clinical correlates

Results of correlation analysis demonstrated that there were no significant correlations between migraine clinical characteristics (age, headache history, attack frequency, duration, pain intensity and time from the last attack) and topographic patterns of neural network ($p > 0.05$). There were no significant correlations between migraine clinical characteristics (age, headache history, attack frequency, duration, pain intensity and time from the last attack) and the network parameters (strength, path length and clustering coefficient) ($p > 0.05$).

Discussion

This study has investigated the functional connectivity neural networks in migraineurs from low- (0.1–1 Hz) to high- (80–250 Hz) frequency ranges by using MEG. The functional connectivity topographic patterns and the measurements of graph theory analysis revealed neuromagnetic differences between the migraineurs and controls in distinct frequency ranges.

Most previous studies have investigated migraine by using MEG while patients were performing a task, including visual stimuli task [34], auditory stimuli task [28] and motor stimuli task [35]. However, these methods can only explore the stimulus-activated brain regions and not the entire brain. By contrast, the present resting-state study focused on the entire brain.

Previous MEG studies investigating resting-state migraine typically analyze a small frequency range [36]. These studies have resulted in several observations, such as suppression of spontaneous cortical activity, long-duration field changes, and large amplitude waves of several seconds' duration [37]. This study has focused on the functional brain network in migraineurs in a much wider frequency range, i.e., 0.1–250 Hz, with a high sampling-rate MEG system. By combining multi-frequency analysis of functional connectivity with graph theory method, we were able to systematically reveal the functional organization of brain networks in migraineurs compared with conventional analysis of brain waveforms.

The present data obtained from MEG is in consistent with previous reports with EEG [17] that functional connectivity in migraine is significantly impaired. The topographic patterns of neural network showed that the

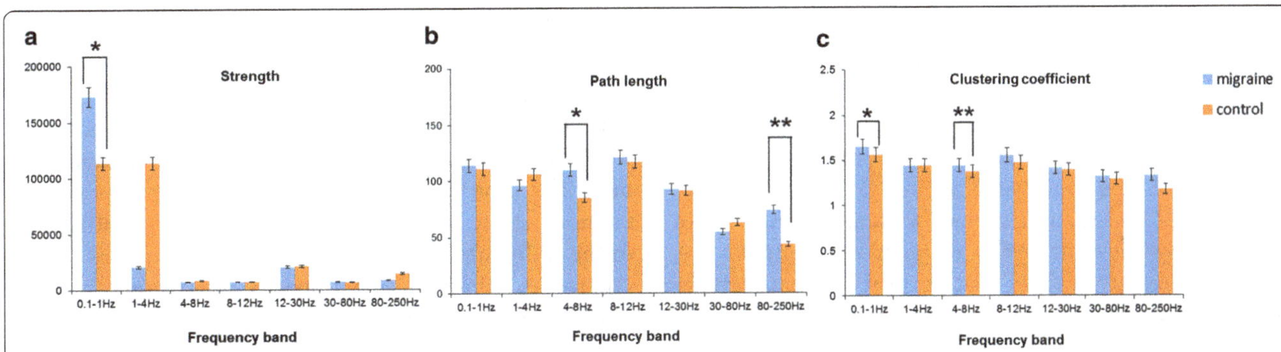

Fig. 5 Diffrences in network parameters (strength, path length, clustering coefficient) between the migraineurs and controls. **a** Comparison of the strength of each frequency band of the migraineurs and controls. **b** Comparison of the path length of each frequency band of the migraineurs and controls. **c** Comparison of the clustering coefficient of each frequency band of the migraineurs and controls (*$p < 0.016$, **$p < 0.005$)

migraineurs had significantly increased functional connectivity in slow wave band as compared with controls. This finding is supported by previous EEG study [16] which has demonstrated an increase in cortical connections during repetitive painful stimulation. However, previous EEG studies [16, 38] mainly focus on low-frequency brain signals (typically < 30 Hz). Therefore, the study of MEG signals above 30 Hz is novel. We consider the study of functional connectivity of neural network in both low- and high-frequency ranges will be important for migraine study.

The analysis of network topographic patterns shows that the migraineurs had significantly increased functional connectivity in the frontal areas than that of the controls in the slow wave (0.1–1 Hz) band. The frontal cortex is one of the most prominent areas associated with brain abnormalities in migraine patients [39, 40]. A recently published paper using MEG has revealed that migraineurs have a high likelihood of neuromagnetic activity in the lateral frontal cortex compared with controls in many frequency ranges [41]. The frontal lobes are responsible for numerous higher order cognitive functions, including planning, decision making, and abstraction, and thus are a primary candidate for dysfunction in many neurodevelopmental and neuropsychiatric disorders [27]. An interictal increase in resting-state functional connectivity in the frontal area may be related to hyperexcitability in the cerebral cortex in migraine. Previous studies have shown a condition of hyperexcitability of pain pathways within the central nervous system, which is thought to represent a crucial event in the neuropathology of migraine [42]. These findings may facilitate to develop new therapeutic strategies for migraine. For example, the repetitive transcranial magnetic stimulation (rTMS) is thought to be effective and well tolerated in the treatment of migraine with aura [43] because high-frequency rTMS increases and low-frequency rTMS decreases the neural excitability of the stimulated cortex [44–46].

The analysis of network topographic patterns also shows that the MwA had significantly increased functional connectivity in the bilateral occipital areas than that of the MwoA and controls in the theta (4–8 Hz) band. These findings suggest a hyperexcitability of the occipital area in the interictal phase of migraineurs with visual aura. Some previous EEG and fMRI studies have also revealed that the migraineurs with aura exhibited an increased resting-state visual network connectivity [19, 47]. These results support that cortical hyperexcitability may play a key role in the cascade of migraine attacks in MwA. This resting-state MEG finding may represent a functional biomarker that could differentiate patients experiencing the aura phenomenon from MwoA, even between migraine attacks.

Quantitative analysis of network using graph theory has revealed that the migraineurs have disrupted organization of brain networks. The disrupted organization of brain networks can be characterized as (1) increased strength in the slow wave (0.1–1 Hz) band; (2) increased path length in the theta (4–8 Hz) and ripple (80–250 Hz) bands; and (3) increased clustering coefficient in the slow wave (0.1–1 Hz) and theta (4–8 Hz) bands. This finding indicated a less optimised topological organization in the intrinsic whole-brain networks of migraineurs. The strength is the sum of weights of connections in the brain areas [13]. An increase of connection strength may indicate a decrease of variations of inter-regional connectivity network. Increased functional connectivity may support the theory of central hyperexcitability in interictal migraine-related brain. The increased path length and clustering coefficient indicated an increased functional segregation and integration of the network topology in migraineurs at the sensor level. Functional segregation in the brain indicates specialised processing within densely interconnected groups of brain regions, whereas functional integration implies rapid combination of specialised information from distributed brain regions [13]. An increase in path length suggests weaker potential for functional integration among brain regions, whereas a higher clustering coefficient corresponds to increased clustering degree of brain regions. As both changes are characterized by a regular topology, we conclude that brain networks in patients with migraine move toward a regular network organization. This finding can advance our understanding of how repeated headache attacks affect the brain topology in migraineurs.

To identify the clinical significance of aberrant MEG parameters in migraineurs, we further calculated the correlations between the abnormal MEG parameters in migraineurs and migraine clinical characteristics. We did not find significant correlations between the network parameters and clinical characteristics in the present study. We speculate that interictal neuromagnetic signals (MEG data recorded during headache free period) might not be able to reflect the headache abnormalities. We noted a previous fMRI study in migraine [48] showed that the clustering coefficient was positively correlated with the duration of migraine in the patients' functional networks. The discrepancy between the results of this previous study and the present study can be attributed to the different frequency bands used for analysis. Biases inherent to differences in density among networks or differences in the clinical features of patients with migraine may also affect the results.

We noted that this study has some limitations. The first limitation of this study is the number of participants. Given that high-frequency MEG analysis requires a high sampling rate of MEG data, considerable time is needed to compute these MEG data. This limitation is common to many MEG studies; however, with the development of computer technology, the problem will be solved in the future. Another limitation is that neural network analysis was performed only at the sensor level. Given that many network studies with MEG have been performed only at the sensor level [12, 49, 50], source-level analysis may improve the signal-to-noise of the reconstructed time series. In the future research, source-level analysis will be added to compare the difference between the two methods.

Conclusions

This study has demonstrated that migraine is associated with frequency-specific alterations of functional connectivity networks. Increased functional connectivity in the frontal area was more than likely to play a role in migraine and the increased functional connectivity of occipital was probably related to visual aura. Furthermore, the migraineurs showed a dysregulated brain topology, characterized by increased strength, path, and clustering coefficient. The findings support the notion that cerebral hyperexcitability plays an important role in the cascade of migraine attacks. This resting-state MEG finding may represent a functional biomarker that could provide valuable insights into the underlying pathophysiology resulting from migraine.

Competing interests

The authors declare that they have no competing interests.

Author' contributions

XW, DW and JX conceived and designed the experiments. DW, YZ, HL, TW and QC performed the experiments. DW, JX, SH and LT analyzed the data. XW, DW, JX, YZ and LT wrote the paper. All authors read and approved the final manuscript.

Acknowledgments

The authors gratefully acknowledge the support of Department of Neurology, Nanjing Brain Hospital Nanjing Medical University. This study was financed based on a National Natural Science Foundation of China grant (grant number 81271440) and a Science and Technology Development Project of Nanjing grant (grant number 201503040).

Author details

[1]Department of Neurology, Nanjing Brain Hospital, Nanjing Medical University, 264 Guangzhou Road, Nanjing, Jiangsu 210029, China. [2]MEG Center, Division of Neurology, Cincinnati Children's Hospital Medical Center, 3333 Burnet Avenue, Cincinnati, OH 45220, USA. [3]MEG Center, Nanjing Brain Hospital, Nanjing, Jiangsu 210029, China.

References

1. Hershey AD, Kabbouche MA, Powers SW (2006) Chronic daily headaches in children. Curr Pain Headache Rep 10(5):370–376
2. Goadsby PJ (2009) Pathophysiology of migraine. Neurol Clin 27(2):335–360. doi:10.1016/j.ncl.2008.11.012
3. Sprenger T, Goadsby PJ (2009) Migraine pathogenesis and state of pharmacological treatment options. BMC Med 7:71. doi:10.1186/1741-7015-7-71
4. Mainero C, Boshyan J, Hadjikhani N (2011) Altered functional magnetic resonance imaging resting-state connectivity in periaqueductal gray networks in migraine. Ann Neurol 70(5):838–845. doi:10.1002/ana.22537
5. Yuan K, Zhao L, Cheng P, Yu D, Zhao L, Dong T, Xing L, Bi Y, Yang X, von Deneen KM, Liang F, Gong Q, Qin W, Tian J (2013) Altered structure and resting-state functional connectivity of the basal ganglia in migraine patients without aura. J Pain 14(8):836–844. doi:10.1016/j.jpain.2013.02.010
6. Schwedt TJ, Schlaggar BL, Mar S, Nolan T, Coalson RS, Nardos B, Benzinger T, Larson-Prior LJ (2013) Atypical resting-state functional connectivity of affective pain regions in chronic migraine. Headache 53(5):737–751. doi:10.1111/head.12081
7. Jin C, Yuan K, Zhao L, Zhao L, Yu D, von Deneen KM, Zhang M, Qin W, Sun W, Tian J (2012) Structural and functional abnormalities in migraine patients without aura. NMR in Biomedicine. doi:10.1002/nbm.2819
8. Moulton EA, Becerra L, Johnson A, Burstein R, Borsook D (2014) Altered hypothalamic functional connectivity with autonomic circuits and the locus coeruleus in migraine. PLoS One 9(4):e95508. doi:10.1371/journal.pone.0095508
9. Sporns O, Chialvo DR, Kaiser M, Hilgetag CC (2004) Organization, development and function of complex brain networks. Trends Cogn Sci 8(9):418–425. doi:10.1016/j.tics.2004.07.008
10. Seeley WW, Crawford RK, Zhou J, Miller BL, Greicius MD (2009) Neurodegenerative diseases target large-scale human brain networks. Neuron 62(1):42–52. doi:10.1016/j.neuron.2009.03.024
11. Pizzella V, Marzetti L, Della Penna S, de Pasquale F, Zappasodi F, Romani GL (2014) Magnetoencephalography in the study of brain dynamics. Funct Neurol 29(4):241
12. Stam CJ, de Haan W, Daffertshofer A, Jones BF, Manshanden I, van Cappellen van Walsum AM, Montez T, Verbunt JP, de Munck JC, van Dijk BW, Berendse HW, Scheltens P (2009) Graph theoretical analysis of magnetoencephalographic functional connectivity in Alzheimer's disease. Brain 132(Pt 1):213–224. doi:10.1093/brain/awn262
13. Rubinov M, Sporns O (2010) Complex network measures of brain connectivity: uses and interpretations. Neuroimage 52(3):1059–1069. doi:10.1016/j.neuroimage.2009.10.003
14. Bullmore E, Sporns O (2009) Complex brain networks: graph theoretical analysis of structural and functional systems. Nat Rev Neurol 10(3):186–198. doi:10.1038/nrn2575
15. Buldu JM, Bajo R, Maestu F, Castellanos N, Leyva I, Gil P, Sendina-Nadal I, Almendral JA, Nevado A, del-Pozo F, Boccaletti S (2011) Reorganization of functional networks in mild cognitive impairment. PLoS One 6(5):e19584. doi:10.1371/journal.pone.0019584
16. de Tommaso M, Trotta G, Vecchio E, Ricci K, Van de Steen F, Montemurno A, Lorenzo M, Marinazzo D, Bellotti R, Stramaglia S (2015) Functional Connectivity of EEG Signals Under Laser Stimulation in Migraine. Front Hum Neurosci 9:640. doi:10.3389/fnhum.2015.00640
17. Thomas E, Sandor PS, Ambrosini A, Schoenen J (2002) A neural network model of sensitization of evoked cortical responses in migraine. Cephalalgia 22(1):48–53
18. de Tommaso M, Stramaglia S, Marinazzo D, Trotta G, Pellicoro M (2013) Functional and effective connectivity in EEG alpha and beta bands during intermittent flash stimulation in migraine with and without aura. Cephalalgia 33(11):938–947. doi:10.1177/0333102413477741
19. Tedeschi G, Russo A, Conte F, Corbo D, Caiazzo G, Giordano A, Conforti R, Esposito F, Tessitore A (2016) Increased interictal visual network connectivity in patients with migraine with aura. Cephalalgia 36(2):139–147. doi:10.1177/0333102415584360
20. Mickleborough MJ, Ekstrand C, Gould L, Lorentz EJ, Ellchuk T, Babyn P, Borowsky R (2015) Attentional Network Differences Between Migraineurs and Non-migraine Controls: fMRI Evidence. Brain Topogr. doi:10.1007/s10548-015-0459-x
21. Wang T, Chen N, Zhan W, Liu J, Zhang J, Liu Q, Huang H, He L, Zhang J, Gong Q (2015) Altered effective connectivity of posterior thalamus in migraine with cutaneous allodynia: a resting-state fMRI study with granger causality analysis. J Headache Pain 17(1):17. doi:10.1186/s10194-016-0610-4
22. Hamalainen MS (1992) Magnetoencephalography: a tool for functional brain imaging. Brain Topogr 5(2):95–102
23. Barkley GL, Baumgartner C (2003) MEG and EEG in epilepsy. J Clin Neurophysiol 20(3):163–178
24. Wheless JW, Castillo E, Maggio V, Kim HL, Breier JI, Simos PG, Papanicolaou AC (2004) Magnetoencephalography (MEG) and magnetic source imaging (MSI). Neurologist 10(3):138–153

25. Maldjian JA, Davenport EM, Whitlow CT (2014) Graph theoretical analysis of resting-state MEG data: Identifying interhemispheric connectivity and the default mode. Neuroimage 96:88–94. doi:10.1016/j.neuroimage.2014.03.065
26. Olde Dubbelink KT, Hillebrand A, Stoffers D, Deijen JB, Twisk JW, Stam CJ, Berendse HW (2014) Disrupted brain network topology in Parkinson's disease: a longitudinal magnetoencephalography study. Brain 137(Pt 1):197–207. doi:10.1093/brain/awt316
27. Ye AX, Leung RC, Schafer CB, Taylor MJ, Doesburg SM (2014) Atypical resting synchrony in autism spectrum disorder. Hum Brain Mapp 35(12): 6049–6066. doi:10.1002/hbm.22604
28. Korostenskaja M, Pardos M, Kujala T, Rose DF, Brown D, Horn P, Wang Y, Fujiwara H, Xiang J, Kabbouche MA, Powers SW, Hershey AD (2011) Impaired auditory information processing during acute migraine: a magnetoencephalography study. Int J Neurosci 121(7):355–365. doi:10.3109/00207454.2011.560312
29. Huo X, Xiang J, Wang Y, Kirtman EG, Kotecha R, Fujiwara H, Hemasilpin N, Rose DF, Degrauw T (2010) Gamma oscillations in the primary motor cortex studied with MEG. Brain Dev 32(8):619–624. doi:10.1016/j.braindev.2009.09.021
30. Xiang J, deGrauw X, Korostenskaja M, Korman AM, O'Brien HL, Kabbouche MA, Powers SW, Hershey AD (2013) Altered cortical activation in adolescents with acute migraine: a magnetoencephalography study. J Pain 14(12):1553–1563. doi:10.1016/j.jpain.2013.04.009
31. Guo X, Xiang J, Wang Y, O'Brien H, Kabbouche M, Horn P, Powers SW, Hershey AD (2012) Aberrant neuromagnetic activation in the motor cortex in children with acute migraine: a magnetoencephalography study. PLoS One 7(11):e50095. doi:10.1371/journal.pone.0050095
32. Xiang J, Korman A, Samarasinghe KM, Wang X, Zhang F, Qiao H, Sun B, Wang F, Fan HH, Thompson EA (2015) Volumetric imaging of brain activity with spatial-frequency decoding of neuromagnetic signals. J Neurosci Methods 239:114–128. doi:10.1016/j.jneumeth.2014.10.007
33. Xiang J, Luo Q, Kotecha R, Korman A, Zhang F, Luo H, Fujiwara H, Hemasilpin N, Rose DF (2014) Accumulated source imaging of brain activity with both low and high-frequency neuromagnetic signals. Front Neuroinformatics 8(57):1–17. doi:10.3389/fninf.2014.00057
34. Vincent M, Pedra E, Mourao-Miranda J, Bramati IE, Henrique AR, Moll J (2003) Enhanced interictal responsiveness of the migraineous visual cortex to incongruent bar stimulation: a functional MRI visual activation study. Cephalalgia 23(9):860–868
35. Xiang J, Degrauw X, Korman AM, Allen JR, O'Brien HL, Kabbouche MA, Powers SW, Hershey AD (2013) Neuromagnetic abnormality of motor cortical activation and phases of headache attacks in childhood migraine. PLoS One 8(12):e83669. doi:10.1371/journal.pone.0083669
36. Chen WT, Wang SJ, Fuh JL, Ko YC, Lee YC, Hamalainen MS, Lin YY (2012) Visual cortex excitability and plasticity associated with remission from chronic to episodic migraine. Cephalalgia 32(7):537–543. doi:10.1177/0333102412443337
37. Barkley GL, Tepley N, Nagel-Leiby S, Moran JE, Simkins RT, Welch KM (1990) Magnetoencephalographic studies of migraine. Headache 30(7):428–434
38. Clemens B, Bank J, Piros P, Bessenyei M, Veto S, Toth M, Kondakor I (2008) Three-dimensional localization of abnormal EEG activity in migraine: a low resolution electromagnetic tomography (LORETA) study of migraine patients in the pain-free interval. Brain Topogr 21(1):36–42. doi:10.1007/s10548-008-0061-6
39. Schwedt TJ, Dodick DW (2009) Advanced neuroimaging of migraine. Lancet Neurol 8(6):560–568. doi:10.1016/S1474-4422(09)70107-3
40. Schmitz N, Admiraal-Behloul F, Arkink EB, Kruit MC, Schoonman GG, Ferrari MD, van Buchem MA (2008) Attack frequency and disease duration as indicators for brain damage in migraine. Headache 48(7):1044–1055. doi:10.1111/j.1526-4610.2008.01133.x
41. Liu H, Ge H, Xiang J, Miao A, Tang L, Wu T, Chen Q, Yang L, Wang X (2015) Resting state brain activity in patients with migraine: a magnetoencephalography study. J Headache Pain 16:525. doi:10.1186/s10194-015-0525-5
42. Aurora SK, Wilkinson F (2007) The brain is hyperexcitable in migraine. Cephalalgia 27(12):1442–1453. doi:10.1111/j.1468-2982.2007.01502.x
43. Bhola R, Kinsella E, Giffin N, Lipscombe S, Ahmed F, Weatherall M, Goadsby PJ (2015) Single-pulse transcranial magnetic stimulation (sTMS) for the acute treatment of migraine: evaluation of outcome data for the UK post market pilot program. J Headache Pain 16:535. doi:10.1186/s10194-015-0535-3
44. Brigo F, Storti M, Nardone R, Fiaschi A, Bongiovanni LG, Tezzon F, Manganotti P (2012) Transcranial magnetic stimulation of visual cortex in migraine patients: a systematic review with meta-analysis. J Headache Pain 13(5):339–349. doi:10.1007/s10194-012-0445-6
45. Teepker M, Hotzel J, Timmesfeld N, Reis J, Mylius V, Haag A, Oertel WH, Rosenow F, Schepelmann K (2010) Low-frequency rTMS of the vertex in the prophylactic treatment of migraine. Cephalalgia 30(2):137–144. doi:10.1111/j.1468-2982.2009.01911.x
46. Minks E, Kopickova M, Marecek R, Streitova H, Bares M (2010) Transcranial magnetic stimulation of the cerebellum. Biomed Pap Med Fac Univ Palacky Olomouc Czech Repub 154(2):133–139
47. Hougaard A (2015) Investigations of functional and structural changes in migraine with aura by magnetic resonance imaging. Danish Med J 62(8):B5129
48. Liu J, Zhao L, Li G, Xiong S, Nan J, Li J, Yuan K, von Deneen KM, Liang F, Qin W, Tian J (2012) Hierarchical alteration of brain structural and functional networks in female migraine sufferers. PLoS One 7(12):e51250. doi:10.1371/journal.pone.0051250
49. Yang CY, Lin CP (2015) Time-Varying Network Measures in Resting and Task States Using Graph Theoretical Analysis. Brain Topogr 28(4):529–540. doi:10.1007/s10548-015-0432-8
50. Dimitriadis SI, Laskaris NA, Simos PG, Micheloyannis S, Fletcher JM, Rezaie R, Papanicolaou AC (2013) Altered temporal correlations in resting-state connectivity fluctuations in children with reading difficulties detected via MEG. Neuroimage 83:307–317. doi:10.1016/j.neuroimage.2013.06.036

24

Increased prevalence of depression and anxiety in patients with migraine and interictal photophobia

Stephanie M. Llop[1], Jonathan E. Frandsen[2], Kathleen B. Digre[2,3], Bradley J. Katz[2,3], Alison V. Crum[2,3], Chong Zhang[4] and Judith E. A. Warner[2,3*]

Abstract

Background: Most patients with migraine report photophobia associated with headache; a subset report interictal photophobia. These patients are light sensitive even during headache-free periods. The objective of this case–control study was to assess the prevalence of symptoms of anxiety and depression in migraine patients with and without interictal photophobia.

Methods: We recruited 16 subjects with migraine and interictal photophobia, 16 age- and gender-matched migraine subjects without interictal photophobia, and 16 age- and gender- matched controls. Migraine subjects met International Headache Society classification criteria. Participants completed a photophobia questionnaire, Beck Depression Inventory (BDI-II), and Beck Anxiety Inventory (BAI). Chi-square analyses and two-tailed Wilcoxon rank sum tests were used for the analyses.

Results: Subjects with interictal photophobia had significantly higher scores on the photophobia questionnaire compared to subjects without interictal photophobia. Subjects with interictal photophobia had significantly higher scores on the BDI-II and BAI compared to subjects without interictal photophobia.

Conclusions: Migraine patients with interictal photophobia are more likely to manifest symptoms of depression and anxiety compared to migraine patients without interictal photophobia. Care providers should be aware of increased prevalence of these symptoms in this population and consider appropriate referrals. Future research could assess whether treatment of photophobia leads to improvements in symptoms of depression and anxiety in migraine patients.

Keywords: Photophobia, Migraine, Depression, Anxiety, Sleep disorders, Intrinsically photosensitive retinal ganglion cells

Background

Photophobia is a general term used to describe light sensitivity or abnormal intolerance of light. Patients with photophobia avoid light because of pain or discomfort. In normal subjects, photophobia appears to serve the function of protecting the retina from damage due to photo-toxicity [1]. However, patients with an underlying disorder like migraine have been shown to display considerably greater light sensitivity when compared to controls [2]. Nearly all patients with migraine report photophobia during headache episodes, but a subset of these patients report photophobia all the time ("interictal photophobia"), even during headache–free periods [3]. Furthermore, interictal photophobia associated with migraine may have a negative, and sometimes disabling, impact on quality of life and social functioning, with the highest prevalence between the ages of 25 and 55 years, potentially the most productive period of life [4].

Several studies demonstrate that the presence of psychiatric co-morbidities is increased in people with

* Correspondence: Judith.warner@hsc.utah.edu
[2]Department of Ophthalmology and Visual Sciences, John A. Moran Eye Center, University of Utah Health Sciences Center, 65 N. Mario Capecchi Drive, Salt Lake City, UT 84132, USA
[3]Department of Neurology, University of Utah Health Sciences Center, 175 North Medical Drive East, Salt Lake City, UT 84132, USA
Full list of author information is available at the end of the article

migraine, especially depression and anxiety [5–10]. There seems to be a bi-directional relationship between migraine and depression, with each disorder increasing the risk of the other [11, 12]. Photophobia also was reported in patients with depression [13], but the nature of this relationship has not been rigorously studied. To the best of our knowledge, the relationship between interictal photophobia associated with migraine and depression and anxiety has never been investigated. In this observational pilot study we wished to better understand the relationships between interictal photophobia, depression and anxiety. We hypothesized that individuals with interictal photophobia and episodic migraine would have more anxiety and depression than those without interictal photophobia. We approached this question by determining the prevalence of symptoms of depression and anxiety in migraine patients with interictal photophobia, migraine patients without interictal photophobia and a control group.

Methods

University of Utah IRB approved this study (IRB # 35510). All authors had full access to all study data. Potential participants were recruited from the clinics of three investigators (BJK, JEAW, KBD). Recruitment and collection of study data took place between July 2009 and June 2011. After sending potential participants an introductory letter, one of the investigators (SML, JEF) contacted each participant by phone to discuss the study. Subsequently, participants signed the informed consent document during a clinic visit, and before completing the study questionnaires. Over a 3 month time we recruited a total of 48 subjects: 16 participants with episodic migraine and interictal photophobia, 16 age-and gender-matched migraine subjects without interictal photophobia, and 16 age- and gender-matched subjects with neither migraine nor photophobia. All migraine subjects met the International Classification of Headache Disorders (ICHD) (second edition) criteria for episodic migraine with or without aura (i.e., headaches less than 15 days/month) [14]. None were wearing sunglasses indoors, or spectacles that were specifically tinted for migraine and/or photophobia. None were being treated for interictal photophobia. We excluded potential subjects with chronic migraine, medication overuse headache, or chronic tension type headache. We did not specifically include or exclude subjects with a known history of depression or anxiety.

We asked each migraine subject whether she/he had light sensitivity between migraine attacks. If a subject answered affirmatively, the subject was assigned to the "migraine with interictal photophobia" group. If they answered negatively, the subject was placed in the "migraine without interictal photophobia" group. Control subjects were recruited from family members and others who accompanied study subjects, and from clinic patients without episodic migraine. All control subjects were matched to the other two groups according to age and gender.

To assess the presence and impact of photophobia, subjects completed a photophobia questionnaire (Fig. 1). We developed this questionnaire from questionnaires that have been used to assess photophobia in previous investigations [15, 16]. During the same session, subjects also completed the Beck Depression Inventory II (BDI-II) and the Beck Anxiety Inventory (BAI), validated methods to assess for symptoms of depression and anxiety, respectively [17–20]. The BDI-II consists of 21 questions, each with a score between 0 and 3. The minimum score is 0 and the maximum score is 63. Scores between 0 and 13 are scored as "minimal" depression, scores between 14 and 19 are scored as "mild" depression, scores between 20 and 28 are scored as "moderate" depression and scores 29 and above are considered to be consistent with "severe" depression. The BAI also consists of 21 questions, each with a score between 0 and 3. Scores between 0 and 21 are interpreted as low anxiety, scores between 22 and 35 are consistent with moderate anxiety, and scores greater than or equal to 36 are interpreted as evidence of severe anxiety.

Statistical analysis

We used Microsoft Excel 2010 and R 3.2.2 for the analyses. Pearson chi-square analyses and Wilcoxon rank sum tests were used to compare the cohorts. A P value of < 0.05 was considered significant. All tests were two sided. The sample size was determined by the number of patients that were seen for photophobia or light sensitivity while the study was open for enrollment.

Results

The mean age of subjects was 51.5 years and all three groups consisted of 2 men and 14 women. Using the photophobia questionnaire, subjects with interictal photophobia obtained a mean score of 7.9 (standard deviation [S.D.] = 3.9), migraine subjects without interictal photophobia obtained a mean score of 0.9 (S.D. = 0.5) and control subjects had a mean score of 1.0 (S.D. = 0.7). The differences between the migraine with interictal photophobia group and the migraine without interictal photophobia group ($P < 0.001$) and the control group ($P < 0.001$) were both statistically significant. The photophobia scores for the migraine without interictal photophobia group and the control group were similar ($P = 0.756$)

The averaged depression inventory total score (i.e., the sum of the scores of all the subsets) was higher for patients with migraine with interictal photophobia (mean = 13; S.D. = 10) than for both migraine patients without interictal photophobia (mean = 6; S.D. = 4.7; $P = 0.021$) and controls

LIGHT SENSITIVITY QUESTIONNAIRE

1. Do you currently drive? Yes No (Not scored)

If you do not drive, is it because of light sensitivity? Yes (Score=4) No (Score=0)

If you do drive, does light sensitivity affect your ability to drive? Yes (Scored below) No (Score=0)

Choose the sentence that most accurately describes the effect of light sensitivity on your ability to drive:

a. _____ Cannot drive at night because of light sensitivity (Score=1)
b. _____ Cannot drive in daytime, but need to prop eyelids open (Score=2)
c. _____ Can drive only short distances because of light sensitivity (Score=3)

2. Which of the following best describes your current ability to read?

a. _____ No limitation (Score=0)
b. _____ Uncomfortable because of light sensitivity, but no limitation (Score=1)
c. _____ Mild to moderate discomfort because of light sensitivity (Score=2)
d. _____ Marked limitation because of light sensitivity (Score=3)

3. Which of the following best describes your current ability to watch television?

a. _____ No limitation (Score=0)
b. _____ Uncomfortable because of light sensitivity, but no limitation (Score=1)
c. _____ Mild to moderate discomfort because of light sensitivity (Score=2)
d. _____ Marked limitation because of light sensitivity (Score=3)

4. Which of the following best describes your ability to watch movies in a theater?

a. _____ No limitation (Score=0)
b. _____ Uncomfortable because of light sensitivity, but no limitation (Score=1)
c. _____ Mild to moderate discomfort because of light sensitivity (Score=2)
d. _____ Marked limitation because of light sensitivity (Score=3)

5. Which of the following best describes your ability to go shopping (i.e. grocery and department stores)?

a. _____ No limitation (Score=0)
b. _____ Uncomfortable because of light sensitivity, but no limitation (Score=1)
c. _____ Mild to moderate discomfort because of light sensitivity (Score=2)
d. _____ Marked limitation because of light sensitivity (Score=3)

6. Which of the following best describes your current ability to do housework or to work outside the home?

a. _____ No limitation (Score=0)
b. _____ Uncomfortable because of light sensitivity, but no limitation (Score=1)
c. _____ Mild to moderate discomfort because of light sensitivity (Score=2)
d. _____ Marked limitation because of light sensitivity (Score=3)

7. Which of the following best describes your ability to walk about?

a. _____ No limitation (Score=0)
b. _____ Uncomfortable because of light sensitivity, but no limitation (Score=1)
c. _____ Difficulty walking in crowds because of light sensitivity (Score=2)
d. _____ Not able to walk alone outside because of light sensitivity (Score=3)
e. _____ Not able to walk unassisted indoors because of light sensitivity (Score=4)

Fig. 1 Photophobia questionnaire. This questionnaire was developed based on previous work by our group and by other groups for the assessment of photophobia in migraine and benign essential blepharospasm, two neurologic disorders that are strongly associated with photophobia. We developed this version to quantify the severity of light sensitivity and assess its effect on some activities of daily living

(mean = 6; S.D. = 8.8; $P = 0.0245$). Seven interictal photophobia subjects had depression inventory total scores that indicated symptoms of depression that were mild, moderate or severe. One migraine subject had mild symptoms of depression. Two control subjects had mild symptoms of depression and one control subject had symptoms of severe depression (Fig. 2).

The averaged anxiety inventory total score was significantly higher for patients with migraine and interictal photophobia (mean = 16; S.D. = 9.8) than for both migraine patients without interictal photophobia (mean = 4; S.D. = 3.4; $P < 0.001$ compared to interictal photophobia) and controls (mean = 5; S.D. = 6.9; $P < 0.001$ compared to interictal photophobia). Figure 3 illustrates the marked differences between interictal photophobia and the other two groups. Thirteen migraine subjects with interictal photophobia had symptoms of anxiety that were mild, moderate or severe. One migraine subject without interictal photophobia had symptoms of mild anxiety; one control subject had symptoms of mild

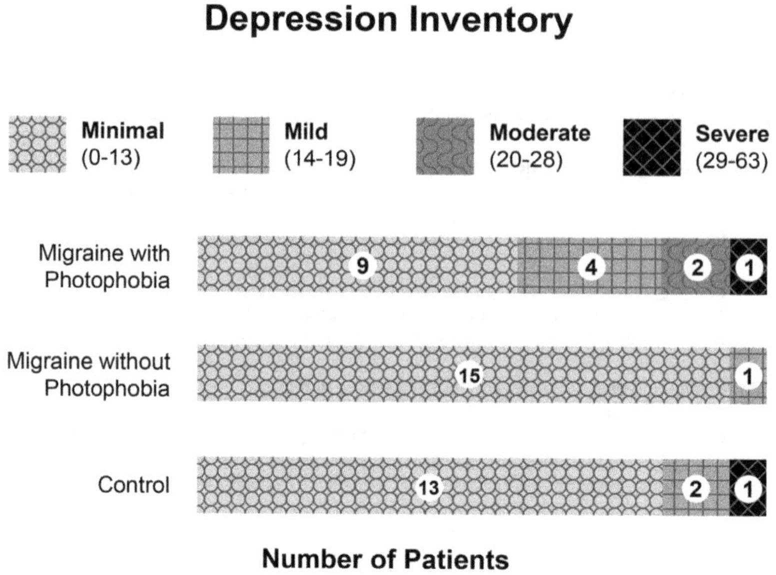

Fig. 2 Depression Inventory scores in migraine subjects with interictal photophobia, migraine subjects without interictal photophobia and a control group. Subjects with interictal photophobia were more likely to have depression inventory scores consistent with mild, moderate or severe depression compared to the other two groups

anxiety and one control subject had symptoms of severe anxiety.

In the process of analyzing the data from the depression inventory, we noticed a marked difference in the prevalence of self-reported sleep problems among the three groups. Twelve of the 16 migraine with interictal photophobia subjects (75 %) reported changes in sleeping patterns (hypersomnia or insomnia) compared to seven control subjects (43.75 %) and six migraine without interictal photophobia subjects (37.5 %). This difference was statistically significant ($P = 0.012$).

Discussion

Subjects who were assigned to the migraine with interictal photophobia group scored higher on the photophobia questionnaire than the other two groups. This result

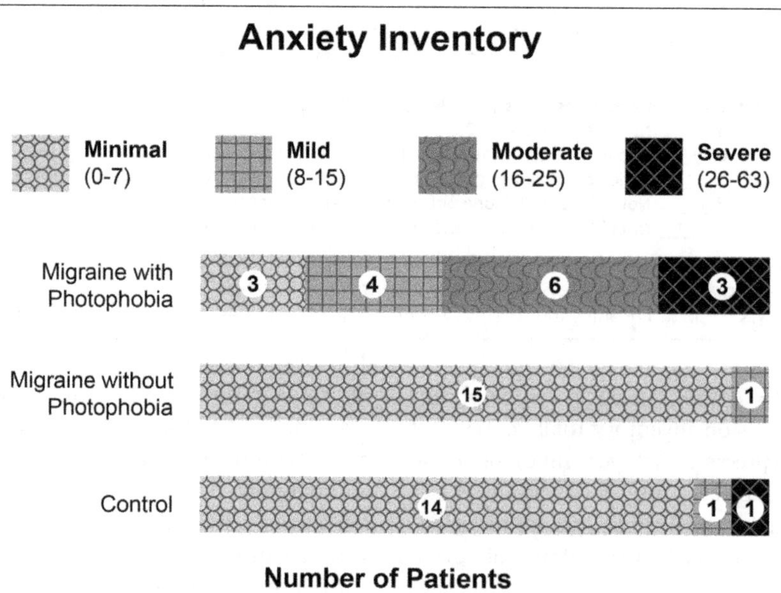

Fig. 3 Anxiety Inventory scores in migraine subjects with interictal photophobia, migraine subjects without interictal photophobia, and a control group. Subjects with interictal photophobia were far more likely to have anxiety inventory scores consistent with mild, moderate or severe anxiety compared to the other two groups

indicates that migraine subjects with interictal photophobia were appropriately assigned to this group based on the clinical interview. Subjects with migraine without interictal photophobia had photophobia questionnaire scores similar to the control group, also indicating that the migraine subjects without photophobia were assigned to the appropriate group based on the clinical interview.

Previous studies have demonstrated an association between migraine, anxiety and depression [5–10]. Researchers have proposed that the relationship between migraine, depression and anxiety is bi-directional, that is that they both influence each other [11, 12]. Previous work has also demonstrated that migraine patients are more light sensitive ("photophobic") than control subjects [15, 21–23], in some cases even between attacks [3]. Here we have demonstrated that symptoms of depression and anxiety are more prevalent among patients with migraine with interictal photophobia. We did not specifically include or exclude subjects with a known history of depression or anxiety. Photophobia may be a marker of more severe migraine (although in this study, not chronic migraine). The mean age of our subjects was 51 years, perhaps an indication of inter-ictal photophobia acquired over years of migraine. Interictal photophobia could represent central sensitization due to a lengthy migraine history.

Our study suggests that the relationship between migraine with interictal photophobia, anxiety and depression may indeed be multidirectional, with each of these entities influencing the other. To our knowledge, there have been no studies of anxiety or depression in other conditions characterized by interictal photophobia (such as iritis). One study of subjects with tinnitus, another distressing subjective neuro-sensory symptom, indicated that report of poor quality of life was mediated by anxiety and depression [24].

Our final observation, that subjects with migraine with interictal photophobia are more likely to report sleep problems was marked, but perhaps not unexpected, given the concomitant symptoms of depression and anxiety. Animal models also suggest a connection between emotional brain centers and light sensitivity. Delwig et al. found that in neonatal mice, which have no formed vision, light evoked vocalizations similar to vocalizations interpreted as anxiety of being isolated from the mother, and patterns of neural activation of the central amygdala and the posterior thalamic group, brain regions that are involved in pain processing and photophobia [25, 26]. The correlation between sleep disorders and migraine with interictal photophobia may be related to the neural circuits that underlie photophobia [27]. Circadian rhythms are entrained by the intrinsically photosensitive retinal ganglion cells of the eye [28]. These same cells appear to be the origin of a neural pathway that mediates the exacerbation of migraine pain by light [26].

We propose that patients who have migraine and interictal photophobia may harbor an abnormality in these neural circuits that results in both photophobia and disturbances of the sleep cycle. If the link between symptoms of anxiety and depression and migraine with interictal photophobia is confirmed by larger studies, this may offer avenues for treatment. There is good evidence that treating migraine improves depression and anxiety and that treating depression and anxiety favorably influences the treatment of migraine [12, 29–31]. What remains to be shown is if treatment of photophobia improves depression and/or anxiety?

Our study group was small and recruited from a tertiary care center, and these limitations should be taken into consideration when extrapolating our results to other patients with migraine and interictal photophobia. Nonetheless, we feel that the results we observed in this small sample merit additional investigation into the interaction between migraine, aura, photophobia, depression and anxiety, particularly by including a larger sample size from primary care settings that serve a variety of ethnic populations. Previous studies have documented differences in the clinical course of those who are members of ethnic or racial groups other than the Caucasian population we encounter in our clinics [32–38]. The photophobia questionnaire we used for this study will provide a valuable tool for further definition and assessment of these potentially important differences. We look forward to such investigations in the future, and we are optimistic that this line of research will improve our ability to care for these patients.

Conclusions

Most migraine specialists are aware of the increased prevalence of depression and anxiety in some of their patients. Our results indicate that if a migraine patient reports light sensitivity between attacks, they are at higher risk for these two mental health disorders. Physicians should consider having such patients evaluated and if necessary, treated for depression and anxiety. Because of the higher prevalence of self-reported sleep problems in this group and because of the adverse influence of poor sleep on migraine, physicians may also wish to consider inquiring about sleep problems and then recommend further evaluation or treatment in this group of patients.

Competing interests

Dr. Digre is listed as an inventor on a patent pending for thin-film coatings designed for the treatment of photophobia; she could receive royalties on any commercial sales of these coatings.

Dr. Katz has a leadership position and an equity interest in Axon Optics, LLC, an internet-based company that markets therapeutic eyewear for light sensitivity and migraine. Dr. Katz is listed as an inventor on a patent pending

for thin-film coatings designed for the treatment of photophobia; he could receive royalties on any commercial sales of these coatings.
Dr. Warner is listed as an inventor on a patent pending for thin-film coatings designed for the treatment of photophobia; she could receive royalties on any commercial sales of these coatings.
Dr. Llop, Dr. Frandsen, and Dr. Crum declare that they have no competing interests.

Authors' contributions

SML recruited subjects, acquired data, analyzed data, and drafted the manuscript. JEF recruited subjects, acquired data, analyzed data and drafted the manuscript. KBD conceived and designed the study and revised the manuscript critically for important intellectual content. BJK analyzed data and revised the manuscript critically for important intellectual content. AVC revised the manuscript critically for important intellectual content. CZ analyzed the data. JEAW conceived and designed the study and revised the manuscript critically for important intellectual content. All authors have given final approval of the version to be published and agree to be accountable for all aspects of the work in ensuring that questions related to the accuracy or integrity of any part of the work are appropriately investigated and resolved.

Acknowledgements

Permission for use of the test products was given by NCS Pearson, Inc., Bloomington, MN, USA.
Susan Schulman, University of Utah School of Medicine, provided assistance with manuscript preparation.

Funding

This project was supported by a grant to the Department of Ophthalmology and Visual Sciences from Research to Prevent Blindness, Inc., New York, NY, USA.
SML and JEF were supported by an NIH/NHLBI Short-Term Training: Students in Health Professional Schools Training Grant T35 HL007744 (PI Jerry Kaplan, PhD) and by University of Utah Institutional Support.
This investigation was supported by the University of Utah Study Design and Biostatistics Center, with funding in part from the National Center for Research Resources and the National Center for Advancing Translational Sciences, National Institutes of Health, through Grant 5UL1TR001067-02 (formerly 8UL1TR000105 and UL1RR025764).
The funding bodies had no role in the study design; in the collection, analysis and interpretation of data; in the writing of the manuscript; and in the decision to submit the manuscript for publication.

Author details

[1]Department of Ophthalmology, University of Puerto Rico School of Medicine, PO Box 365067, San Juan, Puerto Rico 00936, USA. [2]Department of Ophthalmology and Visual Sciences, John A. Moran Eye Center, University of Utah Health Sciences Center, 65 N. Mario Capecchi Drive, Salt Lake City, UT 84132, USA. [3]Department of Neurology, University of Utah Health Sciences Center, 175 North Medical Drive East, Salt Lake City, UT 84132, USA. [4]Division of Epidemiology, Department of Internal Medicine, University of Utah Health Sciences Center, 30 N 1900 East, Salt Lake City, UT 84132, USA.

References

1. Stringham JM, Fuld K, Wenzel AJ (2004) Spatial properties of photophobia. Invest Ophthalmol Vis Sci 45:3838–3848
2. Mulleners WM, Aurora SK, Chronicle EP, Stewart R, Gopal S, Koehler PJ (2001) Self-reported photophobic symptoms in migraineurs and controls are reliable and predict diagnostic category accurately. Headache 41:31–39
3. Main A, Dowson A, Gross M (1997) Photophobia and phonophobia in migraineurs between attacks. Headache 37:492–495
4. Wang SJ, Chen PK, Fuh JL (2010) Comorbidities of migraine. Front Neurol 1: 16. doi:10.3389/fneur.2010.00016
5. Lipton RB, Hamelsky SW, Kolodner KB, Steiner TJ, Stewart WF (2000) Migraine, quality of life, and depression: a population-based case–control study. Neurology 55:629–635
6. Breslau N, Lipton RB, Stewart WF, Schultz LR, Welch KM (2003) Comorbidity of migraine and depression: Investigating potential etiology and prognosis. Neurology 60:1308–1312
7. Galego JC, Cipullo JP, Cordeiro JA, Tognola WA (2004) Depression and migraine. Arq Neuropsiquiatr 62:774–777
8. Antonaci F, Nappi G, Galli F, Manzoni GC, Calabresi P, Costa A (2011) Migraine and psychiatric comorbidity: a review of clinical findings. J Headache Pain 12:115–125. doi:10.1007/s10194-010-0282-4
9. Sevillano-Garcia MD, Manso-Calderón R, Cacabelos-Pérez P (2007) Comorbidity in the migraine: depression, anxiety, stress and insomnia. Rev Neurol 45:400–405
10. Cardona-Castrillon GP, Isaza R, Zapata-Soto AP, Franco JG, Gonzalez-Berrio C, Tamayo-Diaz CP (2007) The comorbidity of major depressive disorder, dysthymic disorder and anxiety disorders with migraine. Rev Neurol 45:272–275
11. Domingues RB, Costa EA, Jr SA, Domingues SA, Leal JC, Gomez RS et al (2008) Correlation between migraine subtypes and depression. Arq Neuropsiquiatr 66:485–487
12. Hamelsky SW, Lipton RB (2006) Psychiatric comorbidity of migraine. Headache 46:1327–1333
13. Seggie J, Canny C, Mai F, McCrank E, Waring E (1989) Antidepressant medication reverses increased sensitivity to light in depression: preliminary report. Prog Neuropsychopharmacol Biol Psychiatry 13:537–541
14. Headache Classification Subcommittee of the International Headache Society (2004) The International Classification of Headache Disorders: 2nd edition. Cephalalgia 24(Suppl 1):9–160
15. Adams WH, Digre KB, Patel BC, Anderson RL, Warner JE, Katz BJ (2006) The evaluation of light sensitivity in benign essential blepharospasm. Am J Ophthalmol 142:82–87
16. Choi JY, Oh K, Kim BJ, Chung CS, Koh SB, Park KW (2009) Usefulness of a photophobia questionnaire in patients with migraine. Cephalalgia 29:953–959. doi:10.1111/j.1468-2982.2008.01822.x
17. Beck AT, Steer RA, Brown GK (1996) Manual for the Beck Depression Inventory-II. Psychological Corporation, San Antonio, TX
18. Beck AT, Epstein N, Brown G, Steer RA (1988) An inventory for measuring clinical anxiety: psychometric properties. J Consulting Clin Psychol 56:893–897
19. Whisman MA, Perez JE, Ramel W (2000) Factor structure of the Beck Depression Inventory-Second Edition (BDI-II) in a student sample. J Clin Psychol 56:545–551
20. Lasa L, Ayuso-Mateos JL, Vazquez-Barquero JL, Díez-Manrique FJ, Dowrick CF (2000) The use of the Beck Depression Inventory to screen for depression in the general population: a preliminary analysis. J Affect Disord 57:261–265
21. Woodhouse A, Drummond PD (1993) Mechanisms of increased sensitivity to noise and light in migraine headache. Cephalalgia 13:417–421
22. Vanagaite J, Pareja JA, Støren O, White LR, Sand T, Stovner LJ (1997) Light-induced discomfort and pain in migraine. Cephalalgia 17:733–741
23. Main A, Vlachonikolis I, Dowson A (2000) The wavelength of light causing photophobia in migraine and tension-type headache between attacks. Headache 40:194–199
24. Bartels H, Pedersen SS, van der Laan BF, Staal MJ, Albers FW, Middel B (2010) The impact of Type D personality on health-related quality of life in tinnitus patients is mainly mediated by anxiety and depression. Otol Neurotol 31:11–8. doi:10.1097/MAO.0b013e3181bc3dd1
25. Delwig A, Logan AM, Copenhagen DR, Ahn AH (2012) Light evokes melanopsin-dependent vocalization and neural activation associated with aversive experience in neonatal mice. PLoS One 7, e43787. doi:10.1371/journal.pone.0043787
26. Noseda R, Kainz V, Jakubowski M, Gooley JJ, Saper CB, Digre K et al (2010) A neural mechanism for exacerbation of headache by light. Nat Neurosci 13:239–245. doi:10.1038/nn.2475
27. Digre KB, Brennan KC (2012) Shedding Light on Photophobia. J Neuroophthalmol 32:68–81. doi:10.1097/WNO.0b013e3182474548
28. Berson DM, Dunn FA, Takao M (2002) Phototransduction by retinal ganglion cells that set the circadian clock. Science 295:1070–1073
29. Boudreau GP, Grosberg BM, McAllister PJ, Lipton RB, Buse DC (2015) Prophylactic Onabotulinumtoxin A in patients with chronic migraine and comorbid depression: An open-label, multicenter, pilot study of efficacy, safety and effect on headache-related disability, depression, and anxiety. Int J Gen Med 9:79–86. doi:10.2147/IJGM.S70456
30. Ligthart L, Gerrits MM, Boomsma DI, Penninx BW (2013) Anxiety and depression are associated with migraine and pain in general: an investigation of the interrelationships. J Pain 14:363–370. doi:10.1016/j.jpain.2012.12.006
31. Moon JS, Smith JH, Lahr BD, Cutrer FM (2013) Longitudinal associations of migraine and depressive symptoms: a cohort analysis. Psychosomatics 54:317–327. doi:10.1016/j.psym.2012.10.010

32. Peterlin BL, Rosso AL, Williams MA, Rosenberg JR, Haythornthwaite JA, Merikangas KR et al (2013) Episodic migraine and obesity and the influence of age, race, and sex. Neurology 81:1314–1321. doi:10.1212/WNL.0b013e3182a824f7
33. Gelaye B, Peterlin BL, Lemma S, Tesfaye M, Berhane Y, Williams MA (2013) Migraine and psychiatric comorbidities among sub-saharan african adults. Headache 53:310–321. doi:10.1111/j.1526-4610.2012.02259.x
34. Heckman BD, Berlin KS, Watakakosol R, St Pierre V (2011) Psychosocial headache measures in Caucasian and African American headache patients: psychometric attributes and measurement invariance. Cephalalgia 31:222–234. doi:10.1177/0333102410372429
35. Heckman BD, Merrill JC, Anderson T (2013) Race, psychiatric comorbidity, and headache characteristics in patients in headache subspecialty treatment clinics. Ethn Health 18:34–52. doi:10.1080/13557858.2012.682219
36. Tietjen GE, Peterlin BL, Brandes JL, Hafeez F, Hutchinson S, Martin VT et al (2007) Depression and anxiety: effect on the migraine-obesity relationship. Headache 47:866–875
37. Stewart WF, Lipton RB, Liberman J (1996) Variation in migraine prevalence by race. Neurology 47:52–59
38. Stewart WF, Roy J, Lipton RB (2013) Migraine prevalence, socioeconomic status, and social causation. Neurology 81:948–955. doi:10.1212/WNL.0b013e3182a43b32

25

Impact of migraine on fibromyalgia symptoms

Maria Adele Giamberardino[1*], Giannapia Affaitati[1], Paolo Martelletti[2], Claudio Tana[3], Andrea Negro[2], Domenico Lapenna[4], Martina Curto[2], Cosima Schiavone[4], Luisa Stellin[4], Francesco Cipollone[1] and Raffaele Costantini[5]

Abstract

Background: Fibromyalgia (FMS) and high frequency episodic/chronic migraine (M) very frequently co-occur, suggesting common pathophysiological mechanisms; both conditions display generalized somatic hyperalgesia. In FMS-M comorbidity we assessed if: a different level of hyperalgesia is present compared to one condition only; hyperalgesia is a function of migraine frequency; migraine attacks trigger FMS symptoms.

Methods: Female patients with fibromyalgia (FMS)(n.40), high frequency episodic migraine (M1)(n.41), chronic migraine (M2)(n.40), FMS + M1 (n.42) and FMS + M2 (n.40) underwent recording of: −electrical pain thresholds in skin, subcutis and muscle and pressure pain thresholds in control sites, −pressure pain thresholds in tender points (TePs), −number of monthly migraine attacks and fibromyalgia flares (3-month diary). Migraine and FMS parameters were evaluated before and after migraine prophylaxis, or no prophylaxis, for 3 months with calcium-channel blockers, in two further FMS + H1 groups (n.49, n.39). 1-way ANOVA was applied to test trends among groups, Student's *t*-test for paired samples was used to compare pre and post-treatment values.

Results: The lowest electrical and pressure thresholds at all sites and tissues were found in FMS + M2, followed by FMS + H1, FMS, M2 and M1 (trend: $p < 0.0001$). FMS monthly flares were progressively higher in FMS, FMS + M1 and FMS + M2 ($p < 0.0001$); most flares (86–87 %) occurred within 12 h from a migraine attack in co-morbid patients ($p < 0.0001$). Effective migraine prophylaxis vs no prophylaxis also produced a significant improvement of FMS symptoms (decreased monthly flares, increased pain thresholds)($0.0001 < p < 0.003$).

Conclusions: Co-morbidity between fibromyalgia and migraine involves heightened somatic hyperalgesia compared to one condition only. Increased migraine frequency – with shift towards chronicity – enhances both hyperalgesia and spontaneous FMS pain, which is reversed by effective migraine prophylaxis. These results suggest different levels of central sensitization in patients with migraine, fibromyalgia or both conditions and a role for migraine as a triggering factor for FMS.

Keywords: Migraine, Fibromyalgia, Pain thresholds, Tender points, Hyperalgesia, Central sensitization

Background

Fibromyalgia Syndrome (FMS) is a chronic pain condition whose prevalence in the general population ranges from 4 to 7 %, with a net female predominance [1, 2]. According to the 1990 ACR criteria, the syndrome is diagnosed if 2 main conditions are fulfilled: 1) presence of diffuse musculoskeletal pain of at least 3 months' duration and 2) positivity of at least 11 out of 18 predetermined body sites (9 symmetrical) called tender points (TePs), i.e., tenderness for an applied standard pressure of 4 kg-f exerted either manually or via a pressure algometer [3]. These criteria were revised in 2010 [4], with preliminary new criteria no longer taking into account the TeP count, while introducing more clinical requisites in addition to the diffuse muscle pain, e.g., the presence of sleep disorders, affective dysfunction, headache or visceral pains [5–9]. FMS has, indeed, a high

* Correspondence: mag@unich.it
[1]Fibromyalgia and Headache Center, Geriatrics Clinics, Department of Medicine and Science of Aging and Ce.S.I., "G. D'Annunzio" University of Chieti, via dei Vestini s.n., 66100 Chieti, Italy
Full list of author information is available at the end of the article

degree of comorbidity with a number of other medical conditions, among which headache, especially with an elevated number of attacks or chronic, is particularly frequent [10, 11]. Though tension-type headache is the most prevalent type in FMS, there is also a high co-occurrence between the syndrome and migraine [12]. A recent large epidemiologic study, in fact, evidenced a 55.8 % prevalence of migraine among fibromyalgia patients [13], while other studies showed the prevalence of fibromyalgia in migraine patients to be over 30 % [14, 15]. Although the pathophysiology of FMS is still incompletely known, a crucial role in the syndrome is believed to be played by central mechanisms of sensitization, secondary to an imbalance of neuromediators involved in nociceptive transmission/control in the Central Nervous System (CNS), in genetically predisposed subjects [16-18]. Clinical evidence of sensitization is provided by the generalized decrease in pain thresholds to different modalities of stimuli at somatic level not only in spontaneous painful areas but also in control, nonpainful sites, which has been widely documented in the syndrome [6, 19, 20]. High frequency and chronic headache have also been found to display increased sensitivity to pain in somatic areas outside the cephalic region, although to a lesser extent with respect to fibromyalgia [21–28]. These observations have raised the question as to whether the association of FMS with headache involves higher degrees of central sensitization with respect to one condition only. Clinical observations also report that FMS patients with concurrent headache, particularly migraine, often present an exacerbation of their typical FMS symptomatology in concomitance with or immediately subsequent to a headache attack, suggesting that headache may represent a triggering factor for fibromyalgia pain. However, in spite of the high degree of co-occurrence between headache and fibromyalgia, no systematic studies appear to have been conducted so far to evaluate the implications of this co-morbidity not only for the spontaneous FMS symptoms but also for the general sensory asset of the patients. This kind of study is instead important not only to better investigate the underlying mechanisms of these chronic pain co-morbidities, but also for therapeutic purposes, as the specific treatment of one condition could have a significant impact upon the symptoms of the other. On this basis, the aim of the present study was to verify: firstly, if the association of FMS with migraine involves different levels of pain hypersensitivity with respect to one condition only; secondly if, in co-morbid patients, the hypersensitivity level is a function of migraine frequency; thirdly, if migraine attacks act as a triggering factor for FMS symptoms. Quantitative sensory tests were carried out in both painful and nonpainful sites and the correlation was explored between occurrence and frequency of migraine attacks and fibromyalgia exacerbations (flares). In addition, the effects were investigated of reducing migraine frequency via specific prophylaxis, on the degree of FMS pain and hyperalgesia.

Preliminary results have already been published in abstract forms [25, 26].

Methods

The study was subdivided into two phases. The first phase evaluated the impact of migraine co-morbidity on somatic pain sensitivity and fibromyalgia pain. The second phase explored, in co-morbid patients, the effects of migraine prophylaxis on fibromyalgia symptoms. All patients attended the Headache and Fibromyalgia Center of the "G D'Annunzio" University of Chieti. The protocol adhered to the principles expressed in the Declaration of Helsinki and received ethic approval by the Institutional Review Board - Department of Medicine and Science of Aging – of the same University. A written informed consent was obtained from all patients (see inclusion criteria below).

Phase 1

Patients affected with fibromyalgia and/or migraine were considered for the study, subdivided into five groups: a) fibromyalgia (FMS), b) high frequency episodic migraine (8–14 days/month)(M1); c) chronic migraine (≥15 days/month)(M2); d) fibromyalgia plus high frequency episodic migraine (FMS + M1); and e) fibromyalgia plus chronic migraine (FMS + M2). *Inclusion criteria for FMS* were: female sex; age 18–65 years; a diagnosis of fibromyalgia performed by a specialist 2–5 years previously (according to ACR 1990 criteria, with subsequent confirmation by 2010 criteria), with start of symptoms not before 6 years preceding their first visit to the Center, average intensity of diffuse musculoskeletal pain between 50 and 70 mm of VAS, under a stable dose of amitriptyline (10 mg/day) in the preceding 3 months (the vast majority of FMS patients attending our Center already are under some form of pharmacologic basal treatment for the continuous and intense nature of their condition. Since it would have been unethical to suspend it for the purpose of the study, we chose to minimize the effects of this treatment on the evaluated parameters by setting a homogeneous treatment regimen with low doses of amitriptyline, for all FMS groups, see below); exclusion of any concurrent pathology able to interfere with the sensory evaluation (e.g., hypertension, diabetes) [29, 30]; exclusion of any other chronic pain condition except fibromyalgia; a negative clinical history of any form of acute pain (except fibromyalgia flares) in the preceding 6 months; exclusion of major psychiatric disorders at specialistic psychiatric examination; written, informed consent to participate in the study.

Inclusion criteria for M1 and M2 were: female sex, age 18–65 years, a diagnosis of migraine according to ICHD criteria (2004 criteria, confirmed by 2013 ICHD-3 beta criteria) [31, 32] with start of symptoms not before 12 years preceding the visit to the Center, and a number of migraine days ≥ 8 in the preceding 3 months; exclusion of any concurrent pathology able to interfere with the sensory evaluation (e.g., hypertension, diabetes); exclusion of any other chronic pain condition except migraine; a negative clinical history of any form of acute pain in the preceding 6 months; exclusion of major psychiatric disorders at specialistic psychiatric examination; informed, written consent to participate in the study.

Inclusion criteria for FMS + M1 and FMS + M2 were: female sex; age 18–65 years; a diagnosis of fibromyalgia as for the FMS group and of migraine as for the M1 and M2 groups; exclusion of any other chronic pain condition except fibromyalgia and migraine; exclusion of any concurrent pathology able to interfere with the sensory evaluation (e.g., hypertension, diabetes); a negative clinical history of any form of acute pain in the preceding 6 months; exclusion of major psychiatric disorders at specialistic psychiatric examination; informed, written consent to participate in the study.

Out of a total of 325 examined patients, n. 203 meeting the inclusion criteria were selected: a) FMS (n. 40; 39.92 ± 6.17SD years); b) M1 (n.41; 38.15 ± 5.37 years); c) M2 (n. 40; 36.9 ± 5.61 years); d) FMS + M1 (n. 42; 38.74 ± 5.93 years); e) FMS + M2 (n.40; 37.17 ± 5.73 years). The five groups did not differ in mean age.

In all groups: pain thresholds to electrical stimulation in skin, subcutis and muscle were measured in multiple, nonpainful, body sites (deltoid, trapezius and quadriceps of one side)(control sites); muscle pressure pain thresholds were evaluated in the same locations and in the 18 TePs. Recording was also performed of: number of monthly migraine attacks in all migraine patients (3-month evaluation in an ad-hoc migraine diary); number of monthly fibromyalgia peak pain episodes ("flares") in all FMS patients (3-month evaluation in an ad-hoc fibromyalgia diary); temporal relationship of FMS flares with migraine attacks in co-morbid groups (comparison of the two diaries; 3-month period).

Phase 2

Patients affected with fibromyalgia plus high frequency episodic migraine (8-14 days/month) were considered (FMS + M1), subdivided into two groups: patients to be subjected to migraine prophylaxis (FMS + M1 *with* prophylaxis) and patients not to be subjected to prophylaxis (FMS + M1 *without* prophylaxis).

Inclusion criteria for FMS + M1 with prophylaxis were the same as for the FMS + M1 group of phase 1, plus: habitual acute medication for fibromyalgia flares represented by paracetamol 1 g; willingness to undergo migraine prophylaxis with calcium-channel blockers; no contraindications to treatment with this drug class [33, 34].

Calcium-channel blockers were selected as preventative treatment because they have no known direct influence on pain symptoms. Other preventative migraine options were discarded for different reasons: beta-blockers for their potential interference with cardiovascular reactivity, already particularly unstable in FMS patients e.g., postural hypotension, and antiepileptics for their direct impact onto pain perception. Further antidepressants were excluded since all patients were already under amitriptyline treatment. Among calcium-channel blockers, flunarizine was chosen as, according to guidelines, it represents the molecule with the highest level of evidence of efficacy [35–37].

Inclusion criteria for FMS + M1 without prophylaxis were the same as for the FMS + M1 group of phase 1, plus habitual acute medication for fibromyalgia flares represented by paracetamol 1 g; unwillingness to undergo any migraine prophylaxis in the immediate future (i.e., unwillingness to add a further prophylactic treatment for migraine to their already existing chronic treatment regimen with amitriptyline).

Out of 145 examined patients, n. 86 were selected who met the inclusion criteria: 47 patients for the treatment group (38.2 ± 6.2 years) and 39 for the non-treatment group (39.1 ± 5.1 years). The two groups did not differ in mean age. In basal conditions all patients underwent the following recordings: monthly number of migraine attacks and fibromyalgic flares (retrospective evaluation relative to the preceding 3 months); monthly analgesic consumption for the fibromyalgia flares (retrospective evaluation relative to the preceding 3 months); pain thresholds to electrical stimulation in skin, subcutis and muscle and pressure pain thresholds in multiple, non-painful, body sites (deltoid, trapezius and quadriceps of one side)(control sites); pain thresholds to pressure stimulation at the 18 tender points (to calculate the mean threshold at TeP level). Patients of both groups were maintained on their standard chronic therapy for fibromyalgia with amitriptyline 10 mg/day. Patients of the FMS + M1 *with* prophylaxis group, but not those of the *without* prophylaxis group, were prescribed additional migraine prophylaxis with flunarizine (5 mg/die) for 3 months. Symptomatic treatment of fibromyalgia flares with paracetamol 1 g continued to be allowed.

All patients were requested to note, in ad-hoc diaries, the number of migraine attacks, fibromyalgia "flares" and rescue medications taken for fibromyalgia flares during the 3-month period of migraine prophylaxis, at the end of which pain thresholds were re-evaluated at both control areas and TeP level.

Pain threshold assessment to pressure stimulation

A standard pressure dynamometer was used for the evaluation (Fischer's algometer, Pain Diagnostic and Treatment, Inc., Great Neck, NY) [38]. The 1-cm diameter rounded probe of the instrument was placed perpendicularly on each evaluation site, pressure was increased by 0.1 kg-f/s until the first report of a painful sensation by the patient, the corresponding kg-f value was noted as the pressure pain threshold for that site. Thresholds were measured at the 18 TePs and in the trapezius, deltoid and quadriceps of one side (control sites). In each of these three muscles, two different points were evaluated (lateral and medial for trapezius – upper and lower for deltoid and quadriceps).

Pain threshold assessment to electrical stimulation

A computerized constant current electrical stimulator (R.S.D. Stimulator, prototype, Florence 1997) delivered 18-ms trains of 0.5-ms monophasic square wave pulses, frequency 310 Hz, automatically every 2 s, to the skin via surface electrodes and to the subcutaneous tissue and the muscle through needle electrodes. Skin electrodes consisted of a 10-mm diameter circular plate in Ag/AgCl (reference electrode) and a cylinder in Ag/AgCl with a 0.3 mm-diameter base (stimulating electrode), placed 1 cm apart on the skin surface with interposition of conductor paste. Subcutis/muscle electrodes were two monopolar needles, 0.3 mm in diameter (teflon isolation except for 2 mm at the tip), inserted vertically, 1.5 cm apart, just below the skin surface for subcutis measurement and deep under the fascia for muscle measurement (intramuscular position verified by observing electrode movement under voluntary contraction and/or low-intensity electrical stimulation). Evaluated sites were the: lateral aspect of the upper border of the trapezius (not coinciding with the TeP site, electrodes placed in the horizontal direction), lower half of the deltoid and lowest third of the quadriceps (anterior aspect of the thigh). Measurement of thresholds in each tissue was performed by the method of the limits, to record typical pain sensations in each tissue (pricking pain for skin, linearly radiating prickling pain for subcutis, cramplike pain for muscle) according to a procedure already described in detail in previous publications [39–41].

Measurements were always performed at the same time of day (10:00– 12:00 a.m.), in the pain-free interval. During all measurements, patients lay comfortably on an adjustable examination bed in a quiet room. The experimenters evaluating thresholds were not aware of the group the patient belonged to.

Statistical analysis

Phase 1

For each patient, the mean threshold was calculated of values recorded at the 18 TePs as the reference value for the specific FMS painful sites, and the mean threshold of the 6 values recorded in trapezius, deltoid and quadriceps as the reference value for the control sites. Means ± Standard Deviation (SD) were calculated of all parameters. Comparison among all groups for each parameter was performed via 1-way ANOVA.

To assess the temporal relationship between the occurrence of migraine attacks and fibromyalgic flares, for each patient the percentage was calculated of flares occurring within 12 h after a migraine attack vs occurrence of flares in any other period. Means ± SD were calculated of these percentages for each fibromyalgia patient group. The comparison between percentages of flares occurring within 12 h after a migraine attack and those of flares occurring at other time points in each group was performed via Wilcoxon matched-pairs signed-ranks test.

Phase 2

Means ± SD were calculated of all parameters. The comparison between treated and untreated groups was performed via Student's *t*-test for unpaired samples. The comparison of parameters before and after prophylaxis in the treated group, and at comparable time points in the non-treated group, was performed via Student's *t*-test for paired samples.

The level of significance was established at $p < 0.05$.

Results and discussion

Phase 1

Pain thresholds in control areas

The lowest electrical thresholds at all body sites and all tissues and lowest muscle pressure pain thresholds were found in FMS + M2 followed by FMS + M1, FMS, M2 and M1. The trend for variation among groups was significant for all parameters ($p < 0.0001$) (Fig. 1 and Fig. 2 left).

Pain thresholds in TePs

The lowest mean pressure pain thresholds at tender point site were found in FMS + M2 followed by FMS + M1, FMS, M2 and M1. The trend for variation among groups was significant ($p < 0.0001$) (Fig. 2 right).

Fibromyalgia vs migraine symptoms

The mean number of monthly FMS flares was significantly and progressively higher in FMS, FMS + M1 and FMS + M2 groups (Fig. 3).

In co-morbid patients, the mean number of monthly migraine attacks was: 11.7 ± 2.1 in the FMS + H1 group

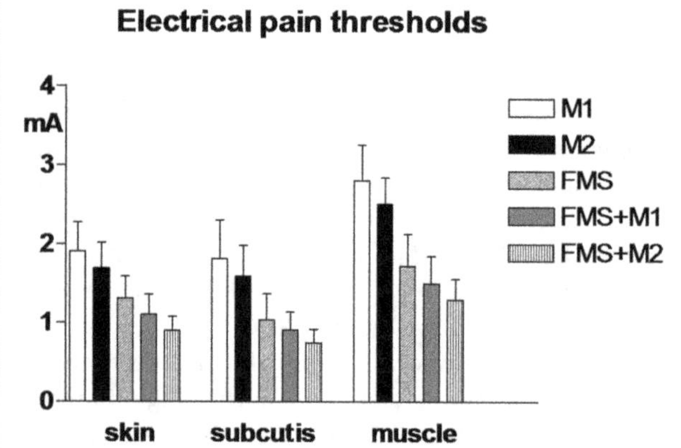

Fig. 1 Pain thresholds to electrical stimulation in control areas (mean values recorded in trapezius, deltoid and quadriceps muscles and overlying subcutis and skin) in patients with high frequency episodic migraine (n. 41)(M1), chronic migraine (n.40)(M2), fibromyalgia (FMS)(n.40), fibromyalgia plus high frequency episodic migraine (n.42)(FMS + M1), fibromyalgia + chronic migraine (n.40)(FMS + M2)(Means ± SD). * = $p < 0.05$; ** = $p < 0.01$; *** = $p < 0.001$. 1-way ANOVA = significant trend for the three tissues, ***. Internal comparisons = for skin, M1 vs M2: **; M1 vs FMS, FMS + M1, FMS + M2: ***; M2 vs FMS, FMS + M1, FMS + M2: ***; FMS vs FMS + M1: *; FMS vs FMS + M2: ***; FMS + M1 vs FMS + M2: * for subcutis, M1 vs M2: *; M1 vs FMS, FMS + M1, FMS + M2: ***; M2 vs FMS, FMS + M1, FMS + M2: ***; FMS vs FMS + M2: *** for muscle, M1 vs M2: *; M1 vs FMS, FMS + M1, FMS + M2: ***; M2 vs FMS, FMS + M1, FMS + M2: ***; FMS vs FMS + M2: ***

and 19.4 ± 3.2 in the FMS + M2 group. The majority of FMS flares occurred within 12 h after a migraine attack, i.e., in 87 % of the cases in FMS + M1 and 86 % in FMS + M2. The difference with respect to flares occurring at a longer time distance from an attack was highly significant ($p < 0.0001$).

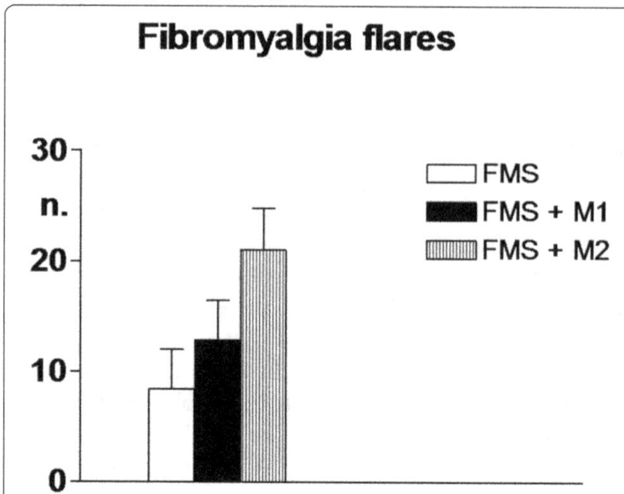

Fig. 3 Mean monthly number of fibromyalgia flares in the three groups of fibromyalgia patients: fibromyalgia only (FMS; n. 40), fibromyalgia plus high frequency episodic migraine (FMS + M1, n. 42), fibromyalgia plus chronic migraine (FMS + M2, n. 40). Means ± SD. 1-way ANOVA = significant trend, ***. Internal comparisons = FMS vs FMS + M1 and FMS + M2: ***; FMS + M1 vs FMS + M2: ***

Phase 2

Spontaneous pain

In patients undergoing migraine prophylaxis, the mean monthly number of migraine attacks was significantly reduced as compared with pre-treatment ($p < 0.0001$), while in patients not subjected to prophylaxis evaluated at comparable time points it did not vary significantly. In patients with prophylaxis but not in those without, also the mean monthly number of fibromyalgia flares and the number of rescue medications taken to treat them were significantly reduced ($p < 0.0001$) (Figs. 4 and 5).

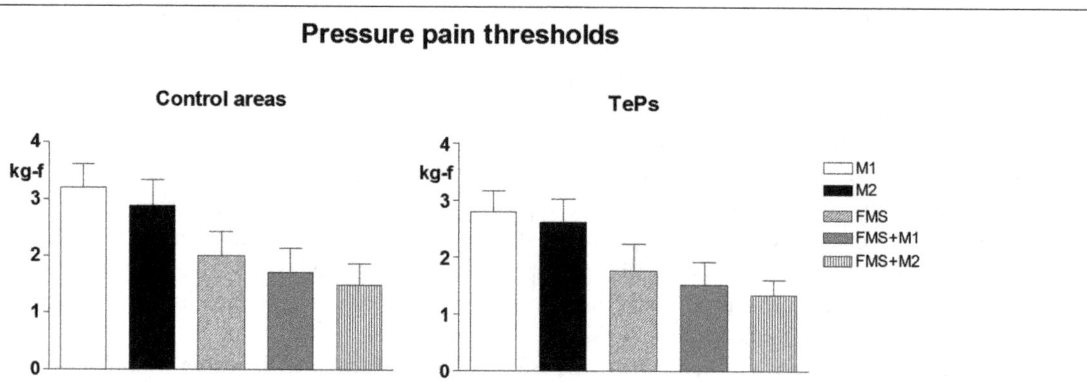

Fig. 2 Pain thresholds to pressure stimulation in control areas (mean values recorded in trapezius, deltoid and quadriceps muscles and overlying subcutis and skin) (*left*) and in tender points (TePs) (mean values recorded at all 18 points)(*right*) in the same patient groups as for Fig. 1. 1-way ANOVA = significant trend for both control areas and TePs, ***. Internal comparisons for control areas = M1 vs M2: **; M1 vs FMS, FMS + M1 and FMS + M2: ***; M2 vs FMS, FMS + M1 and FMS + M2: ***; FMS vs FMS + M1: *; FMS vs FMS + M2:***. Internal comparisons for TePs = M1 vs FMS, FMS + M1 and FMS + M2: ***; M2 vs FMS, FMS + M1 and FMS + M2: ***; FMS vs FMS + M1: *; FMS vs FMS + H2:***

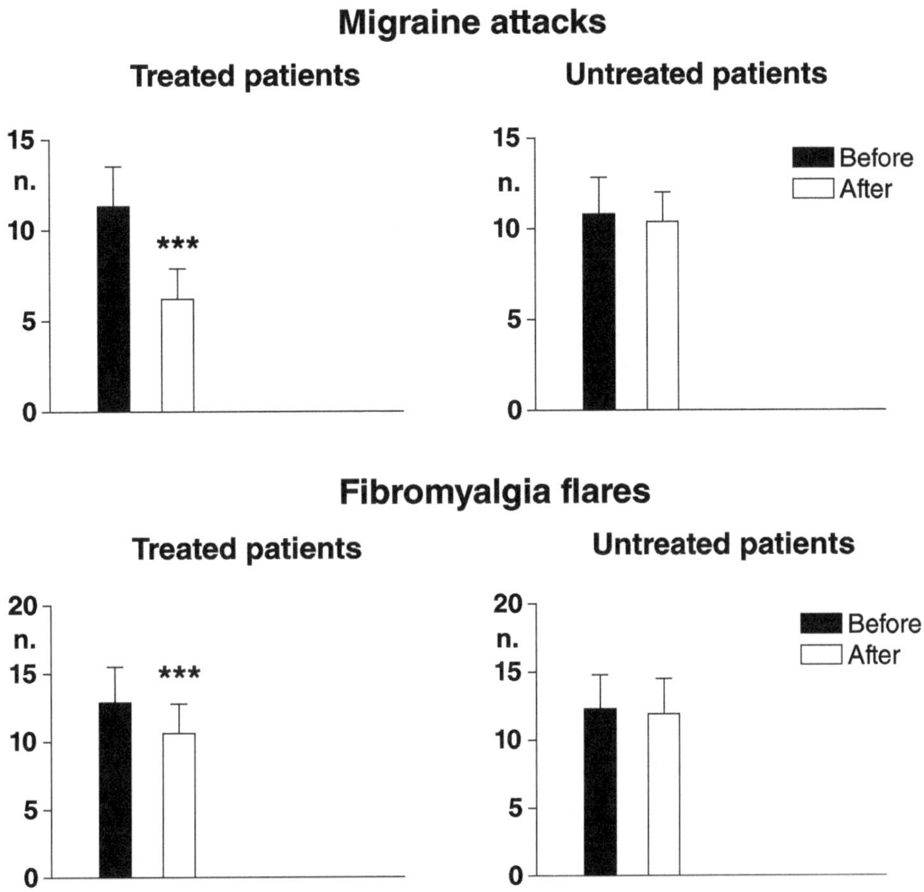

Fig. 4 Mean monthly number of migraine attacks (*upper graphs*) and fibromyalgia flares (*lower graphs*) in two groups of patients with fibromyalgia plus high frequency episodic migraine (FMS + M1) undergoing migraine prophylaxis with flunarizine for 3 months (treated patients, n. 47) and not undergoing migraine prophylaxis (untreated patients, n. 39)(Means ± SD). Before: evaluation relative to the 3 months preceding start of treatment. After: evaluation relative to the 3 months of treatment. Asterisks above SD bars refer to comparison of before vs after values. *** = $p < 0.001$

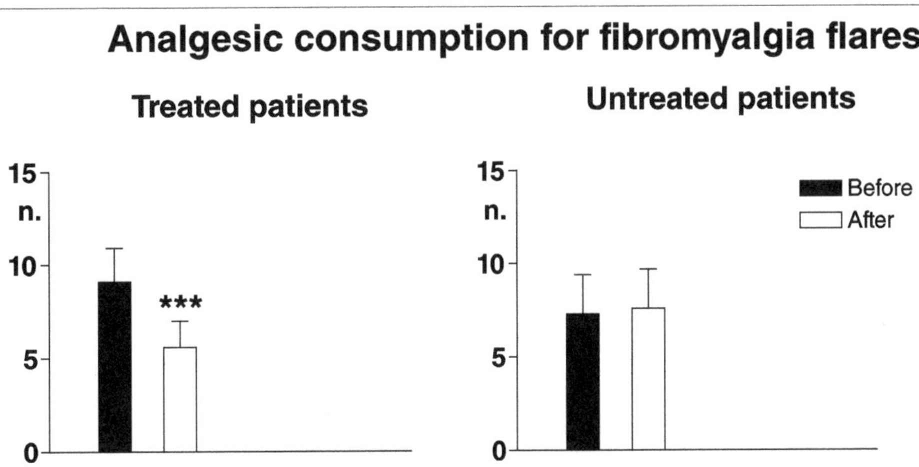

Fig. 5 Mean monthly number of analgesic consumption for fibromyalgia flares. Legend as for Fig. 4

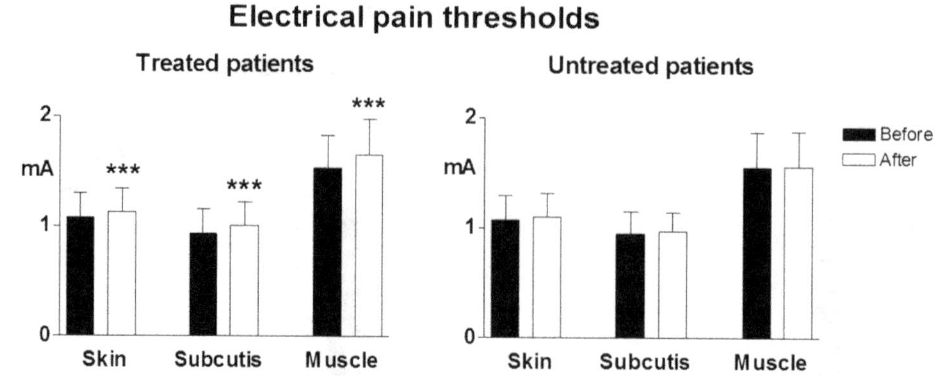

Fig. 6 Pain thresholds to electrical stimulation in skin, subcutis and muscle in control areas. Legend as for Fig. 4

Pain sensitivity

In treated patients electrical pain thresholds in control areas significantly increased in all tissues ($p < 0.003$ for skin, $p < 0.0001$ for subcutis and muscle) and pressure pain thresholds also significantly increased in both control areas ($p < 0.0008$) and TePs ($p < 0.0005$). No significant threshold changes were recorded in non-treated patients (Figs. 6 and 7).

A number of considerations can be made on the results of the study in regard to the co-morbidity of fibromyalgia with migraine. The first phase of the investigation shows firstly that the co-occurrence of both conditions involves

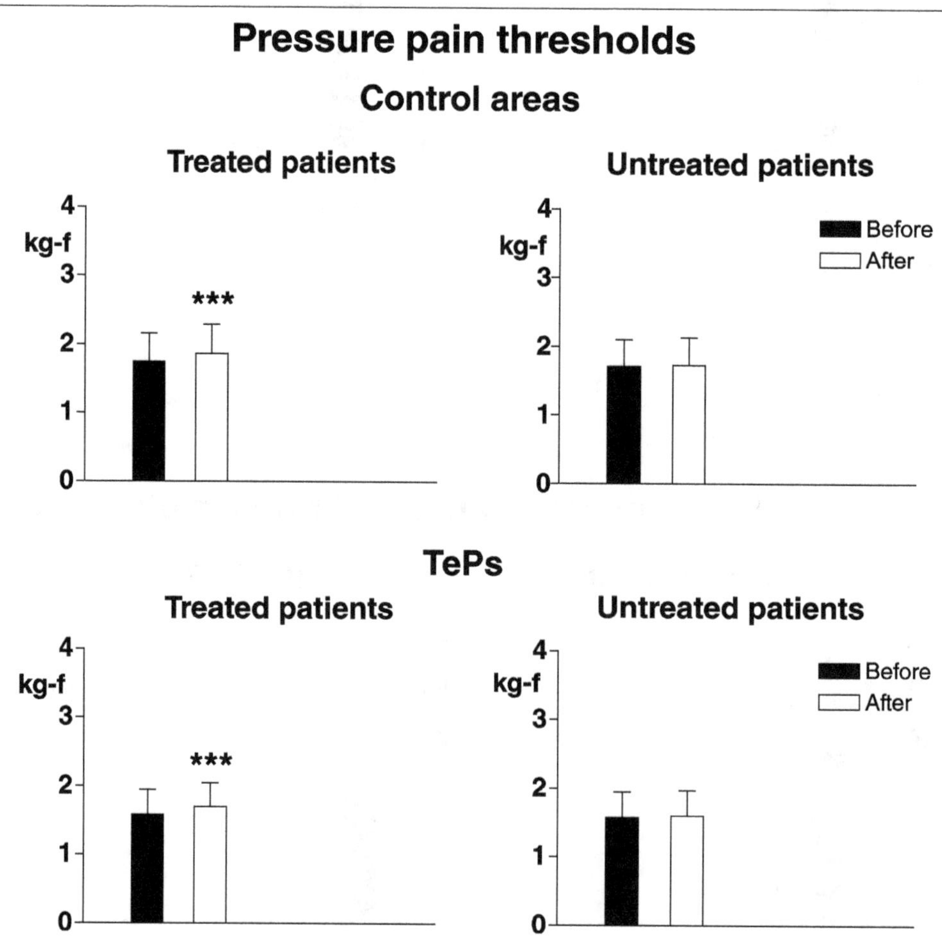

Fig. 7 Pain thresholds to pressure stimulation in control areas (*upper graphs*) and in tender points (*lower graphs*). Legend as for Fig. 4

a higher level of generalized hypersensitivity to pain at somatic level with respect to migraine only and fibromyalgia only, as testified by significantly lower pain thresholds in both painful and control areas. All FMS, but not non-FMS, patients were under stable basal amitriptyline treatment; though in very low doses, this treatment could have potentially influenced pain sensitivity in FMS, by increasing the pain threshold [35, 42]. However, even in this case, the outcome here found of a higher pain sensitivity in FMS vs non-FMS would not have changed without treatment; in contrast, the hypersensitivity difference would probably have been more pronounced.

The first phase of our study secondly shows that the hypersensitivity level is a function of the number of migraine attacks, with thresholds being lower in chronic than high frequency episodic migraine in both migraine-only patients and migraine patients plus fibromyalgia, confirming and extending previous results by de Tommaso et al. who showed that pain at tender points was significantly correlated with headache frequency in co-morbid patients [43].

Thirdly, in co-morbid patients it shows a high degree of temporal correlation between the occurrence of migraine and of FMS pain, with the vast majority of the fibromyalgia flares manifesting within 12 h after a migraine attack. On one hand these results reinforce the notion of a common pathophysiological mechanism in high frequency/chronic migraine and FMS, i.e., the central sensitization process. On the other hand they suggest that the algogenic input to the central nervous system due to the migraine attack is a triggering factor for a further enhancement of the existing hyperexcitability in the sensory compartment at the basis of fibromyalgia, similarly to what has already been documented for other pain generators in FMS, namely myofascial pain syndromes and painful joints [19, 44–46].

The second phase of the investigation further evidences the link between migraine and FMS symptoms. An effective reduction of the number of migraine attacks with a specific prophylaxis is, in fact, paralleled by a reduction also of the spontaneous (number of flares) and evoked (diffuse hyperalgesia) FMS symptoms. Such a result, obtained with a drug class (calcium-channel) not able to directly influence pain symptoms in fibromyalgia, with both patient groups under exactly the same stable dose of amitriptyline basal treatment, is probably due to the reduction of the central effect of nociceptive inputs from the cephalic area onto sensory neurons [33, 34]. Future additional studies will be necessary for confirmation, particularly as regards the effects of migraine prophylaxis, introducing a group of placebo-treated patients and a longer period of symptom assessment (beyond the 3-month duration of the migraine preventative regimen). To the best of our knowledge, however, the present investigation is the first to document the worsening impact of migraine pain on fibromyalgia symptoms in standardized conditions, suggesting that an effective control of the migraine co-morbidity is an important therapeutic measure also for FMS.

Conclusions

In conclusion, co-morbidity between migraine and fibromyalgia involves a higher state of generalized somatic hypersensitivity towards painful stimuli with respect to one condition only. The increase in migraine frequency – with shift towards chronicity – promotes an enhancement of the hypersensitivity and of the spontaneous FMS pain.

These results suggest different levels of central sensitization in patients with migraine, fibromyalgia or both conditions and a role for migraine as a triggering factor for FMS. Prevention of headache chronification in migraine patients would thus appear crucial also for preventing the development of fibromyalgia in predisposed individuals or its worsening in co-morbid patients.

Abbreviations

CNS: central nervous system; FMS: fibromyalgia; M1: high frequency episodic migraine; M2: chronic migraine; TePs: tender points.

Competing interests

MAG received research funding from Epitech Group, honoraria from Bayer, IBSA Institute Biochimique and Helsinn Healthcare, and Royalties from IASP Press.
GA received honoraria from Helsinn Healthcare and Epitech group.
PM received honoraria from Allergan, Bayer, Teva and Mylan.
AN received honoraria from Allergan and Medtronic.
CT, DL, MC, CS, LS, FC and RC declare no competing interests.

Authors' contributions

MAG, PM, FC and RC participated in the conception and design of the study, statistical evaluation of the results and writing of the paper. GA, CT, AN, DL, MC, CS and LS performed the experiments and reviewed the background literature. All authors read and approved the final manuscript.

Author details

[1]Fibromyalgia and Headache Center, Geriatrics Clinics, Department of Medicine and Science of Aging and Ce.S.I., "G. D'Annunzio" University of Chieti, via dei Vestini s.n., 66100 Chieti, Italy. [2]Department of Clinical and Molecular Medicine, Regional Referral Headache Centre, "Sant'Andrea" Hospital, "Sapienza" University, Rome, Italy. [3]Internal Medicine Unit, Guastalla Hospital, AUSL Reggio Emilia, Reggio Emilia, Italy. [4]Department of Medicine and Science of Aging, "G. D'Annunzio" University of Chieti, Chieti, Italy. [5]Institute of Surgical Pathology, "G. D'Annunzio" University of Chieti, Chieti, Italy.

References

1. Hawkins RA (2013) Fibromyalgia: a clinical update. J Am Osteopath Assoc 113:680–9
2. Queiroz LP (2013) Worldwide epidemiology of fibromyalgia. Curr Pain Headache Rep 17:356
3. Wolfe F, Smythe HA, Yunus MB, Bennett RM, Bombardier C, Goldenberg DL, Tugwell P, Campbell SM, Abeles M, Clark P et al (1990) The American College of Rheumatology 1990 criteria for the classification of fibromyalgia. Report of the multicenter criteria committee. Arthritis Rheum 33:160–72
4. Wolfe F, Clauw DJ, Fitzcharles MA, Goldenberg DL, Katz RS, Mease P, Russell AS, Russell IJ, Winfield JB, Yunus MB (2010) The American College of Rheumatology

preliminary diagnostic criteria for fibromyalgia and measurement of symptom severity. Arthritis Care Res (Hoboken) 62:600–10
5. Bernik M, Sampaio TP, Gandarela L (2013) Fibromyalgia comorbid with anxiety disorders and depression: combined medical and psychological treatment. Curr Pain Headache Rep 17:358
6. Caldarella MP, Giamberardino MA, Sacco F, Affaitati G, Milano A, Lerza R, Balatsinou C, Laterza F, Pierdomenico SD, Cuccurullo F, Neri M (2006) Sensitivity disturbances in patients with irritable bowel syndrome and fibromyalgia. Am J Gastroenterol 101:2782–9
7. Giamberardino MA, Affaitati G, Costantini R (2006) Chapter 24. Referred pain from internal organs. Handb Clin Neurol 81:343–61
8. Giamberardino MA, Affaitati G, Costantini R (2010) Visceral referred pain. J Musculoske Pain 18:403–10
9. Kato K, Sullivan PF, Evengård B, Pedersen NL (2006) Chronic widespread pain and its comorbidities: a population-based study. Arch Intern Med 166:1649–54
10. de Tommaso M (2012) Prevalence, clinical features and potential therapies for fibromyalgia in primary headaches. Expert Rev Neurother 12:287–95
11. Sacco S, Ricci S, Carolei A (2011) Tension-type headache and systemic medical disorders. Curr Pain Headache Rep 15:438–43
12. de Tommaso M, Federici A, Loiacono A, Delussi M, Todarello O (2014) Personality profiles and coping styles in migraine patients with fibromyalgia comorbidity. Compr Psychiatry 55:80–6
13. Vij B, Whipple MO, Tepper SJ, Mohabbat AB, Stillman M, Vincent A (2015) Frequency of migraine headaches in patients with fibromyalgia. Headache 55:860–5
14. Küçükşen S, Genç E, Yılmaz H, Sallı A, Gezer İA, Karahan AY, Salbaş E, Cingöz HT, Nas Ö, Uğurlu H (2013) The prevalence of fibromyalgia and its relation with headache characteristics in episodic migraine. Clin Rheumatol 32:983–90
15. Marcus DA, Bhowmick A (2013) Fibromyalgia comorbidity in a community sample of adults with migraine. Clin Rheumatol 32:1553–6
16. Abeles AM, Pillinger MH, Solitar BM, Abeles M (2007) Narrative review: the pathophysiology of fibromyalgia. Ann Int Med 146:726–34
17. Ablin JN, Buskila D (2015) Update on the genetics of the fibromyalgia syndrome. Best Pract Res Clin Rheumatol 29:20–8
18. Clauw DJ (2015) Fibromyalgia and related conditions. Mayo Clin Proc 90:680–92
19. Affaitati G, Costantini R, Fabrizio A, Lapenna D, Tafuri E, Giamberardino MA (2011) Effects of treatment of peripheral pain generators in fibromyalgia patients. Eur J Pain 15:61–9
20. Vecchiet L, Giamberardino MA, de Bigontina P, Dragani L (1994) Comparative sensory evaluation of parietal tissues in painful and nonpainful areas in fibromyalgia and myofascial pain syndrome. In: Gebhart GF, Hansmond DL, Jensen TS (eds) Proceedings of the 7th world congress on pain, progress in pain research and management, vol 2. IASP Press, Seattle
21. Bezov D, Ashina S, Jensen R, Bendtsen L (2011) Pain perception studies in tension-type headache. Headache 51:262–71
22. Coppola G, Di Lorenzo C, Schoenen J, Pierelli F (2013) Habituation and sensitization in primary headaches. J Headache Pain 14:65
23. de Tommaso M, Sardaro M, Vecchio E, Serpino C, Stasi M, Ranieri M (2008) Central sensitisation phenomena in primary headaches: overview of a preventive therapeutic approach. CNS Neurol Disord Drug Targets 7:524–35
24. Filatova E, Latysheva N, Kurenkov A (2008) Evidence of persistent central sensitization in chronic headaches: a multi-method study. J Headache Pain 9:295–300
25. Giamberardino MA, Tafuri E, Di Fabio S, Tana C, Costa A, Fabrizio A, Affaitati G (2011) Chronic headache and fibromyalgia. J Headache Pain 12:13
26. Savini A, Tafuri E, Affaitati G, Fabrizio A, Lerza R, Sidonio G, Giamberardino MA (2008) Sensory evaluation in fibromyalgia and headache. J Headache Pain 9:25
27. Schmidt-Hansen PT, Svensson P, Bendtsen L, Graven-Nielsen T, Bach FW (2007) Increased muscle pain sensitivity in patients with tension-type headache. Pain 129:113–21
28. Zohsel K, Hohmeister J, Oelkers-Ax R, Flor H, Hermann C (2006) Quantitative sensory testing in children with migraine: preliminary evidence for enhanced sensitivity to painful stimuli especially in girls. Pain 123:10–8
29. Obrosova IG (2009) Diabetic painful and insensate neuropathy: pathogenesis and potential treatments. Neurotherapeutics 6:638–47
30. Viggiano A, Zagaria N, Passavanti MB, Pace MC, Paladini A, Aurilio C, Tedesco MA, Natale F, Calabrò R, Monda M, De Luca E (2009) New and low-cost auto-algometry for screening hypertension-associated hypoalgesia. Pain Pract 9:260–5
31. Headache Classification Subcommittee of the International Headache Society (2004) The international classification of headache disorders, 2nd edition. Cephalalgia 24:1–150
32. Headache Classification of the International Headache Society (2013) The international classification of headache disorders, 3rd edition (beta version). Cephalalgia 33:627–808
33. Giamberardino MA, Martelletti P (2015) Emerging drugs for migraine treatment. Expert Opin Emerg Drugs 20:137–47
34. Martelletti P (2015) The therapeutic armamentarium in migraine is quite elderly. Expert Opin Drug Metab Toxicol 11:175–7
35. Jagla G, Mika J, Makuch W, Obara I, Wordliczek J, Przewlocka B (2014) Analgesic effects of antidepressants alone and after their local co-administration with morphine in a rat model of neuropathic pain. Pharmacol Rep 66:459–65
36. Silberstein SD (2015) Preventive migraine treatment. Continuum (Minneap Minn). Headache 21:973–89
37. Sinclair AJ, Sturrock A, Davies B, Matharu M (2015) Headache management: pharmacological approaches. Pract Neurol 15:411–23
38. Fischer AA (1998) Muscle pain syndromes and fibromyalgia. Pressure algometry for quantification of diagnosis and treatment outcome. J Musculoskelet Pain 6:152–7
39. Giamberardino MA, Affaitati G, Lerza R, Lapenna D, Costantini R, Vecchiet L (2005) Relationship between pain symptoms and referred sensory and trophic changes in patients with gallbladder pathology. Pain 114:239–49
40. Giamberardino MA, Costantini R, Affaitati G, Fabrizio A, Lapenna D, Tafuri E, Mezzetti A (2010) Viscero-visceral hyperalgesia: characterization in different clinical models. Pain 151:307–22
41. Giamberardino MA, Tana C, Costantini R (2014) Pain thresholds in women with chronic pelvic pain. Curr Opin Obstet Gynecol 26:253–9
42. Ángel García D, Martínez Nicolás I, Saturno Hernández PJ. Clinical approach to fibromyalgia: synthesis of evidence-based recommendations, a systematic review. Reumatol Clin. 2015; [Epub ahead of print]
43. de Tommaso M, Sardaro M, Serpino C, Costantini F, Vecchio E, Prudenzano MP, Lamberti P, Livrea P (2009) Fibromyalgia comorbidity in primary headaches. Cephalalgia 29:453–64
44. Gerwin R (2013) Are peripheral pain generators important in fibromyalgia and chronic widespread pain? Pain Med 14:777–8
45. Giamberardino MA, Affaitati G, Fabrizio A, Costantini R (2011) Effects of treatment of myofascial trigger points on the pain of fibromyalgia. Curr Pain Headache Rep 15:393–9
46. Giamberardino MA, Affaitati G, Fabrizio A, Costantini R (2011) Myofascial pain syndromes and their evaluation. Best Pract Res Clin Rheumatol 25:185–98

26

Phenotypic features of chronic migraine

Osman Özgür Yalın[1*], Derya Uluduz[2], Aynur Özge[3], Mehmet Ali Sungur[4], Macit Selekler[5] and Aksel Siva[2]

Abstract

Background: Chronic migraine is a disabling, under-recognized, and undertreated disorder that increases health burdens. The aim of this study was to evaluate phenotypic features and the relevance of accompanying symptoms of migraine attacks in chronic migraine.

Method: This study was conducted as part of an ongoing Turkish Headache Database Study investigating the clinical characteristics and outcomes of headache syndromes in the Turkish population. The electronic database was examined retrospectively, and 835 patients with chronic migraine were included.

Results: Patient group consisted of 710 women and 125 men (85 and 15 %, respectively). Mean patient age was 36.8 ± 13.5 years, median value of migraine onset was 60 months (18–120), median headache frequency was 25 days per month (16–30), median of attack duration was 12 h (4–24), and median of intensity was eight (7–9). Increasing headache days per month were inversely related with the presence of nausea, vomiting, phonophobia, and photophobia. Longer duration of headache (months) and higher visual analog scale (VAS) for headache intensity were associated with all accompanying symptoms. Phonophobia, nausea, photophobia, and vomiting were the most frequent accompanying symptoms (experienced by 80.2, 77.6, 71.2, and 40.9 % of patients, respectively). Osmophobia was also frequent in chronic migraine patients (53.4 %) and was closely associated with other accompanying symptoms. Vertigo and dizziness were observed less frequently, and they were not associated with accompanying symptoms.

Conclusion: Phenotype of chronic migraine may be associated with the course of chronification. Duration of illness and attack intensity were closely related with the presence of accompanying symptoms, although headache frequency was found to be inversely related to the presence of accompanying symptoms. Osmophobia was also a frequent symptom and was closely related with other accompanied symptoms, unlike vertigo and dizziness. Inclusion of osmophobia into the diagnostic criteria might improve accurate diagnosis of chronic migraine.

Keywords: Chronic migraine, Phenotype, Accompanying symptoms, Chronification

Background

Chronic migraine (CM) is defined by the presence of headache attacks on 15 days or more per month for at least three months of which 8 or more days meet criteria for migraine [1]. A prevalence rate of 2 % for CM has been estimated [2–4]. Although CM is much less common than episodic migraine (EM), it is substantially more debilitating, with a greater negative effect on quality of life, and it is a challenging disorder for practitioners [4, 5]. Despite the substantial personal and social consequences of CM, its diagnostic criteria are still evolving [6]. The third edition of the International Classification of Headache Disorders (ICHD-3 beta) [1], published in 2013, has comprehensively described primary chronic headache disorders, such as CM, chronic tension-type headache, new daily persistent headache, and chronic hemicrania continua [1]. In this new edition, medication overuse headache is not an exclusion criterion; therefore, CM now represents a broader patient group.

CM is a disabling, underdiagnosed, and undertreated disorder [6]. CM patients constitute the most debilitated subgroup of the migraine population, and may therefore represent a clinically distinct group [7]. According to the American Migraine Prevalence and Prevention study, patients with CM were twice as likely to develop depression,

* Correspondence: osmanozguryalin@yahoo.com
[1]Neurology Department, Istanbul Education and Research Hospital, Kasap İlyas Mah. Org. Abdurrahman, Nafiz Gürman Cd, PK: 34098 Fatih, Istanbul, Turkey
Full list of author information is available at the end of the article

anxiety, and chronic pain than those with EM [8]. Cutaneous allodynia, anxiety, disability, and depression are frequently considered as predictors of chronification [9, 10].

The explicit mechanisms of CM are not fully understood. Atypical modulation of pain may play a role in its pathogenesis [11]. Pain modulatory pathway alterations have been identified in CM [12]. A suggested mechanism for chronification of migraine is that repeated migraine attacks could have cumulative structural effects on the trigeminovascular pathway [13]. This theory is supported by the evidence of iron deposition in the periaqueductal gray matter of patients with a long history of migraine [14]. In addition, CM is associated with a greater degree of impairment in cortical processing of sensory stimuli [15]. Therefore, proposed structural changes in the excitability of the trigeminovascular pathway and/or other brainstem pain modulating systems could result in different phenotypes of the disease.

According to the ICHD-3 beta diagnostic criteria of migraine, accompanying symptoms item (D) require either (1) nausea and/or vomiting and/or (2) photophobia and phonophobia. Although osmophobia is mentioned as an accompanying symptom in the appendix-definitions section, it has not been included in the diagnostic criteria. Osmophobia refers to an increased sensitivity to odors during migraine attacks, and it seems to be a distinguishing feature of migraine [16]. Association between osmophobia and allodynia has also been investigated recently, and it is also proposed as a shared central sensitization mechanism [17].

To the best of our knowledge, the association between headache characteristics and accompanying symptoms of CM has not been reported yet. The aims of this study are (1) to determine the clinical characteristics of headache attacks and to investigate the relevance of associated symptoms such as nausea, vomiting, phonophobia, and photophobia; (2) to investigate other associated symptoms that could improve diagnostic certainty, including osmophobia, dizziness, and vertigo; and (3) to analyze relationships among associated symptoms.

Methods

This retrospective observational study was a part of ongoing Turkish Headache Database (THD) Study. THD investigating the clinical characteristics and outcomes of primary and secondary headache syndromes in Turkish population is supported by Turkish Neurological Society. Out of tertiary headache centers in THD, patients diagnosed with CM based on ICHD-2 criteria between the years 2008 and 2012 in Mersin University, Istanbul University and Kocaeli University were enrolled to this study. The Human Ethical Committee of Mersin University (MEU. 0.01.00.06/265, 20.10.2008) approved this nonprofit study. Subjects meeting the inclusion criteria were enrolled into the study after giving written consent. Diagnosis of migraine was done by headache experts with face-to-face examinations according to ICHD-2 criteria [18]. Subjects younger than 18 years of age and those older than 80 years of age ($n = 123$ subjects), those who had received a headache diagnosis other than CM ($n = 2850$ episodic migraine subjects), and patients with chronic TTH, hemicrania continua, medication overuse headache and patients who had TTH attacks more frequently than migraine attacks ($n = 385$ subjects) were excluded. Data on socio-demographic and clinical characteristics, including age at onset, headache duration, headache frequency, presence of aura, headache characteristics, localization, intensity of pain, triggering factors, associated features, comorbidity, and medical and family history were gathered from a web-based database. Accompanying symptoms of CM were evaluated based on ICHD-2 criteria. Presence of vertigo, dizziness and osmophobia were also analyzed retrospectively taking into consideration of ICHD-3 beta criteria. Vertigo and dizziness is stated when related with migraine attacks. Vertigo definition based to clinical features: internal/external vertigo, positional, occurring during head motion. Similarly dizziness defined sensation of disequilibrium occurring during headache attack, discrimination is particularly based to clinical examination of experts.

When extracting data from the electronic database, we excluded all missing data, including missing data on accompanying symptoms. Therefore, we obtained a reduced number of subjects in osmophobia assessments. Although this could limit the power of the analysis, it also increased the reliability of the data and prevented errors that could be attributed to the retrospective design of the study. The visual analog scale (VAS) was used for assessment of pain intensity.

Statistical analysis

Data were entered and analyzed in the statistical analysis program PASW v.18 (SPSS Inc. Released 2009, PASW Statistics for Windows, Version 18.0. Chicago: SPSS Inc.) statistical package. Distributions of data were examined with the Shapiro-Wilk test, and independent samples t test and one-way ANOVA or non-parametric alternatives (Mann–Whitney U and Kruskal-Wallis tests) were used to compare groups according to the distribution of dependent variables. Continuous variables were summarized as mean ± standard deviation or median (25–75 %) according to the distribution, and categorical variables were summarized as frequency and percentile. Spearman non-parametric correlations were used to analyze relationships among headache properties. Pearson-Chi square or Fisher's exact test were used according to the expected count rule for categorical data. Two-tailed $p < 0.05$ was accepted as significant.

Results

The study group consisted of 835 CM patients, 710 female (85 %), mean age 36.8 ± 13.5 years. The median value of migraine onset was 60 months (18–120), median headache duration was 12 h (4–24) and median headache intensity was eight (7–9). Seventy-seven percent of CM patients described throbbing headache followed by pressing (13.7 %) and dull (5.5 %) headache. The localization of headache was predominantly unilateral (39.5 %), followed by bifrontal (10.7 %), generalized (14.8 %), and sub-occipital (13.6 %). Phonophobia (80.2 %) was the most common accompanying symptom, followed by nausea (77.6 %) and photophobia (71.2 %). Vomiting was present in 40.9 % of patients. Osmophobia was observed in 53.4 % of patients, and dizziness and vertigo was present in 17.5 % and 14.4 % of patients respectively. Characteristics of study patients is summarized at Table 1. The most common triggering factor was emotional stress (79.2 %), followed by skipping meals (57.0 %), menstruation (36.7 %), and seasonal factors (23.0 %). Most of the patients reported no intraday-difference, but for 31.4 % of patients, headaches were most intense in the evening. Headache frequency did not change with age. Headache frequency was inversely related with headache onset ($r = -0.131$, $p < 0.001$), attack duration ($r = -0.110$, $p = 0.002$), and intensity of headache ($r = -0.118$, $p = 0.002$). When correlation analysis adjusted according to gender and age covariates; correlation of headache onset disappeared, headache frequency was inversely related with attack duration ($r = -0.083$, $p = 0.032$), and intensity of headache ($r = -0.139$, $p < 0.001$). Analysis of gender effects revealed no difference between males and females in terms of headache frequency ($p = 0.589$), duration of illness ($p = 0.054$), or intensity ($p = 0.559$). Attack duration (hours) was significantly longer for females ($p < 0.001$) (Table 2).

To reveal the phenotypic features of CM, we compared headache frequency, duration of attack, intensity, and duration of illness according to the presence of accompanying symptoms. First, we compared headache frequency (headache days per month) in terms of the presence of accompanying symptoms. We observed that the presence of nausea, vomiting, phonophobia, and photophobia were significantly associated with fewer headache days per month (Table 3). When we investigated attack duration, we observed that vomiting, phonophobia, and photophobia were associated with longer duration of attack (Table 4). Greater headache intensity (VAS) and longer duration of illness (in months) were significantly associated with the existence of all accompanying symptoms, including nausea, vomiting, phonophobia, photophobia, dizziness, vertigo, and osmophobia (see Tables 5 and 6 for intensity and duration, respectively).

We also analyzed the associations of accompanying symptoms with each other (Table 7). The diagnostic accompanying symptoms described in ICHD-2 and also in ICHD-3 beta are nausea, vomiting, phonophobia, and photophobia, and these symptoms were found to be closely related with each other ($p = 0.001$). The crosstab analysis revealed that osmophobia and dizziness were significantly correlated with the presence of other diagnostic accompanying symptoms. By using x^2 tests, we found that osmophobia was associated with more frequent incidences of nausea ($p = 0.006$), vomiting ($p = 0.013$), phonophobia ($p = 0.001$), and photophobia ($p = 0.001$). Dizziness was associated with more frequent incidences of nausea ($p = 0.008$), vomiting (0.001), phonophobia ($p = 0.001$), and photophobia ($p = 0.001$). The presence of vertigo was

Table 1 Headache characteristics of study group

Gender	Female	710 (85 %)
	Male	125 (15 %)
Age	Age	36,8 ± 13,5
Headache characteristics	Duration of illness (months)	60 (18–120)
	Headache frequency (days/month)	25 (16–30)
	Headache duration (hours)	12 (4–24)
	Headache intensity (VAS)	8 (7–9)
Quality of headache (*n* = 817)	Throbbing headache	631 (77.2 %)
	Pressing	112 (13.7 %)
	Dull	45 (5.5 %)
	Others	29 (3.5 %)
Headache localization (*n* = 811)	Unilateral	320 (39.5 %)
	Bifrontal	87 (10.7 %)
	Generalized	120 (14.8 %)
	Sub-occipital	110 (13.6 %)
	Others	198 (21.4 %)
Accompanying symptoms	Phonophobia (*n* = 792)	635 (80.2 %)
	Nausea (*n* = 789)	612 (77.6 %)
	Photophobia (n = 787)	560 (71.2 %)
	Vomiting (*n* = 738)	302 (40.9 %)
	Osmophobia (*n* = 238)	127 (53.4 %)
	Dizziness (*n* = 661)	116 (17.5 %)
	Vertigo (*n* = 641)	92 (14.4 %)

VAS visual analog scale

Table 2 Headache characteristics according to gender

	Male (*n* = 125)	Female (*n* = 710)	*p*
Headache frequency (days/month)	20 [16–30]	25 [16–30]	0.589
Duration of illness (months)	48 [12–120]	60 [24–132]	0.054
Headache duration (hours)	7 [2–24]	12 [4–24]	<0.001
Headache intensity (VAS)	8 [7–9]	8 [7–9]	0.559

VAS visual analog scale

Table 3 Headache frequency (days/month) according to accompanying symptoms

Accompanying symptoms		Number of subjects (*n*)	Headache days/month	*P* value
Nausea	Present	612	20 [15–30]	*0.008*
	Absent	177	30 [16–30]	
Vomiting	Present	302	20 [15–30]	*<0.001*
	Absent	436	30 [18–30]	
Phonophobia	Present	635	20 [15–30]	*0.002*
	Absent	157	30 [20–30]	
Photophobia	Present	560	20 [15–30]	*<0.001*
	Absent	227	30 [20–30]	
Dizziness	Present	116	25 [16–30]	0.056
	Absent	545	20 [16–30]	
Vertigo	Present	92	25 [16–30]	0.440
	Absent	549	24 [16–30]	
Osmophobia	Present	127	20 [16–30]	0.371
	Absent	111	20 [15–30]	

Table 5 Headache intensity (VAS) according to accompanying symptoms

Accompanying symptoms		Number of subjects (*n*)	Headache intensity (VAS)	*P* value
Nausea	Present	612	8 [7–10]	*<0.001*
	Absent	177	7 [6–9]	
Vomiting	Present	302	8 [7–10]	*<0.001*
	Absent	436	7 [6–9]	
Phonophobia	Present	635	8 [7–10]	*<0.010*
	Absent	157	7 [6–8]	
Photophobia	Present	560	8 [7–10]	*<0.001*
	Absent	227	7 [6–8]	
Dizziness	Present	116	8 [7–10]	*0.004*
	Absent	545	8 [7–9]	
Vertigo	Present	92	8 [7–10]	*0.006*
	Absent	549	8 [7–9]	
Osmophobia	Present	127	8 [7–10]	*0.032*
	Absent	111	8 [7–9]	

not associated with nausea ($p = 0.445$), vomiting ($p = 0.142$), or photophobia ($p = 0.063$). A detailed analysis of the accompanying symptoms is presented in Table 7.

Discussion

Our study revealed that the presence of diagnostic accompanying symptoms (nausea, vomiting, phonophobia, and photophobia) lessened with higher numbers of headache days per month. This finding is compatible with the literature. Migraine characteristics, especially accompanying symptoms, are less prominent in the CM population [19]. This could be important for two reasons: first the absence of accompanying symptoms could lead to underdiagnosis of CM. Second, this observation could point to cumulative effects of frequent headaches. CM is described as an altered entity, and there is growing evidence of chronicity-related structural effects in pain pathways [20]. Interestingly, in our population, headache frequency did not change with age or gender. Duration of illness and intensity scores (VAS) were also similar for both genders. However, headache duration was significantly longer in females. Slater et al. reported longer headache duration

Table 4 Headache duration (hours) according to accompanying symptoms

Accompanying symptoms		Number of subjects (*n*)	Headache duration (hours)	*P* value
Nausea	Present	612	12 [4–24]	0.056
	Absent	177	12 [3–24]	
Vomiting	Present	302	19 [6–24]	*<0.001*
	Absent	436	12 [3–24]	
Phonophobia	Present	635	12 [4–24]	*0.010*
	Absent	157	11 [4–24]	
Photophobia	Present	560	12 [4–24]	*0.003*
	Absent	227	10 [3–24]	
Dizziness	Present	116	12 [6–24]	0.148
	Absent	545	12 [4–24]	
Vertigo	Present	92	12 [5–24]	0.826
	Absent	549	12 [4–24]	
Osmophobia	Present	127	12 [7–24]	0.219
	Absent	111	12 [4–24]	

Table 6 Duration of illness (months) according to accompanying symptoms

Accompanying symptoms		Number of subjects (*n*)	Duration of illness (months)	*P* value
Nausea	Present	612	60 [24–156]	*<0.001*
	Absent	177	36 [10–114]	
Vomiting	Present	302	108 [36–180]	*<0.001*
	Absent	436	36 [12–120]	
Phonophobia	Present	635	60 [24–156]	*<0.001*
	Absent	157	36 [9–96]	
Photophobia	Present	560	72 [24–166]	*<0.001*
	Absent	227	36 [12–96]	
Dizziness	Present	116	114 [36–240]	*<0.001*
	Absent	545	48 [12–120]	
Vertigo	Present	92	82 [24–180]	*0.015*
	Absent	549	48 [12–120]	
Osmophobia	Present	127	120 [48–240]	*<0.001*
	Absent	111	48 [12–120]	

Table 7 Associations of accompanying symptoms with each other

		Nausea	Vomiting	Phonophobia	Photophobia	Dizziness	Vertigo	Osmophobia
Nausea	+		51.2	86.1	77.4	19.7	14.9	57.8
	-		7.9	58.0	47.4	10.6	12.4	35.4
	p		*0.001*	*0.001*	*0.001*	*0.008*	0.445	*0.006*
Vomiting	+	95.3		88.2	83.1	25.0	16.5	59.8
	-	62.6		71.9	59.4	12.6	12.4	43.1
	p	*0.001*		*0.001*	*0.001*	*0.001*	0.142	*0.013*
Phonophobia	+	83.5	45.5		82.1	20.4	16.8	59.6
	-	52.9	22.3		27.4	6.6	6.6	19.5
	p	*0.001*	*0.001*		*0.001*	*0.001*	*0.002*	*0.001*
Photophobia	+	84.7	48.8	92.3		21.2	16.0	59.7
	-	59.3	22.1	49.6		9.3	10.5	28.0
	p	*0.001*	*0.001*	*0.001*		*0.001*	0.063	*0.001*
Dizziness	+	85.2	55.3	91.2	85.2		50.0	71.3
	-	73.5	34.7	73.9	64.0		6.2	32.0
	p	*0.008*	*0.001*	*0.001*	*0.001*		*0.001*	*0.001*
Vertigo	+	78.0	44.9	89.1	75.8	59.3		65.7
	-	74.3	36.8	74.3	65.9	8.8		39.9
	p	0.445	0.142	*0.002*	0.063	*0.001*		*0.001*
Osmophobia	+	86.4	53.5	93.5	88.8	60.8	43.6	
	-	71.8	36.9	70.3	67.6	22.7	21.1	
	p	*0.006*	*0.013*	*0.001*	*0.001*	*0.001*	*0.001*	

In this table, + lines indicate subjects who had related symptoms, and – lines indicate subjects who did not have related symptoms

in females in childhood migraine [21]. Adult population studies also report longer headache duration in females [22, 23], suggesting a female gender tendency in CM.

Both duration of illness (months) and headache intensity (VAS) scores were found to be significantly associated with the presence of all accompanying symptoms, including nausea, vomiting, phonophobia, photophobia, dizziness, vertigo, and osmophobia. Although our study covered only CM patients, our results indicate that duration of illness and headache intensity are closely related with accompanying symptoms. Kelman et al. reported that headache intensity was correlated with nausea, vomiting, photophobia, phonophobia, and dizziness, and headache duration was correlated with osmophobia and taste abnormalities [23]. In our results, accompanying symptoms were present as hallmarks of duration of illness and attack intensity in the CM population.

Attack duration was found to be related to the presence of vomiting, phonophobia, and photophobia. However, the presence of other accompanying symptoms—including nausea, osmophobia, vertigo, and dizziness—did not change with varying attack duration. Conversely, Kelman and Tanis reported a correlation between attack duration and osmophobia and taste abnormalities. However, their study also covered EM patients [23]. This difference could point to the effects of chronification on attack phenotype.

Finally, we analyzed the relationships of associated symptoms with each other. The results revealed that nausea, vomiting, phonophobia, and photophobia are closely correlated with each other. Osmophobia (53.4 %) was also a common accompanying symptom. In addition, the presence of osmophobia was significantly associated with other diagnostic accompanying symptoms. Because ICHD-3 beta did not include other common symptoms accompanying diagnostic criteria, there is insufficient data investigating the predictive value of such symptoms. The diagnostic utility of osmophobia was proposed previously by some authors, especially for Asian migraineurs, in whom photophobia is less common [16]. Similarly, Silva-Neto et al. reported that osmophobia may be a specific marker for migraine and suggested its inclusion within the diagnostic criteria [24]. According to a recent study, the prevalence of both allodynia and osmophobia were higher in chronic than in episodic migraineurs [17]. Same study also reported a relationship between duration of headache and osmophobia.

This study has some limitations. First, the retrospective study design limited our data to monitoring blood pressure, body mass index, and educational-socioeconomic status. Second, this study did not include EM patients, so we could not compare our findings with those of EM sufferers. Due to the retrospective design of this study some missing values of the parameters was one of our limitations. But even so power analysis of the data is mostly estimated 80–99 % for variables. However, this study gives us clues about the determinants of phenotype in CM populations.

Conclusion

In conclusion, our study supports and expands the literature and could be summarized as follows: (1) CM is defined as 15–30 headache days per month, and in our study population, higher numbers of headache days were found to be correlated with less prominent nausea, vomiting, photophobia, and phonophobia; (2) long duration of headache (months) and higher attack intensity (VAS) were found to be correlated with more frequent incidences of all accompanying symptoms investigated; (3) longer attack duration (hours) was found to be correlated with the presence of vomiting and phono-photophobia; (4) duration of headache and attack intensity are the most relevant determinants of CM attack phenotype; (5) osmophobia is also common in CM and is associated with diagnostic accompanying symptoms; and (6) dizziness and vertigo were less frequent in the CM population and do not have a prominent relationship with other diagnostic accompanying symptoms.

Future studies focusing on clinical presentation and accompanying symptoms could provide additional data to shed light on the phenotypes, classifications, and pathophysiological pathways of chronicity.

Abbreviations

CM: chronic migraine; ICHD-3 beta: the third edition of the International Classification of Headache Disorders; VAS: visual analogue scale.

Competing interests

The authors declare that they have no competing interests.

Authors' contributions

OÖY, DU, AÖ, MS, and MAS participated in the alignment and drafted the manuscript. OÖY, DUİ, AÖ, MAS, AS participated in the design of the study and performed the statistical analysis. DU, AO conceived of the study, and participated in its design and coordination and helped to draft the manuscript. All authors read and approved the final manuscript.

Acknowledgements

This study is conducted as a part of Turkish Headache Database Project. Turkish Headache Database Project is supported by Turkish Neurological Society and unsolicited grant from Allergan INC.

Author details

[1]Neurology Department, Istanbul Education and Research Hospital, Kasap İlyas Mah. Org. Abdurrahman, Nafiz Gürman Cd, PK: 34098 Fatih, Istanbul, Turkey. [2]Neurology Department, Istanbul University Cerrahpasa School of Medicine, İstanbul, Turkey. [3]Neurology Department, Mersin University School of Medicine, Mersin, Turkey. [4]Biostatistics Department, Düzce University School of Medicine, Düzce, Turkey. [5]Neurology Department, Kocaeli University School of Medicine, Kocaeli, Turkey.

References

1. Headache Classification Committee of the International Headache Society (IHS) (2013) The International classification of headache disorders, 3rd ed. (beta version). Cephalalgia 33(9):629–808
2. Natoli JL, Manack A, Dean B, Turkel CC, Stovner L, Lipton RB (2009) Global prevalence of chronic migraine: a systematic review. Cephalalgia 31:1116–1130
3. Bigal ME, Serrano D, Buse D, Scher A, Stewart WF, Lipton RB (2008) Acute migraine medications and evolution from episodic to chronic migraine: a longitudinal population-based study. Headache 48(8):1157–1168
4. Buse DC, Manack AN, Fanning KM, Serrano D, Reed ML, Turkel CC, Lipton RB (2012) Chronic migraine prevalence, disability, and sociodemographic factors: results from the American Migraine Prevalence and Prevention Study. Headache 52(10):1456–1470
5. Ertas M, Baykan B, Orhan EK, Zarifoglu M, Karli N, Saip S, Siva A (2012) One-year prevalence and the impact of migraine and tension-type headache in Turkey: a nationwide home-based study in adults. Headache 13(2):147–157
6. Lipton RB, Silberstein SD (2015) Episodic and chronic migraine headache: breaking down barriers to optimal treatment and prevention. Headache 55(S2):103–122
7. Sanderson JC, Devine EB, Lipton RB, Bloudek LM, Varon SF, Blumenfeld AM, Sullivan SD (2013) Headache-related health resource utilisation in chronic and episodic migraine across six countries. J Neurol Neurosurg Psychiatry 84:1309–1317
8. Buse DC, Manack A, Serrano D, Turkel C, Lipton RB (2010) Sociodemographic and comorbidity profiles of chronic migraine and episodic migraine sufferers. J Neurol Neurosurg Psychiatry 81:428–432
9. Lipton RB (2011) Chronic migraine, classification, differential diagnosis, and epidemiology. Headache 51(S2):77–78
10. Bigal ME, Lipton RB (2006) Modifiable risk factors for migraine progression. Headache 46(9):1334–1343
11. Schwedt TJ (2014) Chronic migraine. BMJ 348:g1416
12. Aurora SK, Barrodale PM, Tipton RL, Khodavirdi A (2007) Brainstem dysfunction in chronic migraine as evidenced by neurophysiological and positron emission tomography studies. Headache 47(7):996–1003
13. Noseda R, Burstein R (2013) Migraine pathophysiology: anatomy of the trigeminovascular pathway and associated neurological symptoms, cortical spreading depression, sensitization, and modulation of pain. Pain. 154:44–53.
14. Welch KMA, Nagesh V, Aurora SK, Gelman N (2001) Periaqueductal gray matter dysfunction in migraine: cause or the burden of illness? Headache 41(7):629–637
15. Aurora SK (2009) Spectrum of illness: understanding biological patterns and relationships in chronic migraine. Neurology 72(5):8–13
16. Wang YF, Fuh JL, Chen SP, Wu JC, Wang SJ (2012) Clinical correlates and diagnostic utility of osmophobia in migraine. Cephalalgia 32(16):1180–1188
17. Lovati C, Giani L, Castoldi D, D'Alessandro CM, DeAngeli F, Capiluppi E, Mariani C (2015) Osmophobia in allodynic migraineurs: cause or consequence of central sensitization? J Neurol Sci 36(1):145–147
18. Olesen J, Steiner TJ (2004) The International classification of headache disorders, 2nd edn (ICDH-II). J Neurol Neurosurg Psychiatry 75(6):808–811
19. Kelman L (2006) Pain characteristics of acute migraine attack. Headache 46(6):942–953
20. Bernstein C, Burstein R (2012) Sensitization of the trigeminovascular pathway: perspective and implications to migraine pathophysiology. J Clin Neurol 8:89–99
21. Slater S, Crawford MJ, Kabbouche MA, LeCates SL, Cherney S, Vaughan P, Hershey AD (2009) Effects of gender and age on paediatric headache. Cephalalgia 29(9):969–973
22. Bolay H, Ozge A, Saginc P, Orekici G, Uludüz D, Yalın O, Siva A, Bıçakçi Ş, Karakurum B, Öztürk M (2015) Gender influences headache characteristics with increasing age in migraine patients. Cephalalgia 35(9):792–800
23. Kelman L, Tanis D (2006) The relationship between migraine pain and other associated symptoms. Cephalalgia 26(5):548–553
24. Silva-Néto RB, Peres MFP, Valença MM (2014) Accuracy of osmophobia in the differential diagnosis between migraine and tension-type headache. J Clin Neurol 339:118–122

Permissions

All chapters in this book were first published in TJHP, by Springer; hereby published with permission under the Creative Commons Attribution License or equivalent. Every chapter published in this book has been scrutinized by our experts. Their significance has been extensively debated. The topics covered herein carry significant findings which will fuel the growth of the discipline. They may even be implemented as practical applications or may be referred to as a beginning point for another development.

The contributors of this book come from diverse backgrounds, making this book a truly international effort. This book will bring forth new frontiers with its revolutionizing research information and detailed analysis of the nascent developments around the world.

We would like to thank all the contributing authors for lending their expertise to make the book truly unique. They have played a crucial role in the development of this book. Without their invaluable contributions this book wouldn't have been possible. They have made vital efforts to compile up to date information on the varied aspects of this subject to make this book a valuable addition to the collection of many professionals and students.

This book was conceptualized with the vision of imparting up-to-date information and advanced data in this field. To ensure the same, a matchless editorial board was set up. Every individual on the board went through rigorous rounds of assessment to prove their worth. After which they invested a large part of their time researching and compiling the most relevant data for our readers.

The editorial board has been involved in producing this book since its inception. They have spent rigorous hours researching and exploring the diverse topics which have resulted in the successful publishing of this book. They have passed on their knowledge of decades through this book. To expedite this challenging task, the publisher supported the team at every step. A small team of assistant editors was also appointed to further simplify the editing procedure and attain best results for the readers.

Apart from the editorial board, the designing team has also invested a significant amount of their time in understanding the subject and creating the most relevant covers. They scrutinized every image to scout for the most suitable representation of the subject and create an appropriate cover for the book.

The publishing team has been an ardent support to the editorial, designing and production team. Their endless efforts to recruit the best for this project, has resulted in the accomplishment of this book. They are a veteran in the field of academics and their pool of knowledge is as vast as their experience in printing. Their expertise and guidance has proved useful at every step. Their uncompromising quality standards have made this book an exceptional effort. Their encouragement from time to time has been an inspiration for everyone.

The publisher and the editorial board hope that this book will prove to be a valuable piece of knowledge for researchers, students, practitioners and scholars across the globe.

List of Contributors

Jie Fang, Xingkai An, Zhenzhen Yu and Hongli Qu
Department of Neurology, The First Affiliated Hospital of Xiamen University, Xiamen, China

Shuai Chen
The First Clinical Medical College of Fujian Medical University, Fuzhou, China

Qilin Ma
Department of Neurology, The First Affiliated Hospital of Xiamen University, Xiamen, China
The First Clinical Medical College of Fujian Medical University, Fuzhou, China

Jong-Hee Sohn, Chul-Ho Kim and Hui-Chul Choi
Department of Neurology, Chuncheon Sacred Heart Hospital, Hallym University College of Medicine, 153 Gyo-dong, Chuncheon-si, Gangwon-do 200-704, Republic of Korea

Kimberly A. Leiken, Emily Curry and Hisako Fujiwara
Division of Neurology, Cincinnati Children's Hospital Medical Center, 3333 Burnet Avenue, MLC 2015, Cincinnati, OH 45220, USA

Jing Xiang, Joanne E. Kacperski, Hope L. O'Brien, Marielle A. Kabbouche, Andrew D. Hershey and Douglas F. Rose
Division of Neurology, Cincinnati Children's Hospital Medical Center, 3333 Burnet Avenue, MLC 2015, Cincinnati, OH 45220, USA
Department of Pediatrics, University of Cincinnati, College of Medicine, Cincinnati, OH, USA

Scott W. Powers
Department of Pediatrics, University of Cincinnati, College of Medicine, Cincinnati, OH, USA
Division of Behavioral Medicine and Clinical Psychology, Cincinnati Children's Hospital Medical Center, Cincinnati, OH, USA

Janelle R. Allen
Division of Behavioral Medicine and Clinical Psychology, Cincinnati Children's Hospital Medical Center, Cincinnati, OH, USA

Jiyoung Kim
Department of Neurology, Bio Medical Research Institute, Pusan National University Hospital, Pusan National University School of Medicine, Busan, South Korea

Soo-Jin Cho
Department of Neurology, Dongtan Sacred Heart Hospital, Hallym University College of Medicine, Hwaseong, South Korea

Won-Joo Kim
Department of Neurology, Gangnam Severance Hospital, Yonsei University College of Medicine, Seoul, South Korea

Kwang Ik Yang
Sleep Disorders Center, Department of Neurology, Soonchunhyang University College of Medicine, Cheonan Hospital, Cheonan, South Korea

Chang-Ho Yun
Clinical Neuroscience Center, Department of Neurology, Seoul National University Bundang Hospital, Seongnam, South Korea

Min Kyung Chu
Department of Neurology, Kangnam Sacred Heart Hospital, Hallym
University College of Medicine, 1 Singil-ro, Yeongdeungpo-gu, Seoul 07441, South Korea

Huahua Jiang, Yong Deng, Yixin Zhang, Jieli Jin, Xueying Kong, Qiuwen Zhu and Jiying Zhou
Department of Neurology, The First Affiliated Hospital of Chongqing Medical University, 1st You Yi Road, Yu Zhong District, Chongqing 400016, China

Kuiyun Wang
Department of Neurology, The first people's Hospital of Jintang County, Sichuan, China

Jiyoung Kim
Department of Neurology, Bio Medical Research Institute, Pusan National University Hospital, Pusan National University School of Medicine, Busan, Republic of Korea

Soo-Jin Cho
Department of Neurology, Dongtan Sacred Heart Hospital, Hallym University College of Medicine, Hwaseong, Republic of Korea

Won-Joo Kim
Department of Neurology, Gangnam Severance Hospital, Yonsei University College of Medicine, Seoul, Republic of Korea

Kwang Ik Yang
Sleep Disorders Center, Department of Neurology, Cheonan Hospital, Soonchunhyang University College of Medicine, Cheonan, Republic of Korea

Chang-Ho Yun
Clinical Neuroscience Center, Department of Neurology, Seoul National University Bundang Hospital, Seongnam, Republic of Korea

Min Kyung Chu
Department of Neurology, Kangnam Sacred Heart Hospital, Hallym University College of Medicine, Seoul, Republic of Korea

Mengqi Liu, Shuangfeng Liu and Lin Ma
Department of Radiology, Chinese PLA General Hospital, 28 Fuxing Road, Beijing 100853, China

Xiaoyan Chen and Shengyuan Yu
Department of Neurology, Chinese PLA General Hospital, 28 Fuxing Road, Beijing 100853, China

Zhiye Chen
Department of Neurology, Chinese PLA General Hospital, 28 Fuxing Road, Beijing 100853, China
Department of Radiology, Chinese PLA General Hospital, 28 Fuxing Road, Beijing 100853, China

Chin-Teng Lin and Chun-Hsiang Chuang
Faculty of Engineering and Information Technology, University of Technology Sydney, Sydney, Australia
Brain Research Center, National Chiao Tung University, Hsinchu, Taiwan

Zehong Cao
Department of Electrical and Computer Engineering, Institute of Electrical Control Engineering, National Chiao Tung University, Hsinchu, Taiwan
Brain Research Center, National Chiao Tung University, Hsinchu, Taiwan
Faculty of Engineering and Information Technology, University of Technology Sydney, Sydney, Australia

Jong-Ling Fuh and Kuan-Lin Lai
Neurological Institute, Taipei Veterans General Hospital, Taipei, Taiwan

Albert C. Yang
Department of Psychiatry, Taipei Veterans General Hospital, Taipei, Taiwan
Faculty of Medicine, National Yang-Ming University School of Medicine, Taipei, Taiwan
Division of Interdisciplinary Medicine and Biotechnology, Beth Israel Deaconess Medical Center/Harvard Medical School, Boston, MA, USA

Shuu-Jiun Wang
Brain Research Center, National Yang-Ming University, Taipei, Taiwan
Faculty of Medicine, National Yang-Ming University School of Medicine, Taipei, Taiwan
Neurological Institute, Taipei Veterans General Hospital, Taipei, Taiwan

Zhiye Chen and Lin Ma
Department of Radiology, Chinese PLA General Hospital, 28 Fuxing Road, Beijing 100853, China
Department of Neurology, Chinese PLA General Hospital, 28 Fuxing Road, Beijing 100853, China
Department of Radiology, Hainan Branch of Chinese PLA General Hospital, Beijing 100853, China

Zhao Dong, Xiaoyan Chen and Shengyuan Yu
Department of Neurology, Chinese PLA General Hospital, 28 Fuxing Road, Beijing 100853, China

Mengqi Liu
Department of Radiology, Hainan Branch of Chinese PLA General Hospital, Beijing 100853, China
Department of Radiology, Chinese PLA General Hospital, 28 Fuxing Road, Beijing 100853, China

Mingjie Zhang, Wenjing Tang, Xiaolin Wang, Zhao Dong and Shengyuan Yu
Department of Neurology, Chinese PLA General Hospital, 28 Fuxing Road, Beijing 100853, People's Republic of China

Yufei Liu
Department of Neurology, Tianjin Third Center Hospital, Tianjin 300170, People's Republic of China

Mangsuo Zhao
Department of Neurology, Yuquan Hospital, Medical Center, Tsinghua University, Beijing 100049, People's Republic of China

Shuangfeng Liu and Lin Ma
Department of Radiology, Chinese PLA General Hospital, 28 Fuxing Road, Beijing 100853, China

Xiaoyan Chen and Shengyuan Yu
Department of Neurology, Chinese PLA General Hospital, 28 Fuxing Road, Beijing 100853, China

Mengqi Liu
Department of Radiology, Hainan Branch of Chinese PLA General Hospital, Sanya 572013, China
Department of Radiology, Chinese PLA General Hospital, 28 Fuxing Road, Beijing 100853, China

Zhiye Chen
Department of Radiology, Chinese PLA General Hospital, 28 Fuxing Road, Beijing 100853, China
Department of Radiology, Hainan Branch of Chinese PLA General Hospital, Sanya 572013, China
Department of Neurology, Chinese PLA General Hospital, 28 Fuxing Road, Beijing 100853, China

Lifang Huang, Hong juan Dong, Xi Wang, Yan Wang and Zheman Xiao
Department of Neurology, Renmin Hospital of Wuhan University, Wuhan
430060, Hubei Province, People's Republic of China

Riccardo Williams and Rita Cerutti
Department of Dynamic and Clinical Psychology, Sapienza University of Rome, Rome, Italy

Luigi Leone
Department of Social and Developmental Psychology, Sapienza University of Rome, Rome, Italy

Noemi Faedda
Phd program in Behavioural Neuroscience, Department of Paediatrics and Child and Adolescent Neuropsychiatry, Sapienza University of Rome, Rome, Italy

Benedetta Bellini, Elisa Salvi, Giulia Natalucci, Paola Verdecchia and Vincenzo Guidetti
Department of Paediatrics and Child and Adolescent Neuropsychiatry, Sapienza University of Rome, Via dei Sabelli 108, 00185 Rome, Italy

Marco Arruda
Glia Institute, Ribeirão Preto, São Paulo, Brazil

Stella Gagliardi, Gaetano Salvatore Grieco, Marialuisa Valente and Cristina Cereda
Genomic and Post-Genomic Center, "C. Mondino" National Neurological Institute, Mondino 2, 27100 Pavia, Italy

Francesca Gualandi and Marcella Neri
Medical Genetics Unit, Department of Medical Sciences and Reproduction and Growth, University-Hospital S'Anna Ferrara, Ferrara, Italy

Luisa Maria Caniatti and Elisabetta Groppo
Neurology Unit, Department of Neuroscience/ Rehabilitation, University-Hospital S'Anna Ferrara, Ferrara, Italy

Giuseppe Nappi
Headache Science Center, C. Mondino National Neurological Institute, Pavia, Italy

Jilei Zhang, Mengxing Wang, Haifeng Lu, Shuai Xu, Zhaoxia Qin, Jianqi Li and Xiaoxia Du
Shanghai Key Laboratory of Magnetic Resonance and Department of Physics, School of Physics and Materials Science, East China Normal University, 3663 North Zhong-Shan Road, 200062 Shanghai, People's Republic of China

Jingjing Su, Qian Yao, Ying Zhao and Qiting Zhang
Department of Neurology and Jiuyuan Municipal Stroke Center, Shanghai Ninth People's Hospital, Shanghai Jiao Tong University School of Medicine, 639 Zhizaoju Road, 200011 Shanghai, People's Republic of China

Ge-Fei Li, Rong Zhao, Yan-Hui Shi, Guo-Hong Cui, Jian-Ren Liu and Yi-Lan Wu
Clinical Research Center, Shanghai Jiao Tong University School of Medicine, Shanghai 200011, China
Department of Neurology and Jiuyuan Municipal Stroke Center, Shanghai Ninth People's Hospital, Shanghai Jiao Tong University School of Medicine, 639 Zhizaoju Road, 200011 Shanghai, People's Republic of China

Daniel Serrano
Endpoint Outcomes, Boston, MA, USA

Richard B. Lipton
The Saul R. Korey Department of Neurology, Albert Einstein College of Medicine, Bronx, NY, USA
Montefiore Headache Center; Department of Neurology and Department of Epidemiology and Population Health, Albert Einstein College of Medicine, Bronx, NY, USA

Ann I. Scher
Department of Preventive Medicine and Biometrics, Uniformed Services University of the Health Sciences, Bethesda, MD, USA

Michael L. Reed
Vedanta Research, Chapel Hill, NC, USA

Walter (Buzz) F. Stewart
Sutter Health, Walnut Creek, CA, USA

Aubrey Manack Adams
Allergan plc, Irvine, CA, USA

Dawn C. Buse
Montefiore Medical Center, Department of Neurology, Albert Einstein College of Medicine, Bronx, NY, USA

Paolo Martelletti
European Headache Federation, Rome, Italy
Department of Clinical and Molecular Medicine, Sapienza University of Rome, Rome, Italy

Todd J. Schwedt
Department of Neurology, Mayo Clinic, 5777 East Mayo Boulevard, Phoenix, AZ 85054, USA

Michel Lanteri-Minet
Département d'Evaluation et Traitement de la Douleur CHU Nice, FHU
InovPain, Université Côte Azur, Nice, France

Rebeca Quintana
GfK EMER, Madrid, Spain

Simon Evans
Migraine Action, Leicester, UK

Pamela Vo, Annik K. Laflamme and Rachel Fink
Novartis Pharma AG, Basel, Switzerland

Donna Walsh
European Federation of Neurological Associations, Brussels, Belgium

Paula Dumas
Migraine Again, Irvine, USA

Petter Moe Omland, Marit Stjern and Trond Sand
Department of Neuromedicine and Movement Science, NTNU, Norwegian University of Science and Technology, Trondheim, Norway
Department of Neurology and Clinical Neurophysiology, St. Olavs Hospital, Trondheim, Norway

Gøril Bruvik Gravdahl
Norwegian Advisory Unit on Headaches, St. Olavs Hospital, Trondheim, Norway

Martin Uglem
NTNU, Faculty of Medicine and Health Sciences, P.B. 8905, N-7491 Trondheim, Norway
Department of Neuromedicine and Movement Science, NTNU, Norwegian University of Science and Technology, Trondheim, Norway

Jan Mehnert and Arne May
Department of Systems Neuroscience, University Medical Center Eppendorf, Martinistraße 52, 20246 Hamburg, Germany

Kerstin Luedtke
Department of Academic Physiotherapy, University of Luebeck, Luebeck, Germany
Department of Systems Neuroscience, University Medical Center Eppendorf, Martinistraße 52, 20246 Hamburg, Germany

Kristian A. Haanes, Alejandro Labastida-Ramírez, Kayi Y. Chan, René de Vries, Alexander H. J. Danser and Antoinette MaassenVanDenBrink
Division of Vascular Medicine and Pharmacology, Department of Internal Medicine, Erasmus MC, Rotterdam, Dr Molewaterplein 50, 3015, GE, Rotterdam, The Netherlands

Jimmy Zhang, Brian Shook, Paul Jackson and Christopher M. Flores
Janssen Research & Development, L.L.C, Welsh and McKean Roads, Spring House, PA 19477, USA

Carlos M. Villalón
Departamento de Farmacobiología, Cinvestav-Coapa, Czda. de los Tenorios 235, Col. Granjas-Coapa, Deleg. Tlalpan, C.P, 14330 Ciudad de México, Mexico

Tomor Harnod
Department of Neurosurgery, Hualien Tzu Chi General Hospital, Buddhist Tzu Chi Medical Foundation, Hualien, Taiwan
College of Medicine, Tzu Chi University, Hualien, Taiwan

Cheng-Li Lin
Management Office for Health Data, China Medical University Hospital, Taichung, Taiwan
College of Medicine, China Medical University, Taichung, Taiwan

Chia-Hung Kao
Graduate Institute of Biomedical Sciences and School of Medicine, College of Medicine, China Medical University, No. 2, Yuh-Der Road, Taichung 404, Taiwan
Department of Nuclear Medicine and PET Center, China Medical University Hospital, Taichung, Taiwan
Department of Bioinformatics and Medical Engineering, Asia University, Taichung, Taiwan

Lena Ohlsson and Lars Edvinsson
Department of Clinical Sciences, Division of Experimental Vascular Research, Lund University, BMC A13, Sölvegatan 17, SE-223 62 Lund, Sweden
Department of Internal Medicine and Neurosurgery, University Hospital, Lund, Sweden

Erik Kronvall
Department of Clinical sciences, Neurosurgery, Skane University Hospital, Lund, Sweden
Department of Internal Medicine and Neurosurgery, University Hospital, Lund, Sweden

Jennifer Stratton
Teva Biologics R&D, Redwood City, California, USA
Department of Internal Medicine and Neurosurgery, University Hospital, Lund, Sweden

Di Wu, Yuchen Zhou, Lu Tang, Hongxing Liu, Shuyang Huang and Xiaoshan Wang
Department of Neurology, Nanjing Brain Hospital, Nanjing Medical University, 264 Guangzhou Road, Nanjing, Jiangsu 210029, China

Jing Xiang
MEG Center, Division of Neurology, Cincinnati Children's Hospital Medical Center, 3333 Burnet Avenue, Cincinnati, OH 45220, USA

Qiqi Chen and Ting Wu
MEG Center, Nanjing Brain Hospital, Nanjing, Jiangsu 210029, China

Stephanie M. Llop
Department of Ophthalmology, University of Puerto Rico School of Medicine, San Juan, Puerto Rico 00936, USA

Jonathan E. Frandsen
Department of Ophthalmology and Visual Sciences, John A. Moran Eye Center, University of Utah Health Sciences Center, 65 N. Mario Capecchi Drive, Salt Lake City, UT 84132, USA

Kathleen B. Digre, Bradley J. Katz, Alison V. Crum and Judith E. A. Warner
Department of Neurology, University of Utah Health Sciences Center, 175 North Medical Drive East, Salt Lake City, UT 84132, USA
Department of Ophthalmology and Visual Sciences, John A. Moran Eye Center, University of Utah Health Sciences Center, 65 N. Mario Capecchi Drive, Salt Lake City, UT 84132, USA

Chong Zhang
Division of Epidemiology, Department of Internal Medicine, University of Utah Health Sciences Center, 30 N 1900 East, Salt Lake City, UT 84132, USA

Maria Adele Giamberardino, Giannapia Affaitati and Francesco Cipollone
Fibromyalgia and Headache Center, Geriatrics Clinics, Department of Medicine and Science of Aging and Ce.S.I., "G. D'Annunzio" University of Chieti, via dei Vestini s.n., 66100 Chieti, Italy

Andrea Negro, Martina Curto and Paolo Martelletti
Department of Clinical and Molecular Medicine, Regional Referral Headache Centre, "Sant'Andrea" Hospital, "Sapienza" University, Rome, Italy

Claudio Tana
Internal Medicine Unit, Guastalla Hospital, AUSL Reggio Emilia, Reggio Emilia, Italy

Cosima Schiavone, Luisa Stellin and Domenico Lapenna
Department of Medicine and Science of Aging, "G. D'Annunzio" University of Chieti, Chieti, Italy

Raffaele Costantini
Institute of Surgical Pathology, "G. D'Annunzio" University of Chieti, Chieti, Italy

Osman Özgür Yalın
Neurology Department, Istanbul Education and Research Hospital, Kasapİlyas Mah. Org. Abdurrahman, Nafiz Gürman Cd, PK: 34098 Fatih, Istanbul, Turkey

Derya Uluduz and Aksel Siva
Neurology Department, Istanbul University Cerrahpasa School of Medicine, İstanbul, Turkey

Aynur Özge
Neurology Department, Mersin University School of Medicine, Mersin, Turkey

Mehmet Ali Sungur
Biostatistics Department, Düzce University School of Medicine, Düzce, Turkey

Macit Selekler
Neurology Department, Kocaeli University School of Medicine, Kocaeli, Turkey

Index